Access Your Online Resources

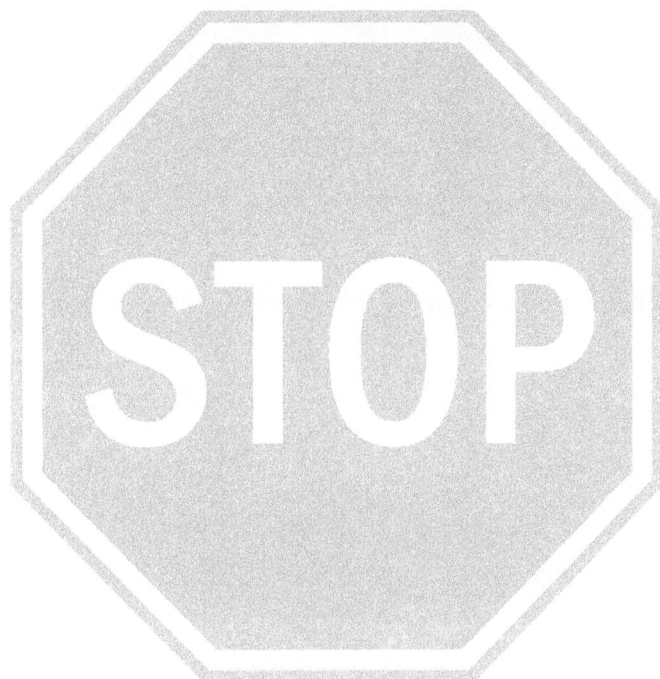

DON'T MISS OUT ON THE ONLINE RESOURCES INCLUDED WITH YOUR PURCHASE!

Your purchase of this product unlocks access to our Online Resources page. Elevate your study experience with our **interactive practice test interface**, along with all of the additional resources that we couldn't include in this book.

Flip to the Online Resources section at the end of this book to find the link and a QR code to get started!

Mometrix
TEST PREPARATION

CWOCN®
Exam
Secrets

Study Guide
Your Key to Exam Success

M✓metrix
TEST PREPARATION

Written and edited by the Mometrix Test Prep

Mometrix offers volume discount pricing to institutions. For more information or a price quote, please contact our sales department at sales@mometrix.com or 888-248-1219.

CWOCN® and WOCNCB® are registered trademarks of the Wound Ostomy Continence Nursing Certification Board. Mometrix Test Preparation is not affiliated with or endorsed by the Wound Ostomy Continence Nursing Certification Board.

Paperback
ISBN 13: 978-1-60971-600-4
ISBN 10: 1-60971-600-0

Ebook
ISBN 13: 978-1-62120-542-5
ISBN 10: 1-62120-542-8

Hardback
ISBN 13: 978-1-5167-0574-0
ISBN 10: 1-5167-0574-2

Dear Future Exam Success Story

First of all, **THANK YOU** for purchasing Mometrix study materials!

Second, congratulations! You are one of the few determined test-takers who are committed to doing whatever it takes to excel on your exam. **You have come to the right place.** We developed these study materials with one goal in mind: to deliver you the information you need in a format that's concise and easy to use.

In addition to optimizing your guide for the content of the test, we've outlined our recommended steps for breaking down the preparation process into small, attainable goals so you can make sure you stay on track.

We've also analyzed the entire test-taking process, identifying the most common pitfalls and showing how you can overcome them and be ready for any curveball the test throws you.

Standardized testing is one of the biggest obstacles on your road to success, which only increases the importance of doing well in the high-pressure, high-stakes environment of test day. Your results on this test could have a significant impact on your future, and this guide provides the information and practical advice to help you achieve your full potential on test day.

Your success is our success

We would love to hear from you! If you would like to share the story of your exam success or if you have any questions or comments in regard to our products, please contact us at **800-673-8175** or **support@mometrix.com**.

Thanks again for your business and we wish you continued success!

Sincerely,
The Mometrix Test Preparation Team

Need more help? Check out our flashcards at:
http://MometrixFlashcards.com/WOCNCB

---

ii

TABLE OF CONTENTS

Introduction

Thank you for purchasing this resource! You have made the choice to prepare yourself for a test that could have a huge impact on your future, and this guide is designed to help you be fully ready for test day. Obviously, it's important to have a solid understanding of the test material, but you also need to be prepared for the unique environment and stressors of the test, so that you can perform to the best of your abilities.

For this purpose, the first section that appears in this guide is the **Secret Keys**. We've devoted countless hours to meticulously researching what works and what doesn't, and we've boiled down our findings to the five most impactful steps you can take to improve your performance on the test. We start at the beginning with study planning and move through the preparation process, all the way to the testing strategies that will help you get the most out of what you know when you're finally sitting in front of the test.

We recommend that you start preparing for your test as far in advance as possible. However, if you've bought this guide as a last-minute study resource and only have a few days before your test, we recommend that you skip over the first two Secret Keys since they address a long-term study plan.

If you struggle with **test anxiety**, we strongly encourage you to check out our recommendations for how you can overcome it. Test anxiety is a formidable foe, but it can be beaten, and we want to make sure you have the tools you need to defeat it.

1

Secret Key #1 – Plan Big, Study Small

There's a lot riding on your performance. If you want to ace this test, you're going to need to keep your skills sharp and the material fresh in your mind. You need a plan that lets you review everything you need to know while still fitting in your schedule. We'll break this strategy down into three categories.

Information Organization

Start with the information you already have: the official test outline. From this, you can make a complete list of all the concepts you need to cover before the test. Organize these concepts into groups that can be studied together, and create a list of any related vocabulary you need to learn so you can brush up on any difficult terms. You'll want to keep this vocabulary list handy once you actually start studying since you may need to add to it along the way.

Time Management

Once you have your set of study concepts, decide how to spread them out over the time you have left before the test. Break your study plan into small, clear goals so you have a manageable task for each day and know exactly what you're doing. Then just focus on one small step at a time. When you manage your time this way, you don't need to spend hours at a time studying. Studying a small block of content for a short period each day helps you retain information better and avoid stressing over how much you have left to do. You can relax knowing that you have a plan to cover everything in time. In order for this strategy to be effective though, you have to start studying early and stick to your schedule. Avoid the exhaustion and futility that comes from last-minute cramming!

Study Environment

The environment you study in has a big impact on your learning. Studying in a coffee shop, while probably more enjoyable, is not likely to be as fruitful as studying in a quiet room. It's important to keep distractions to a minimum. You're only planning to study for a short block of time, so make the most of it. Don't pause to check your phone or get up to find a snack. It's also important to **avoid multitasking**. Research has consistently shown that multitasking will make your studying dramatically less effective. Your study area should also be comfortable and well-lit so you don't have the distraction of straining your eyes or sitting on an uncomfortable chair.

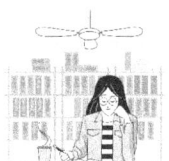

The time of day you study is also important. You want to be rested and alert. Don't wait until just before bedtime. Study when you'll be most likely to comprehend and remember. Even better, if you know what time of day your test will be, set that time aside for study. That way your brain will be used to working on that subject at that specific time and you'll have a better chance of recalling information.

Finally, it can be helpful to team up with others who are studying for the same test. Your actual studying should be done in as isolated an environment as possible, but the work of organizing the information and setting up the study plan can be divided up. In between study sessions, you can discuss with your teammates the concepts that you're all studying and quiz each other on the details. Just be sure that your teammates are as serious about the test as you are. If you find that your study time is being replaced with social time, you might need to find a new team.

Secret Key #2 – Make Your Studying Count

You're devoting a lot of time and effort to preparing for this test, so you want to be absolutely certain it will pay off. This means doing more than just reading the content and hoping you can remember it on test day. It's important to make every minute of study count. There are two main areas you can focus on to make your studying count.

Retention

It doesn't matter how much time you study if you can't remember the material. You need to make sure you are retaining the concepts. To check your retention of the information you're learning, try recalling it at later times with minimal prompting. Try carrying around flashcards and glance at one or two from time to time or ask a friend who's also studying for the test to quiz you.

To enhance your retention, look for ways to put the information into practice so that you can apply it rather than simply recalling it. If you're using the information in practical ways, it will be much easier to remember. Similarly, it helps to solidify a concept in your mind if you're not only reading it to yourself but also explaining it to someone else. Ask a friend to let you teach them about a concept you're a little shaky on (or speak aloud to an imaginary audience if necessary). As you try to summarize, define, give examples, and answer your friend's questions, you'll understand the concepts better and they will stay with you longer. Finally, step back for a big picture view and ask yourself how each piece of information fits with the whole subject. When you link the different concepts together and see them working together as a whole, it's easier to remember the individual components.

Finally, practice showing your work on any multi-step problems, even if you're just studying. Writing out each step you take to solve a problem will help solidify the process in your mind, and you'll be more likely to remember it during the test.

Modality

Modality simply refers to the means or method by which you study. Choosing a study modality that fits your own individual learning style is crucial. No two people learn best in exactly the same way, so it's important to know your strengths and use them to your advantage.

For example, if you learn best by visualization, focus on visualizing a concept in your mind and draw an image or a diagram. Try color-coding your notes, illustrating them, or creating symbols that will trigger your mind to recall a learned concept. If you learn best by hearing or discussing information, find a study partner who learns the same way or read aloud to yourself. Think about how to put the information in your own words. Imagine that you are giving a lecture on the topic and record yourself so you can listen to it later.

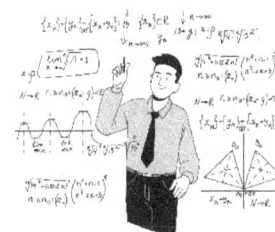

For any learning style, flashcards can be helpful. Organize the information so you can take advantage of spare moments to review. Underline key words or phrases. Use different colors for different categories. Mnemonic devices (such as creating a short list in which every item starts with the same letter) can also help with retention. Find what works best for you and use it to store the information in your mind most effectively and easily.

Secret Key #3 – Practice the Right Way

Your success on test day depends not only on how many hours you put into preparing, but also on whether you prepared the right way. It's good to check along the way to see if your studying is paying off. One of the most effective ways to do this is by taking practice tests to evaluate your progress. Practice tests are useful because they show exactly where you need to improve. Every time you take a practice test, pay special attention to these three groups of questions:

- The questions you got wrong
- The questions you had to guess on, even if you guessed right
- The questions you found difficult or slow to work through

This will show you exactly what your weak areas are, and where you need to devote more study time. Ask yourself why each of these questions gave you trouble. Was it because you didn't understand the material? Was it because you didn't remember the vocabulary? Do you need more repetitions on this type of question to build speed and confidence? Dig into those questions and figure out how you can strengthen your weak areas as you go back to review the material.

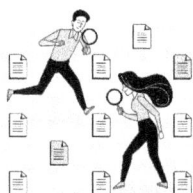

Additionally, many practice tests have a section explaining the answer choices. It can be tempting to read the explanation and think that you now have a good understanding of the concept. However, an explanation likely only covers part of the question's broader context. Even if the explanation makes perfect sense, **go back and investigate** every concept related to the question until you're positive you have a thorough understanding.

As you go along, keep in mind that the practice test is just that: practice. Memorizing these questions and answers will not be very helpful on the actual test because it is unlikely to have any of the same exact questions. If you only know the right answers to the sample questions, you won't be prepared for the real thing. **Study the concepts** until you understand them fully, and then you'll be able to answer any question that shows up on the test.

It's important to wait on the practice tests until you're ready. If you take a test on your first day of study, you may be overwhelmed by the amount of material covered and how much you need to learn. Work up to it gradually.

On test day, you'll need to be prepared for answering questions, managing your time, and using the test-taking strategies you've learned. It's a lot to balance, like a mental marathon that will have a big impact on your future. Like training for a marathon, you'll need to start slowly and work your way up. When test day arrives, you'll be ready.

Start with the strategies you've read in the first two Secret Keys—plan your course and study in the way that works best for you. If you have time, consider using multiple study resources to get different approaches to the same concepts. It can be helpful to see difficult concepts from more than one angle. Then find a good source for practice tests. Many times, the test website will suggest potential study resources or provide sample tests.

Practice Test Strategy

If you're able to find at least three practice tests, we recommend this strategy:

UNTIMED AND OPEN-BOOK PRACTICE

Take the first test with no time constraints and with your notes and study guide handy. Take your time and focus on applying the strategies you've learned.

TIMED AND OPEN-BOOK PRACTICE

Take the second practice test open-book as well, but set a timer and practice pacing yourself to finish in time.

TIMED AND CLOSED-BOOK PRACTICE

Take any other practice tests as if it were test day. Set a timer and put away your study materials. Sit at a table or desk in a quiet room, imagine yourself at the testing center, and answer questions as quickly and accurately as possible.

Keep repeating timed and closed-book tests on a regular basis until you run out of practice tests or it's time for the actual test. Your mind will be ready for the schedule and stress of test day, and you'll be able to focus on recalling the material you've learned.

Secret Key #4 – Pace Yourself

Once you're fully prepared for the material on the test, your biggest challenge on test day will be managing your time. Just knowing that the clock is ticking can make you panic even if you have plenty of time left. Work on pacing yourself so you can build confidence against the time constraints of the exam. Pacing is a difficult skill to master, especially in a high-pressure environment, so **practice is vital**.

Set time expectations for your pace based on how much time is available. For example, if a section has 60 questions and the time limit is 30 minutes, you know you have to average 30 seconds or less per question in order to answer them all. Although 30 seconds is the hard limit, set 25 seconds per question as your goal, so you reserve extra time to spend on harder questions. When you budget extra time for the harder questions, you no longer have any reason to stress when those questions take longer to answer.

Don't let this time expectation distract you from working through the test at a calm, steady pace, but keep it in mind so you don't spend too much time on any one question. Recognize that taking extra time on one question you don't understand may keep you from answering two that you do understand later in the test. If your time limit for a question is up and you're still not sure of the answer, mark it and move on, and come back to it later if the time and the test format allow. If the testing format doesn't allow you to return to earlier questions, just make an educated guess; then put it out of your mind and move on.

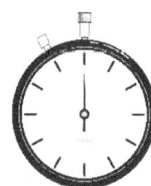

On the easier questions, be careful not to rush. It may seem wise to hurry through them so you have more time for the challenging ones, but it's not worth missing one if you know the concept and just didn't take the time to read the question fully. Work efficiently but make sure you understand the question and have looked at all of the answer choices, since more than one may seem right at first.

Even if you're paying attention to the time, you may find yourself a little behind at some point. You should speed up to get back on track, but do so wisely. Don't panic; just take a few seconds less on each question until you're caught up. Don't guess without thinking, but do look through the answer choices and eliminate any you know are wrong. If you can get down to two choices, it is often worthwhile to guess from those. Once you've chosen an answer, move on and don't dwell on any that you skipped or had to hurry through. If a question was taking too long, chances are it was one of the harder ones, so you weren't as likely to get it right anyway.

On the other hand, if you find yourself getting ahead of schedule, it may be beneficial to slow down a little. The more quickly you work, the more likely you are to make a careless mistake that will affect your score. You've budgeted time for each question, so don't be afraid to spend that time. Practice an efficient but careful pace to get the most out of the time you have.

Secret Key #5 – Have a Plan for Guessing

When you're taking the test, you may find yourself stuck on a question. Some of the answer choices seem better than others, but you don't see the one answer choice that is obviously correct. What do you do?

The scenario described above is very common, yet most test takers have not effectively prepared for it. Developing and practicing a plan for guessing may be one of the single most effective uses of your time as you get ready for the exam.

In developing your plan for guessing, there are three questions to address:

- When should you start the guessing process?
- How should you narrow down the choices?
- Which answer should you choose?

When to Start the Guessing Process

Unless your plan for guessing is to select C every time (which, despite its merits, is not what we recommend), you need to leave yourself enough time to apply your answer elimination strategies. Since you have a limited amount of time for each question, that means that if you're going to give yourself the best shot at guessing correctly, you have to decide quickly whether or not you will guess.

Of course, the best-case scenario is that you don't have to guess at all, so first, see if you can answer the question based on your knowledge of the subject and basic reasoning skills. Focus on the key words in the question and try to jog your memory of related topics. Give yourself a chance to bring the knowledge to mind, but once you realize that you don't have (or you can't access) the knowledge you need to answer the question, it's time to start the guessing process.

It's almost always better to start the guessing process too early than too late. It only takes a few seconds to remember something and answer the question from knowledge. Carefully eliminating wrong answer choices takes longer. Plus, going through the process of eliminating answer choices can actually help jog your memory.

Summary: Start the guessing process as soon as you decide that you can't answer the question based on your knowledge.

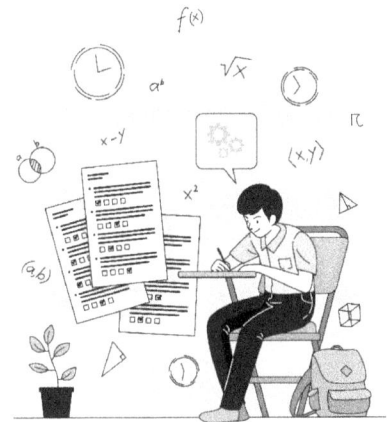

7

How to Narrow Down the Choices

The next chapter in this book (**Test-Taking Strategies**) includes a wide range of strategies for how to approach questions and how to look for answer choices to eliminate. You will definitely want to read those carefully, practice them, and figure out which ones work best for you. Here though, we're going to address a mindset rather than a particular strategy.

Your odds of guessing an answer correctly depend on how many options you are choosing from.

Number of options left	5	4	3	2	1
Odds of guessing correctly	20%	25%	33%	50%	100%

You can see from this chart just how valuable it is to be able to eliminate incorrect answers and make an educated guess, but there are two things that many test takers do that cause them to miss out on the benefits of guessing:

- Accidentally eliminating the correct answer
- Selecting an answer based on an impression

We'll look at the first one here, and the second one in the next section.

To avoid accidentally eliminating the correct answer, we recommend a thought exercise called **the $5 challenge**. In this challenge, you only eliminate an answer choice from contention if you are willing to bet $5 on it being wrong. Why $5? Five dollars is a small but not insignificant amount of money. It's an amount you could afford to lose but wouldn't want to throw away. And while losing $5 once might not hurt too much, doing it twenty times will set you back $100. In the same way, each small decision you make—eliminating a choice here, guessing on a question there—won't by itself impact your score very much, but when you put them all together, they can make a big difference. By holding each answer choice elimination decision to a higher standard, you can reduce the risk of accidentally eliminating the correct answer.

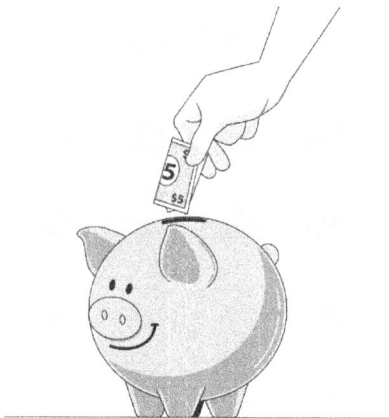

The $5 challenge can also be applied in a positive sense: If you are willing to bet $5 that an answer choice *is* correct, go ahead and mark it as correct.

Summary: Only eliminate an answer choice if you are willing to bet $5 that it is wrong.

Which Answer to Choose

You're taking the test. You've run into a hard question and decided you'll have to guess. You've eliminated all the answer choices you're willing to bet $5 on. Now you have to pick an answer. Why do we even need to talk about this? Why can't you just pick whichever one you feel like when the time comes?

The answer to these questions is that if you don't come into the test with a plan, you'll rely on your impression to select an answer choice, and if you do that, you risk falling into a trap. The test writers know that everyone who takes their test will be guessing on some of the questions, so they intentionally write wrong answer choices to seem plausible. You still have to pick an answer though, and if the wrong answer choices are designed to look right, how can you ever be sure that you're not falling for their trap? The best solution we've found to this dilemma is to take the decision out of your hands entirely. Here is the process we recommend:

Once you've eliminated any choices that you are confident (willing to bet $5) are wrong, select the first remaining choice as your answer.

Whether you choose to select the first remaining choice, the second, or the last, the important thing is that you use some preselected standard. Using this approach guarantees that you will not be enticed into selecting an answer choice that looks right, because you are not basing your decision on how the answer choices look.

A. This is wrong.
B. Also wrong.
C. Maybe?
D. Maybe?

This is not meant to make you question your knowledge. Instead, it is to help you recognize the difference between your knowledge and your impressions. There's a huge difference between thinking an answer is right because of what you know, and thinking an answer is right because it looks or sounds like it should be right.

Summary: To ensure that your selection is appropriately random, make a predetermined selection from among all answer choices you have not eliminated.

9

Test-Taking Strategies

This section contains a list of test-taking strategies that you may find helpful as you work through the test. By taking what you know and applying logical thought, you can maximize your chances of answering any question correctly!

It is very important to realize that every question is different and every person is different: no single strategy will work on every question, and no single strategy will work for every person. That's why we've included all of them here, so you can try them out and determine which ones work best for different types of questions and which ones work best for you.

Question Strategies

⊘ READ CAREFULLY

Read the question and the answer choices carefully. Don't miss the question because you misread the terms. You have plenty of time to read each question thoroughly and make sure you understand what is being asked. Yet a happy medium must be attained, so don't waste too much time. You must read carefully and efficiently.

⊘ CONTEXTUAL CLUES

Look for contextual clues. If the question includes a word you are not familiar with, look at the immediate context for some indication of what the word might mean. Contextual clues can often give you all the information you need to decipher the meaning of an unfamiliar word. Even if you can't determine the meaning, you may be able to narrow down the possibilities enough to make a solid guess at the answer to the question.

⊘ PREFIXES

If you're having trouble with a word in the question or answer choices, try dissecting it. Take advantage of every clue that the word might include. Prefixes can be a huge help. Usually, they allow you to determine a basic meaning. *Pre-* means before, *post-* means after, *pro-* is positive, *de-* is negative. From prefixes, you can get an idea of the general meaning of the word and try to put it into context.

⊘ HEDGE WORDS

Watch out for critical hedge words, such as *likely, may, can, often, almost, mostly, usually, generally, rarely,* and *sometimes.* Question writers insert these hedge phrases to cover every possibility. Often an answer choice will be wrong simply because it leaves no room for exception. Be on guard for answer choices that have definitive words such as *exactly* and *always*.

⊘ SWITCHBACK WORDS

Stay alert for *switchbacks*. These are the words and phrases frequently used to alert you to shifts in thought. The most common switchback words are *but, although,* and *however*. Others include *nevertheless, on the other hand, even though, while, in spite of, despite,* and *regardless of*. Switchback words are important to catch because they can change the direction of the question or an answer choice.

⊘ FACE VALUE

When in doubt, use common sense. Accept the situation in the problem at face value. Don't read too much into it. These problems will not require you to make wild assumptions. If you have to go beyond creativity and warp time or space in order to have an answer choice fit the question, then you should move on and consider the other answer choices. These are normal problems rooted in reality. The applicable relationship or explanation may not be readily apparent, but it is there for you to figure out. Use your common sense to interpret anything that isn't clear.

10

Answer Choice Strategies

⊘ ANSWER SELECTION

The most thorough way to pick an answer choice is to identify and eliminate wrong answers until only one is left, then confirm it is the correct answer. Sometimes an answer choice may immediately seem right, but be careful. The test writers will usually put more than one reasonable answer choice on each question, so take a second to read all of them and make sure that the other choices are not equally obvious. As long as you have time left, it is better to read every answer choice than to pick the first one that looks right without checking the others.

⊘ ANSWER CHOICE FAMILIES

An answer choice family consists of two (in rare cases, three) answer choices that are very similar in construction and cannot all be true at the same time. If you see two answer choices that are direct opposites or parallels, one of them is usually the correct answer. For instance, if one answer choice says that quantity x increases and another either says that quantity x decreases (opposite) or says that quantity y increases (parallel), then those answer choices would fall into the same family. An answer choice that doesn't match the construction of the answer choice family is more likely to be incorrect. Most questions will not have answer choice families, but when they do appear, you should be prepared to recognize them.

⊘ ELIMINATE ANSWERS

Eliminate answer choices as soon as you realize they are wrong, but make sure you consider all possibilities. If you are eliminating answer choices and realize that the last one you are left with is also wrong, don't panic. Start over and consider each choice again. There may be something you missed the first time that you will realize on the second pass.

⊘ AVOID FACT TRAPS

Don't be distracted by an answer choice that is factually true but doesn't answer the question. You are looking for the choice that answers the question. Stay focused on what the question is asking for so you don't accidentally pick an answer that is true but incorrect. Always go back to the question and make sure the answer choice you've selected actually answers the question and is not merely a true statement.

⊘ EXTREME STATEMENTS

In general, you should avoid answers that put forth extreme actions as standard practice or proclaim controversial ideas as established fact. An answer choice that states the "process should be used in certain situations, if…" is much more likely to be correct than one that states the "process should be discontinued completely." The first is a calm rational statement and doesn't even make a definitive, uncompromising stance, using a hedge word *if* to provide wiggle room, whereas the second choice is far more extreme.

⊘ BENCHMARK

As you read through the answer choices and you come across one that seems to answer the question well, mentally select that answer choice. This is not your final answer, but it's the one that will help you evaluate the other answer choices. The one that you selected is your benchmark or standard for judging each of the other answer choices. Every other answer choice must be compared to your benchmark. That choice is correct until proven otherwise by another answer choice beating it. If you find a better answer, then that one becomes your new benchmark. Once you've decided that no other choice answers the question as well as your benchmark, you have your final answer.

⊘ PREDICT THE ANSWER

Before you even start looking at the answer choices, it is often best to try to predict the answer. When you come up with the answer on your own, it is easier to avoid distractions and traps because you will know exactly what to look for. The right answer choice is unlikely to be word-for-word what you came up with, but it should be a close match. Even if you are confident that you have the right answer, you should still take the time to read each option before moving on.

General Strategies

⊘ TOUGH QUESTIONS

If you are stumped on a problem or it appears too hard or too difficult, don't waste time. Move on! Remember though, if you can quickly check for obviously incorrect answer choices, your chances of guessing correctly are greatly improved. Before you completely give up, at least try to knock out a couple of possible answers. Eliminate what you can and then guess at the remaining answer choices before moving on.

⊘ CHECK YOUR WORK

Since you will probably not know every term listed and the answer to every question, it is important that you get credit for the ones that you do know. Don't miss any questions through careless mistakes. If at all possible, try to take a second to look back over your answer selection and make sure you've selected the correct answer choice and haven't made a costly careless mistake (such as marking an answer choice that you didn't mean to mark). This quick double check should more than pay for itself in caught mistakes for the time it costs.

⊘ PACE YOURSELF

It's easy to be overwhelmed when you're looking at a page full of questions; your mind is confused and full of random thoughts, and the clock is ticking down faster than you would like. Calm down and maintain the pace that you have set for yourself. Especially as you get down to the last few minutes of the test, don't let the small numbers on the clock make you panic. As long as you are on track by monitoring your pace, you are guaranteed to have time for each question.

⊘ DON'T RUSH

It is very easy to make errors when you are in a hurry. Maintaining a fast pace in answering questions is pointless if it makes you miss questions that you would have gotten right otherwise. Test writers like to include distracting information and wrong answers that seem right. Taking a little extra time to avoid careless mistakes can make all the difference in your test score. Find a pace that allows you to be confident in the answers that you select.

⊘ KEEP MOVING

Panicking will not help you pass the test, so do your best to stay calm and keep moving. Taking deep breaths and going through the answer elimination steps you practiced can help to break through a stress barrier and keep your pace.

Final Notes

The combination of a solid foundation of content knowledge and the confidence that comes from practicing your plan for applying that knowledge is the key to maximizing your performance on test day. As your foundation of content knowledge is built up and strengthened, you'll find that the strategies included in this chapter become more and more effective in helping you quickly sift through the distractions and traps of the test to isolate the correct answer.

Now that you're preparing to move forward into the test content chapters of this book, be sure to keep your goal in mind. As you read, think about how you will be able to apply this information on the test. If you've already seen sample questions for the test and you have an idea of the question format and style, try to come up with questions of your own that you can answer based on what you're reading. This will give you valuable practice applying your knowledge in the same ways you can expect to on test day.

Good luck and good studying!

Wound Care: Assessment

Patient Interviews

INTERVIEW PROCESS AND TECHNIQUES

The care provider should review previous medical records, have a clear idea of the purpose of the interview, and outline the questions. If possible, the patient should be interviewed alone or should be asked if he or she wants family members present. Both verbal and nonverbal responses should be observed during an interview. Important factors include:

- **Initial introductions**: Make introductions by name and explain roles and the purpose of the interview, asking how the patient wishes to be addressed and avoiding using familiar terms, such as "dear," which may be considered condescending. Stress the confidential nature of the interview and explain who will receive the information.
- **Interview structure**: The interview may be somewhat unstructured, guided by patient responses, or may be very structured with the care provider asking a list of questions, but he or she must remain flexible while still guiding the discussion in order to accommodate different communication styles.
- **Appearance**: The care provider should be professionally dressed and wearing a clear nametag. The patient's appearance should be observed non-judgmentally for clothes (loose/tight clothes may indicate weight change), cleanliness (dirty clothes/skin/hair may indicate cognitive or physical impairment or poverty), and demeanor (calm, fidgeting, nervous).

HISTORY COLLECTION DURING INITIAL PATIENT INTERVIEW

In order to plan for optimal wound management, history collection during the initial patient interview should include as much information about the wound as possible. Information should include:

- Type of wound, size, and location
- Etiology of the wound (known, unknown)
- Duration of wound
- Degree of pain associated with the wound (increasing, decreasing)
- All previous treatments/interventions (both medical and patient-initiated), including types of dressings
- Changes in the wound (increase in size, decrease in size, tunneling, wound edges, and wound color)
- Evidence of necrosis, exudate, edema, granulation tissue, epithelial tissue, induration, erythema, and cyanosis
- Presence of odor (character of odor and amount of exudate)
- Nutritional status, including fluid intake, supplements, vitamins, and usual diet
- Medical history, including diseases, injuries, surgeries, and hospitalizations
- Lifestyle, including homelessness
- Habits, including use of tobacco, alcohol, and illicit substances
- List of medications, including OTC, traditional medicines (such as herbs), and prescribed medications
- Recent laboratory work (CBC, FBS, A1c)
- Mobility issues

ISSUES OF CULTURAL DIVERSITY DURING THE INTERVIEW AND ASSESSMENT

Issues of cultural diversity must be considered during the initial interview and the wound assessment. Individuals vary considerably in their attitudes, so assuming that all members of an ethnic or cultural group share the same values is never valid. The individual must be assessed as well as the group. It is important to take time to observe family dynamics and language barriers, arranging for translators if necessary to ensure that there is adequate communication. In patriarchal cultures, such as the Mexican culture, the eldest male may speak for the patient. In some Muslim cultures, females will resist care by males. Acknowledging biological differences, such as skin color, is important for assessing skin because wounds and bruising may have a different appearance. The attitudes and beliefs of the patient in relation to wound care must be understood, accepted, and treated with respect. In some cases, the use of healers or cultural traditions must be incorporated into a plan of care.

Wound Care: Assessment

Anatomy and Physiology of the Skins

EPIDERMIS

The epidermis is the outer avascular layer of skin. It is composed of stratified squamous epithelial cells (keratinocytes) and regenerates every 4-6 weeks. Layers of the epidermis consist of the following:

- **Stratum corneum**, the outer layer, is flattened dead keratinized cells (corneocytes), providing a waterproof barrier against microorganisms and injury.
- **Stratum lucidum** is 1-5 translucent cells thick and is found in the palms and soles of the feet where the skin is thicker.
- **Stratum granulosum** is 1-5 cells thick and contains keratinocytes with granules that contain proteins.
- **Stratum spinosum** (prickly layers) contains spiny desmosomes that join cube-like cells in multiple layers, providing structure and support.
- **Stratum germinativum/stratum basale** is one layer of active undifferentiated basal cells with a basement membrane zone beneath.

Cells ascend into the stratum spinosum and become keratinocytes. It can take 2-3 weeks for a cell to leave the basal layer and move upward to the stratum corneum, replenishing the various layers. The basal layer contains melanocytes, which provide pigmentation and protection from sunlight.

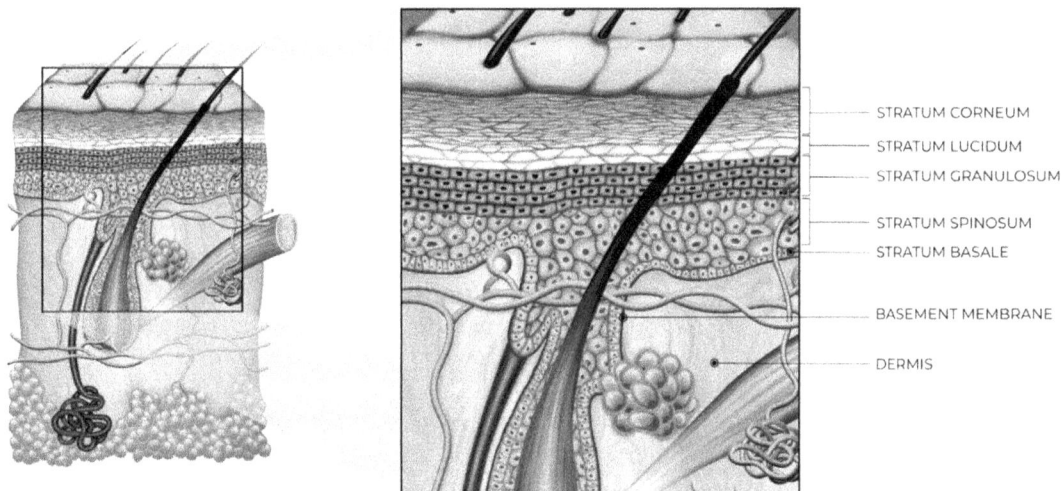

BASEMENT MEMBRANE ZONE

The junction of the epidermis and dermis is the **basement membrane zone** (BMZ), which provides support for the cells above. It comprises two layers:

- **Lamina lucida** (because of translucent electrons) contains glycoprotein laminin.
- **Lamina densa** (because of dense electrons) comprises type IV collagen.

Lamina reticularis (bottom portion) is synthesized by cells in connective tissues beneath and contains fibronectin. It contains Type I, II, III and sometimes IV collagen. It serves as the interface between the basement membrane and the underlying connective tissue.

The anchoring structures are composed of hemidesmosomes, which the basal keratocytes use with anchoring filaments and fibrils to attach. BMZ antibodies have been found that react to various antigens. Langerhans cells are part of the immune system. The BMZ is affected by blister formation and disrupted during healing of wounds. The BMZ is modified in skin with psoriasis, affecting adhesion, migration, proliferation, and differentiation of keratinocytes, interfering with the normal function of the basement membrane.

DERMIS AND HYPODERMIS

The dermis is the layer beneath the epidermis and BMZ. The dermis contains nerves, sebaceous glands, sweat glands, hair follicles, lymphatic vessels, veins, and arteries. Fibroblasts produce the primary proteins of this layer, collagen and elastin, with a protein substance called **ground substance** in the space between them. Mast cells, macrophages, and lymphocytes, which are all involved in the skin immune system (SIS), are also found in the dermis. There are **two areas of the dermis**:

- **Papillary dermis** contains the vascular networks that support the epidermis with oxygen and nutrients. It also functions in thermoregulation by regulating blood flow and contains sensory nerve endings.
- **Reticular dermis** contains the hair follicles and glands and is comprised of connective tissue with collagen and elastic fibers that provides elasticity and strength to the skin. It also contains blood vessels.

The **hypodermis** comprises the layer of subcutaneous tissue below the dermis, providing vasculature, cushioning, and insulation.

FUNCTIONS OF THE SKIN

The primary functions of the skin are the following:

- **Protection**: The skin provides a waterproof barrier to protect against microorganisms, chemicals, and ultraviolet radiation through pigmentation provided by melanocytes.
- **Immunity**: The skin immune system (SIS) with the Langerhans cells protects against foreign antigens. Mast cells and macrophages destroy pathogenic microorganisms as well as promote tissue repair and wound healing.
- **Sensation**: The nerve endings are found in the skin, allowing the person to sense pain, pressure, and temperature. Combinations of sensations detected by nerve receptors translate into sensations of burning, itching, and tickling.
- **Thermoregulation**: The blood vessels within the skin help control body temperature by constricting to retain body heat, or dilating to release heat.
- **Metabolism**: Ultraviolet radiation converts 7-dehydrocholesteral to cholecalciferol, Vitamin D. Vitamin D is synthesized within the skin and then transmits to other parts of the body. It is critical in the metabolism of calcium and phosphate for the formation of bone.
- **Appearance**: Skin provides a cosmetic appearance and communicates identification.

> **Review Video: Integumentary System**
> Visit mometrix.com/academy and enter code: 655980

Wound Care: Assessment

MUSCULOSKELETAL SYSTEM AND THE SKIN

The musculoskeletal system includes 203 bones: long bones (femur), short bones (carpal), and flat bones (sternum). The outer hard shell of the bone is the cortex and the inner porous area is the trabecular bone. The skeletal system is connected by tendons and cartilage and protected, supported, and allowed movement by about 700 soft tissue muscles. Muscles are comprised of muscle fibers. Muscle tissue is contractile and elastic and allows movement of body parts by shortening and lengthening. There are three types of muscles in the human body:

- **Skeletal muscle**: Voluntary muscles that are attached to bones of the head, neck, arms, and legs and facilitate movement
- **Smooth muscle**: Involuntary muscles that make up the walls of blood vessels and hollow organs, such as the bladder
- **Cardiac muscle**: Involuntary muscles comprised of muscle cells found only in the heart

While the skeletal system provides support, it also increases the risk of pressure sores and delays healing when tissue is compressed between bone and surface. The muscles have a high demand for oxygen and are fed by many blood vessels, which are also critical for wound healing. When wounds damage muscles, the blood flow may be interrupted.

VASCULAR SYSTEM AND THE SKIN

The vascular system comprises the venous system and the arterial system. The venous system includes veins, venules, and venous capillaries. Deoxygenated venous blood returns to the heart per the inferior vena cava, superior vena cava, and coronary sinus (bringing blood from the coronary arteries) into the right atrium, then through the tricuspid valve to the right ventricle and through the pulmonic valve into the lungs to exchange carbon dioxide for oxygen. The oxygenated blood returns through the pulmonary veins to the left atrium, through the mitral valve, into the left ventricle, through the aortic valve, and into the aorta and arterial system. The arterial system includes the coronary arteries (which branch from the aorta after it leaves the heart) and arteries, arterioles, and arterial capillaries. In response to a wound, vasoconstriction occurs to reduce bleeding, and clots form to close the wound. This is followed by vasodilation to provide nutrients to the wound and phagocytosis to fight infection and provide growth factors. Angiogenesis increases circulation to healing tissue.

> **Review Video: Cardiovascular System**
> Visit mometrix.com/academy and enter code: 376581

NEUROLOGICAL SYSTEM AND THE SKIN

The neurological (nervous) system consists of the central nervous system (CNS) (brain, spinal cord and nerves) and the peripheral nervous system (PNS) (sensory neurons, ganglia [nerve clusters], and nerves connecting to the central nervous system). The brain consists of the cerebrum (frontal, temporal, parietal, and occipital lobes) the cerebellum, and the brainstem, which is continuous with the spinal cord. The PNS is divided into the autonomic nervous system and the somatic nervous system. The autonomic nervous system, which comprises the parasympathetic and sympathetic nervous systems, controls the body's organs and maintains homeostasis (balance). The SNS plays an important role in angiogenesis, which is critical to wound healing. Functions of the autonomic nervous system include heart rate and function, respiration, digestion, sexual arousal, and other systems. The somatic nervous system comprises cranial and spinal nerves that connect the central nervous system to the skeletal muscles and skin. The somatic nervous system is the voluntarily-controlled component of the peripheral nervous system, and it receives and responds to external sensory stimuli from the skin (such as from pressure or wound pain) and sensory organs.

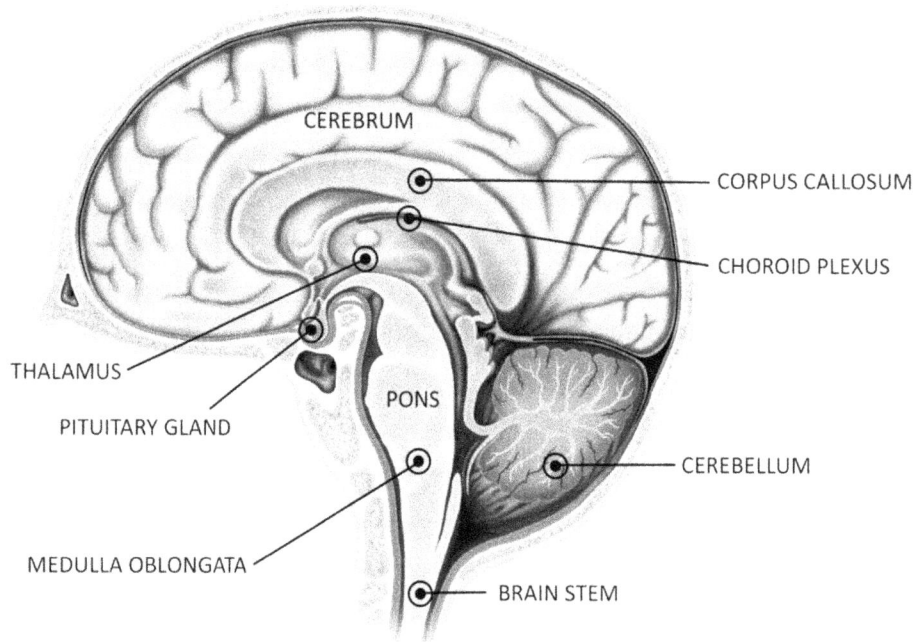

LYMPHATIC SYSTEM AND THE SKIN

The lymphatic system absorbs fluids (lymph) from the blood into the interstitial spaces, carries excess fluids back to the bloodstream, absorbs fatty acids from the intestines, and transports them to the blood. The lymphatic system can also transport cancerous cells from one organ to another. The lymphatic system includes the thymus gland, the spleen, lymph nodes, bone marrow, and lymphatic pathways. The **thymus gland** contains lymphocytes and secretes thymosins, which stimulate maturation of T lymphocytes, a critical cell necessary to fight infections. The **spleen** serves as a reservoir of blood, filters blood, promotes phagocytosis, provides antibodies to strip capsules from bacteria, and produces blood cells if bone marrow not functioning properly). **Lymph nodes** filter harmful particles and provide immune surveillance and are primarily in the cervical, axillary, supratrochlear, thoracic, abdominal, pelvic, and inguinal areas. **Bone marrow** produces blood cells and **lymphatic pathways** (vessels, capillaries, trunks, collecting ducts) carry the lymph through the body. As part of wound healing, lymphatic vessels must regenerate. Lymphatic dysfunction with edema can impair circulation, delay healing, promote bacterial colonization, and result in fibrosis of tissue and chronic inflammation.

Wound Healing

PRIMARY, SECONDARY, AND TERTIARY HEALING

Primary healing (healing by first intention) involves a wound that is surgically closed by suturing, flaps, or split or full-thickness grafts to completely cover the wound. Primary healing is the most common approach used for surgeries or repair of wounds or lacerations, especially when the wound is essentially "clean."

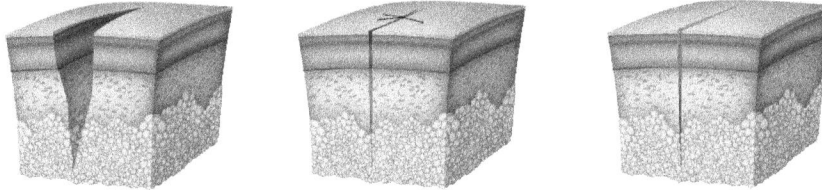

Secondary healing (healing by second intention) involves leaving the wound open and allowing it to close through granulation and epithelialization. Debridement of the wound is done to prepare the wound bed for healing. This approach may be used with contaminated "dirty" or infected wounds to prevent abscess formation and allow the wound to drain.

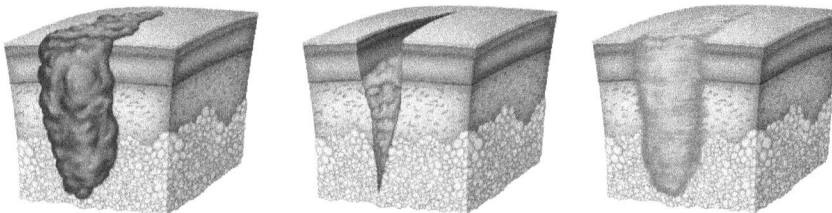

Tertiary healing (healing by third intention) is also sometimes called delayed primary closure because it involves first debriding the wound and allowing it to begin healing while open and then later closing the wound through suturing or grafts. This approach is common with wounds that are contaminated, such as severe animal bites, or wounds related to mixed trauma.

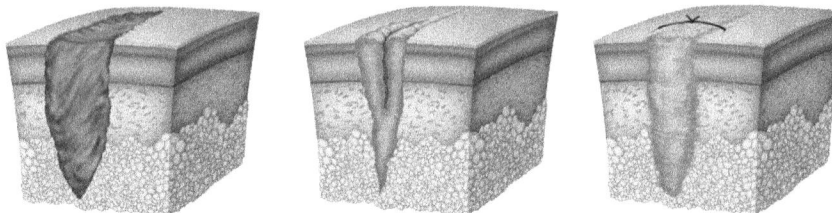

PHASES OF WOUND HEALING

There are **four phases of wound healing**:

1. **Hemostasis** is the first phase of wound healing, occurring within minutes of injury. After the wound occurs, the blood vessels constrict to decrease bleeding. Platelets gather to form a clot and then secrete factors, which cause the production of thrombin. This stimulates fibrin formation from fibrinogen. The resultant clot is a strong one, which becomes the serosanguinous crust (scab) for the wound. Platelets secrete cytokines, including platelet-derived growth factor that begins the healing process.

21

2. The **inflammation phase** occurs next and lasts about four days normally. Blood vessels in the area leak plasma and neutrophils into the wound, causing erythema, edema, and increased warmth. Any debris or microorganisms are destroyed by the neutrophils and localized mast cells through phagocytosis. When fibrin is broken down, it attracts macrophages to the area. They also destroy microorganisms and secrete growth factors to stimulate the next phase of healing.
3. The **proliferative phase** occurs over about days 5-20 in normal healing. During the proliferative phase, fibroblasts secrete collagen to manufacture a framework within the wound. New capillaries sprout from damaged vessel ends in a process called angiogenesis. Keratinocytes cause epithelialization in which new skin cells form at the edges of the wound, migrating inward to meet in the center of the defect. Approximately five days after a wound occurs, the fibroblasts and myofibroblasts contract to bring the wound edges closer, resulting in a smaller defect.
4. **Remodeling or maturation** of a wound begins about 21 days after the wound occurs and continues over the next year. Collagen is deposited, eventually resulting in a stiff, strong scar that has 70-80% of the tensile strength of normal skin. Blood vessels in the newly formed tissues gradually disappear from the scar during this phase.

WOUND HEALING ON THE CELLULAR LEVEL

Cytokines are proteins that serve as soluble mediators and are essential to wound healing. They include growth factors, tumor necrosis factors, interferons, and interleukins. Cytokines are produced from platelets, fibroblasts, monocytes, endothelial cells, and macrophages and facilitate communication between cells and regulate cell proliferation and inflammatory reactions as part of healing. Cytokines also attract neutrophils and macrophages. Cells in the wound produce extracellular matrix proteins. The extracellular matrix includes fibrous and adhesive proteins (collagen, elastin, laminin, fibronectin) and polysaccharides (proteoglycans and glycosaminoglycans [GAGs]). Following injury, platelets aggregate and degranulate, activating factor XII (Hagerman), which promotes formation of a fibrinous clot, which then activates fibrinolysis to break down the clot triggering the complement system. Platelet degranulation triggers release of cytokines into the wound, including:

- **Platelet-derived growth factor (PDGF)**: Activates immune cells and fibroblasts, promotes formation of extracellular matrix and angiogenesis.
- **Fibroblast growth factor (FGF) and epidermal growth factor (EGF)**: Increases proliferation/migration of keratinocytes and extracellular matrix deposition, epithelial cell proliferation, angiogenesis, and formation of granulation tissue.
- **Transforming growth factor (TGFα and TGFβ)**: Promotes formation of extracellular matrix, reduces scarring, increases collagen and tissue inhibitors of metalloproteinase synthesis, decreasing collagen and fibronectin.
- **Tumor necrosis factor α**: Expressed by macrophages to stimulate angiogenesis.

PARTIAL-THICKNESS AND FULL-THICKNESS WOUND HEALING

Partial-thickness wounds involve only the epidermis and the upper parts of the dermis, so the underlying structures that repair skin and provide nutrients, such as the vasculature, and protection, such as the glands, remain intact. Bleeding activates hemostasis and provides a temporary bacterial barrier. Coagulation occurs and fibrin is formed with the clot sealing disrupted vessels. This is followed by fibrinolysis, during which the clot breaks down and repair begins with the inflammatory stage. Healing phase's progress and wounds usually heal within about 2 weeks.

Full-thickness wounds involve the loss of the epidermis and dermis and may also involve loss of underlying tissues, through the fascia, muscle, and to the bone. Full-thickness wounds may be acute or chronic and heal by primary or secondary intention. Those healing by secondary intention are usually surgical wounds that have dehisced or those resulting from underlying morbidities that interfere with normal healing. Bleeding and hemostasis do not occur with healing by secondary intention, compromising the healing process.

ACUTE AND CHRONIC WOUND HEALING

Acute wounds are usually related to an injury and bleed freely because circulation is unimpaired. They heal quickly and continuously, going through the phases of healing in a predictable manner for the size of the wound. There are few if any complications in the healing process.

Chronic wounds are associated with problems in healing, often because of underlying arterial insufficiency. There may not be normal functioning of the components in the healing process or the components may be delayed. For example, the inflammatory phase of healing is usually prolonged. Normal regulatory signals that cause growth to occur may be ignored by the body. There may be repeated injuries to the area, increased inflammation, and poor supply of oxygen and nutrients to the wound. There may be host factors, such as smoking and malnutrition that hamper healing. Genetic and systemic disease can both result in chronic wounds that fail to heal.

MICROENVIRONMENTAL FACTORS THAT AFFECT WOUND HEALING

Wound microenvironment refers to the condition of the wound bed. One problem is that there is often insufficient bleeding in the wound microenvironment initially, so there is less thrombin produced and this impairs production of fibrin. There may be an inadequate supply of growth factors. The lack of growth factors prevents the proliferation of new cells. Lack of innervation may further impair healing. The inflammatory phase is often prolonged, and there is inadequate debridement as phagocytosis is impaired. The presence of infection competes with newly forming skin cells for adequate oxygen and nutrients. The toxins from bacteria further pollute the microenvironment. Moisture is necessary for repair but the presence of excess exudate can restrict cell growth and introduce harmful proteases that further break down growth factors.

SIGNS OF WOUND HEALING

The wound bed must be examined to determine the color of the tissues, amount of moisture present, and degree of epithelialization to demonstrate **signs of healing**:

- Granulation tissue has a granular appearance, is beefy red, feels soft and sponge-like to the touch, bleeds readily when probed, and exhibits no twitch when pinched. It must be distinguished from non-granular tissue, which is smooth and red, and not healing, and hypergranulation, which is soft and spongy and rises above the level of the wound and interferes with epithelialization.
- Epithelialization migrates out from the edges of the wound towards the center. Tissue is usually dry and appears light pink or violet-colored.

The wound bed may show a combination of slough, necrotic tissue, and granular tissue at the same time, so the percentage of each should be determined so that the progress of epithelialization can be demonstrated over time. Pain should be assessed as it may indicate infection.

SCARRING

FACTORS INFLUENCING THE AMOUNT OF SCAR TISSUE FORMED

Deeper wounds produce more scar tissue because a larger amount of granulation tissue is deposited over a longer period of time. The amount of inflammation in a wound also helps to determine the amount of scar tissue formed. Highly pigmented skin produces more scar tissue as does a genetic propensity towards scarring. Tension on a wound during healing causes tissue damage and increased inflammation. This tension is increased in the young versus an older person due to tighter skin and more activity, so children form larger scars than elderly people. Wound location also contributes to scar formation.

EXCESSIVE SCARRING

Excessive scarring includes hypertrophic and keloid scars, which are characterized by raised scars that are erythematous and itchy. Excessive scarring is more common in darkly pigmented skin or in areas where the tissue may stretch, such as over joints. Young or pregnant patients or those with a family history of excessive scarring are at increased risk. There are some distinctions between hypertrophic and keloid scars:

- **Hypertrophic scars** most frequently occur over joints where there is tension on the wound (dorsum of the feet, buttocks, shoulder and upper arms, and upper back). They remain localized to the area of the original wound and may spontaneously regress. Scars that form over joints can cause limited mobility as they contract and may need surgical revision to allow more normal movement.
- **Keloid scars** most frequently occur on the upper back and chest as well as the deltoids and earlobes. They extend beyond the original wound and rarely regress. They usually arise after the wound has healed as raised, shiny, rope-like fibrous scars. They do not result in contracture of the wound. Keloids are most common in those with darker skin and occur due to excess collagen deposition, causing increased growth.

SCARLESS HEALING

Scarless healing occurs in the early-gestation fetus, during the first 2 trimesters, but this ability to heal without scars is lost during the 3rd trimester. This is important for intrauterine surgical procedures, commonly performed during the second trimester when abnormalities become evident. The fetus heals without scarring for a variety of reasons:

- Platelet aggregation is lessened, resulting in less growth factor, such as PDGF.
- The inflammatory response is lessened because of immaturity of the immune system and lack of inflammatory cytokines.
- Wounds move quickly from the inflammatory to the proliferative stage of healing. Fibroblasts, keratinocytes, and endothelial cells, critical to tissue formation, rapidly cover the wound bed. There is no contraction or scarring of the wound.
- Growth factors are balanced so they stimulate growth of connective tissue but prevent excess from forming.
- New and native collagen is indistinguishable, so the new tissue remains flexible.

NON-HEALING WOUNDS

Characteristics of non-healing wounds include:

- **Infection**: Infection increases pro-inflammatory cytokines and prolongs the inflammatory phase of wound healing, sometimes resulting in a non-healing chronic wound. Growth factors may degrade. With infection, granulation tissue may appear dusky. Common pathogens include *Staphylococcus aureus, Pseudomonas aeruginosa,* and β-hemolytic *streptococci.*
- **Biofilm**: A dense thin layer of bacteria in a moist adhesive matrix of secreted polymers that clings to the surface of wounds. Multiple bacteria may be present in a biofilm. The biofilm is resistant to antibiotics and to phagocytosis by white blood cells, resulting in degrading and/or non-healing wounds. Biofilms on the surface of wounds may be mechanically removed.
- **Closed edge**: The wound edges become rolled/curled, dry, and hyperkeratotic and fail to advance, a condition referred to as epibole. Epibole appear light-colored in comparison to surrounding tissue, rounded, and firm. Causes include impaired wound bed, infection, hypoxia, drying, and trauma.

FACTORS THAT AFFECT SKIN'S ABILITY TO HEAL
AGE

Age is an important consideration when evaluating the skin because the characteristics of the skin change as people age.

- An **infant's** skin is thinner than an adult's because, while the epidermis is developed, the dermis layer is only about 60% of that of an adult and continues to develop after birth. The skin of premature infants is especially friable, allowing for transepidermal water loss and evaporative heat loss.
- During **adolescence**, the hair follicles activate, the thickness of the dermis decreases about 20%, and epidermal turnover time increases, so healing slows.
- As people **continue to age**, Langerhans' cells decrease in number, making the skin more prone to cancer, and the inflammatory reactions decrease. The sweat glands, vascularity, and subcutaneous fat all decrease, interfering with thermoregulation and contributing to dryness and irritation of the skin. The epidermal-dermal junction flattens, resulting in skin that is prone to tearing. The elastin in the skin degrades with age and solar exposure. The thinning of the hypodermis can lead to pressure injuries.

> **Review Video: Integumentary System**
> Visit mometrix.com/academy and enter code: 655980

LOTIONS, OILS, AND SOAPS

Lotions, oils, and soaps all have an effect on the skin. Many oils and lotions are used to increase hydration of the skin. These can include oil baths, which have a minimal effect on hydration but do increase the skin-surface lipids. Lipids are the fatty substances that surround skin cells, and those in the outer layer of skin, the stratum corneum, with fatty acids form the water barrier to retain skin hydration and soften skin. Sebum, produced by the sebaceous glands, is also a lipid. Applying lotion increases the hydration of the epidermis, giving the skin a smoother appearance, and moisturizing lotions also increase the lipids, providing some protection. Alkaline soaps, on the other hand, removes the lipid coating of the skin for about 45 minutes after a normal washing and may increase dryness and susceptibility to bacterial infection. Alcohol and acetone also remove the lipid coating and can increase dehydration of the skin. Acidic cleaners are less irritating than either neutral or alkaline cleaners.

SUN EXPOSURE

Sun exposure is one of the primary factors in aging of the skin, referred to as photoaging or dermatoheliosis. Tanning occurs when ultraviolet radiation (UVR) damages the epidermis and stimulates the production of melanin as a protective mechanism to prevent damage to deeper layers of skin. When the melanin is overpowered, sunburn results, damaging the outer layers of the skin and sometimes the DNA of the skin cells, which can lead to cancer. There are several effects of photoaging that should be noted in assessment:

- Decrease in elasticity and strength
- Dry, rough, wrinkled skin
- Fine veins on face and ears
- Freckles and large brown macules (solar lentigines, liver spots) on face, and exposed areas, such as hands and arms and white macules on exposed areas of upper and lower extremities
- Benign lesions, such as actinic and seborrheic keratoses
- Malignant lesions, such as basal cell and squamous cell carcinoma

MEDICATIONS

Medications are a frequent cause of dermatologic effects that can impair the integrity of the skin:

- **Photosensitivity** can be either photoallergic with exposure to ultraviolet radiation causing an allergic reaction, usually with rash, erythema, edema, and pruritus or phototoxic with the drug being converted into a toxin that causes edema, pain, and pronounced erythema. Thiazide diuretics and conjugated estrogens often cause photosensitive reactions.
- **Allergic reactions** may involve rash, urticaria or more complex reactions, such as serum sickness. Amoxicillin alone or with clavulanate causes a high rate of these reactions.
- **Erythema multiforme** has been caused by nifedipine, verapamil, and diltiazem (calcium channel blockers).
- **Toxic epidermal necrolysis** with full-thickness loss of epidermis can be caused by ciprofloxacin.
- **Thinning or atrophy of the skin** because of a loss of collagen and telangiectasia (spider veins) are associated with oral, topical, and inhaled corticosteroids.

LOCAL FACTORS

Local factors that may impact the healing process include:

- **Local infection**: Invasion of the wound by microorganisms, such as *Staphylococcus aureus, MRSA, Pseudomonas,* and *Escherichia coli,* not only slows healing but may cause the wound to erode and increase in size, increasing the risk of systemic infection. Inflammation is a normal part of the healing process, but prolonged inflammation delays healing.
- **Repeat trauma**: If a wound is not adequately protected or if the patient is not positioned correctly, further erosion of the wound may occur.
- **Impaired tissue oxygenation**: Conditions that result in vasoconstriction or low blood flow to the area (such as PAD, blood clot, and hypotension) of the wound can impair healing or worsen the wound. Wounds are typically hypoxic initially because of disruption of blood flow and increased need for oxygen, but this triggers angiogenesis and release of growth factors, which should increase oxygenation unless other factors are present.

SYSTEMIC FACTORS

Systemic factors that may impact the healing process include:

- **Inadequate nutrition**: A diet with adequate nutrition and protein is necessary for healing, so an inadequate diet may slow the healing process.
- **Obesity**: Patients who are overweight are at increased risk of pressure injuries because of compression of tissues, and have slower rates of healing as well as increased risk of infection.
- **Chronic disease**: Some diseases, such as diabetes mellitus and hypertension may impair healing.
- **Systemic infection**: Whether originating from the wound or elsewhere, a systemic infection impairs healing.
- **Decrease in sex hormones** (usually associated with age): Low levels of androgens and estrogen slow healing of wounds.
- **Stress**: Emotional stress increases glucocorticoids and reduces cytokines at the wound, impairing healing.

Diagnostic Studies

LABORATORY TESTS RELEVANT TO WOUND HEALING AND SKIN BREAKDOWN

Wound healing and the prevention of skin breakdown requires an adequate nutritional status. Labs that assess for malnutrition, anemia, and dehydration are done to assess the risk for skin breakdown and delayed wound healing. Tests that are frequently used as part of wound management include the following.

TOTAL PROTEIN AND ALBUMIN

Total protein levels can be influenced by many factors, including stress and infection, but it may be monitored as part of an overall nutritional assessment. Protein is critical for wound healing, and because metabolic rate increases in response to a wound, protein needs increase in wounded patients:

- Normal values: 5-9 g/dL
- Diet requirements for wound healing: 1.25-1.5 g/kg per day

Albumin is a protein that is produced by the liver and is a necessary component for cells and tissues. Levels decrease with renal disease, malnutrition, and severe burns. Albumin levels are the most common screening to determine protein levels. Albumin has a half-life of 18-20 days, so it is more sensitive to long-term protein deficiencies than to short-term.

- Normal values: 3.5-5.5 g/dL
- Mild deficiency: 3-3.5 g/dL
- Moderate deficiency: 2.5-3.0 g/dL
- Severe deficiency: <2.5 g/dL

Levels below 3.2 correlate with increased morbidity and death. Dehydration (poor intake, diarrhea, or vomiting) elevates levels, so adequate hydration is important to ensure meaningful results

TRANSFERRIN

Transferrin, which transports about one-third of the body's iron, is a protein produced by the liver. It transports iron from the intestines to the bone marrow where it is used to produce hemoglobin. The half-life of transferrin is about 8-10 days. It is sometimes used as a measure of nutritional status; however, transferrin levels are sensitive to many different things. Levels rapidly decrease with protein malnutrition. Liver disease and anemia can also depress levels, but a decrease in iron, commonly found with inadequate protein, stimulates the liver to produce more transferrin, which increases levels but also decreases production of albumin and prealbumin. Levels may also increase with pregnancy, use of oral contraceptives, and polycythemia. Thus, transferrin levels alone are not always reliable measurements of nutritional status:

- Normal values: 200-400 mg/dL
- Mild deficiency: 150-200 mg/dL
- Moderate deficiency: 100-150 mg/dL
- Severe deficiency: <100 mg/dL

> **Review Video: Transferrin**
> Visit mometrix.com/academy and enter code: 267479

PREALBUMIN

Prealbumin (transthyretin) is most commonly monitored for acute changes in nutritional status because it has a half-life of only 2-3 days. Prealbumin is a protein produced in the liver, so it is often decreased with liver disease. Oral contraceptives and estrogen can also decrease levels. Levels may rise with Hodgkin's disease or the use of steroids or NSAIDS. Prealbumin is necessary for transportation of both thyroxine and vitamin A throughout the body, so if levels fall, both thyroxine and vitamin A utilization are affected.

- Normal values: 16-40 mg/dL
- Mild deficiency: 10-15 mg/dL
- Moderate deficiency: 5-9 mg/dL
- Severe deficiency: <5 mg/dL

Prealbumin is a good measurement because it quickly decreases when nutrition is inadequate and rises quickly in response to increased protein intake. Protein intake must be adequate to maintain levels of prealbumin. Death rates increase with any decrease in prealbumin levels.

INDICATORS OF HYDRATION
SERUM SODIUM AND OSMOLALITY

Hydration is essential for proper healing and for meaningful results of laboratory measures of nutrition. A number of different tests can be used to monitor hydration.

Serum sodium measures the sodium level in the blood. Some drugs, such as steroids, laxatives, contraceptives, NSAIDS, and IV fluids containing sodium can elevate levels. Other drugs, such as diuretics and vasopressin can reduce levels.

- Normal values: 135-150 mEq/L
- Dehydration: >150 mEq/L

Serum osmolality measures the concentration of ions, such as sodium, chloride, potassium, glucose, and urea, in the blood. Levels increase with dehydration, which stimulates the antidiuretic hormone (AD), resulting in increased water reabsorption and more concentrated urine in an effort to compensate. Changes in osmolality can affect normal cell functioning, eventually destroying the cells if levels remain high.

- Normal levels: 285-295 mOsm/kg H_2O.
- Dehydration: >295 mOsm/kg H_2O.

BLOOD UREA NITROGEN (BUN), BUN-CREATININE RATIO, AND SPECIFIC GRAVITY/URINE

Blood urea nitrogen (BUN), a protein by-product, is excreted by the kidneys. An elevation of both BUN and creatinine indicates kidney disease, but elevated BUN alone may indicate dehydration:

- Normal values: 7-23 mg/dL
- Dehydration: >23 mg/dL

BUN-creatinine ratio monitors renal failure, where there is enhanced reabsorption in the proximal tubules, causing the urea level to rise. Dehydration or conditions that limit fluid into the kidneys increases urea. Increased urea is also an indication of an upper GI bleed where the proteins in the blood are broken down and reabsorbed in the lower intestinal tract.

- Normal value: 10:1
- Dehydration: >25:1

Specific gravity/urine measures the ability of the kidneys to concentrate or dilute the urine according to changes in serum. The most common cause of an increased specific gravity is dehydration. It may also increase with an increased secretion of anti-diuretic hormone (ADH).

- Normal value: 1.003-1.028
- Dehydration: >1.028

GLUCOSE AND HEMOGLOBIN AIC

Glucose is manufactured by the liver from ingested carbohydrates and is stored as glycogen for use by the cells. If intake is inadequate, glucose can be produced from muscle and fat tissue, leading to increased wasting. High levels of glucose are indicative of diabetes mellitus, which predisposes people to skin injuries, slow healing, and infection. Fasting blood glucose levels are used to diagnose and monitor:

- Normal values: 70-99 mg/dL
- Impaired: 100-125 mg/dL
- Diabetes: >125 mg/dL

There are a number of different conditions that can increase glucose levels: stress, renal failure, Cushing syndrome, hyperthyroidism, and pancreas disorders. Medications, such as steroids, estrogens, lithium, phenytoin, diuretics, and tricyclic antidepressants, may increase glucose levels. Other conditions, such as adrenal insufficiency, liver disease, hypothyroidism, and starvation can decrease glucose levels.

Hemoglobin AIC comprises hemoglobin A with a glucose molecule because hemoglobin holds onto excess blood glucose, so it shows the average blood glucose levels over a 2-3 month period and is used primarily to monitor long-term diabetic therapy.

- Normal value: ≤6%
- Elevation: >7%

TOTAL LYMPHOCYTE COUNT

The immune system responds quickly to changes in protein intake because proteins are critical to antibody and lymphocyte production. T lymphocytes develop in the thymus gland and are a part of the cell-mediated immune response. B-lymphocytes develop in the bone marrow and are part of the humoral (antibody-mediated) immune response.

Total lymphocyte count (TLC) can reflect changes in nutritional status because a decrease in protein causes decreased immunity. Lymphocytes are expressed on a differential as a percentage of the white blood count. The TLC is calculated by multiplying the percentage by the total white blood count and then dividing by 100.

- Normal values: 2000 cells/mm^3
- Mild deficiency: 1500-1800 cells/mm^3
- Moderate deficiency: 900-1500 cells/mm^3
- Severe deficiency: <900 cells/mm^3

While low levels may be indicative of malnutrition, levels are also depressed with stress, autoimmune diseases, chemotherapy, infection, and HIV.

COMPLETE BLOOD COUNT WITH RBCS, PLATELETS, HGB AND HCT

The complete blood count with differential and platelet (thrombocyte) count provides information about the blood and other body systems. Red blood cell (erythrocyte) counts and concentrations may vary with anemia, hemorrhage, or various disorders. A decrease in red blood cells may affect healing because of less oxygen to tissues, but changes do not indicate infection.

- **Hemoglobin**, a protein found in erythrocytes, uses iron to bind and transport oxygen. Deficiencies of amino acids, vitamins, or minerals can cause a decrease in hemoglobin, impacting healing and increasing the danger of pressure injuries by reducing oxygen to tissue. Dehydration and severe burns can cause an increase.
  - Normal values: Males, 13-18 g/dL. Females, 12-16 g/dL.

- **Hematocrit** measures the percentage of packed red blood cells in 100 ml of blood. A decrease can indicate blood loss and anemia. An increase may indicate dehydration, and measurements may help to monitor the effects of rehydration.
  - o Normal values: Males, 42-52%. Females, 37-48%.
- **Platelet** normal values of 150,000-400,000 may increase to over a million during acute infection.

COMPLETE BLOOD COUNT WITH WBCs AND DIFFERENTIAL

White blood cell (leukocyte) count is used as an indicator of bacterial and viral infection. WBC is reported as the total number of all white blood cells.

- Normal WBC for adults: 4,800-10,000
- Acute infection: >10,000 (a level of 30,000 or more indicates the infection is severe).
- Viral infection: 4,000 and below

The differential provides the percentage of each different type of leukocyte. An increase in the total white blood cell count is usually related to an increase in one type. Often an increase in immature neutrophils (known as bands) referred to as a "shift to the left," is an indication of an infectious process:

- Normal immature neutrophils (bands): 1-3%. Increase with infection
- Normal segmented neutrophils (segs) for adults: 50-62%. Increase with acute, localized, or systemic bacterial infections.
- Normal eosinophils: 0-3%. Decrease with stress and acute infection.
- Normal basophils: 0-1%. Decrease during acute stage of infection.
- Normal lymphocytes; 25-40%. Increase in some viral and bacterial infections.
- Normal monocytes: 3-7%. Increase during recovery stage of acute infection.

C-REACTIVE PROTEIN AND ERYTHROCYTE SEDIMENTATION RATE

C-reactive protein is an acute-phase reactant produced by the liver in response to an inflammatory response that causes neutrophils, granulocytes, and macrophages to secrete cytokines. Thus, levels of C-reactive protein rise when there is inflammation or infection. It has also been found to be a helpful measurement of response to treatment for pyoderma gangrenosum ulcers:

- Normal values: 2.6-7.6 μg/dL

Erythrocyte sedimentation rate (sed rate) measures the distance erythrocytes fall in a vertical tube of anticoagulated blood in one hour. Because fibrinogen, which increases in response to infection, also increases the rate of the fall, the sed rate can be used as a non-specific test for inflammation when infection is suspected. The sed rate is sensitive to osteomyelitis and may be used to monitor treatment response. Values vary according to gender and age:

- <50: Males 0-15 mm/hr. Females 0-20 mm/hr.
- >50: Males 0-20 mm/hr. Females 0-30 mm/hr.

WOUND CULTURE AND SENSITIVITIES

Wound culture and sensitivities are done when there are signs of infection in a wound or no progress in healing over a two-week period. The wound culture identifies the pathogenic agent and the sensitivities show which antimicrobials are the most affective for treatment. The culture should be done prior to the administration of antibiotics, which may interfere with the results. Sterile technique should be used. A culture area may be done, taking the sample from clean tissue rather than exudate, which may give a false report, showing organisms in the area but not in the tissue itself. There are **three methods of culturing**:

- **Swabbing** the area is the most common method used but the sample is easily contaminated by surface flora.
- **Needle aspiration** of fluid adjacent to the wound may result in underestimation of organisms.
- Culturing by **tissue biopsy** is often most effective method, but not all labs can process these samples and the process disrupts the wound and increases pain.

DIAGNOSTIC IMAGING

Imaging can also be useful when diagnosing and evaluating wounds and vasculature:

- **Magnetic Resonance Angiography (MRA)**: This type of angiography is minimally invasive and may use contrast. Radio waves and a magnetic field produce computer-generated images that are more detailed than with standard angiography.
- **Computed Tomography Angiography (CTA)**: This is a minimally-invasive procedure that may use contrast to enhance vessels. It requires a sophisticated computer program to produce multiple images for computer-generated cross-sectional pictures, but it is becoming more widely available.
- **Computer enhanced angiography**: This is an invasive procedure that requires the insertion of catheters into the femoral artery. Vessel wall injury can occur and clots can be liberated from the vessel walls by accident. The contrast used can damage the kidneys. Angioplasty may be performed during angiography, combining diagnosis with treatment in one procedure. Smaller vessels may not be seen so this test is not conclusive when deciding whether amputation of the limb should take place.

MEASURING VENOUS REFILL

Measuring venous refill is critical to diagnosing the cause and wounds and extent/severity of vascular disease:

- **Photo plethysmography (PPG)** measures venous refill time using light absorption via an infrared light emitting diode that emits light through the skin. PPG measures light absorbed and reflected from the hemoglobin of the blood during the filing of tiny blood vessels to determine changes in blood volume.
- **Light Reflective Rheography (LRR)**, based on PPG, uses infrared light and three light diodes, which reduces reflection of external light and the skin surface to produce a more accurate measure of venous refill than the PPG.
- **String Gauge Plethysmography (SGP)** uses PPG to study venous flow, but also uses a string gauge wrapped around the leg to detect tension changes in the calf during exertion, revealing venous refill and emptying.

DETERMINING ADEQUATE BLOOD FLOW

DOPPLER

Doppler is equipment that provides an ultrasonic evaluation of arterial circulation of the extremities. Doppler evaluation is used when the circulation of the extremity appears impaired (edema, pallor, cyanosis), when pulses cannot be palpated manually, and to determine site for arterial puncture. The procedure is described below:

1. Place conductive gel on the end of the probe or on the skin over the site to be assessed, hold the device at a 45-degree angle to the skin, and move it about the skin until the pulse is heard.
2. Count the pulse rate, describe the intensity, remove the device, wipe away the conductive gel, and then use a marking pen to mark the site.
3. When assessing the sound, the echo heard is at a higher frequency when blood flow is in the direction of the transducer and lower frequency when it is in the opposite direction (representing the Doppler effect/frequency shift).

There are two methods of using doppler to assess blood flow:

- **Continuous wave doppler** is a non-invasive test that uses a pencil-like probe containing a piezoelectric crystal that emits a sound wave that is reflected by the blood vessel back to the probe, producing an audible sound that is analyzed to determine whether blood flow is adequate. The Doppler is also used along with a blood pressure cuff to compare brachial and ankle pressures to diagnose claudication.
- **Laser doppler skin perfusion pressures**: A blood pressure cuff containing a laser probe in the bladder of the cuff is used to measure skin perfusion to detect early limb ischemia. It detects both tissue perfusion and vascular status and is 80% accurate.

DUPLEX ULTRASOUND SCREENING FOR LOWER EXTREMITY ARTERIAL DISEASE

The purpose of duplex ultrasound screening is to evaluate for the presence of atherosclerotic disease, which causes lower extremity arterial disease. This has traditionally been completed by measuring the ankle-brachial index. Duplex ultrasound of the lower extremity, usually the superficial femoral artery, can be accomplished just as easily and is a more sensitive and specific test to identify for the presence of lower extremity arterial disease. Screening can also help to diagnose early disease, before patients are strongly symptomatic. This could enable them to change any modifiable risk factors, such as smoking or obesity, to decrease their odds of developing strong symptoms or complications of lower extremity arterial disease. This can also be an indicator that there may be coronary artery disease present if the atherosclerotic disease is present in the lower extremity arteries.

TRANSCUTANEOUS OXYGEN PRESSURE (TcPO$_2$)

Transcutaneous oxygen pressure (TcPO$_2$) uses non-invasive electrodes placed directly on the skin to measure the oxygen being released from the capillaries. These electrodes are heated slightly to ensure blood flow is promoted to the extremity and to minimize misreads secondary to cold-induced vasoconstriction. TcPO$_2$ measurement can be done as an absolute value in mmHg, or as a ratio that compares the value at the extremity to the value at the chest (with 0.9 being accepted as normal). The normal absolute value for perfusion of the lower extremities is around 60 mmHg and a level of >40 mmHg has been proven sufficient for wound healing. When the perfusion level drops below 30 mmHg, healing is compromised. While pulse oximetry is widely used to measure more systemic oxygenation status, TcPO$_2$ is indicated when the goal is to determine the level of ischemia localized to the extremities or to define the severity of vascular compromise or disease. It is often used in measuring perfusion to an amputation site and in managing foot ulcers.

ULTRASOUND FOR MONITORING WOUND CARE AND HEALING

Ultrasound technology is now used for monitoring wound care and healing as well as promoting healing. Clinical studies are now underway to determine the effectiveness of low-frequency, low-intensity ultrasound treatments for chronic wounds. Some studies indicate that ultrasound stimulation increases the rate of healing. Currently, ultrasound is used primarily for measuring and tracking. For example, Wound Mapping Ultrasound offers three-dimensional measurement, alert notifications, digital imaging, and diagnostic capabilities as well as visualization of blood flow. A special transparent dressing is applied over the wound to protect it from the transducer, so patients may feel pressure or some discomfort. Upon completion of the ultrasound, a report is generated that indicates the size, shape, depth, whether there is undermining or absence presence, and the type of invasion of local tissue that is present (such as to muscle, tendon, bone, and/or joint capsule).

Performing Initial Assessment

ASSESSING ETIOLOGIC FACTORS

Wounds should be evaluated for **etiology** (the origin of the wound) during the initial assessment to ensure proper treatment. Wounds can arise from a number of different etiologies:

- **Pressure**: Wounds that occur over bony prominences, such as the heels and coccyx, may be related to pressure, shear, or friction. The skin should be carefully examined for discolorations or changes in texture that might indicate compromise.
- **Arterial**: Arterial insufficiency is associated with a decrease in pedal pulses, and cool atrophic (shiny, dry) skin. It may result in small punctate-type ulcers, frequently on the dorsum of foot.
- **Venous stasis**: A decrease in venous circulation often results in hemoglobin leaking into the tissues of the lower leg, causing a brown discoloration. Tissue is often edematous, and ulcers are most common near the medial malleolus.
- **Diabetic neuropathy/ischemia**: Neuropathy can result in a lack of sensation to pain so that injuries to the feet may go unnoticed. Diabetes may also cause damage to small vessels, resulting in ischemia that can lead to ulcerations.
- **Trauma**: Injuries resulting from accidents or other types of trauma may vary considerably with some resulting in extensive damage to bones, tissues, organs, and circulation. Additionally, the wounds may be contaminated. Each wound must be assessed individually for multiple factors.
- **Burns**: Burn wounds may be chemical, thermal, or electric and should be assessed according to the area, the percentage of the body burned, and the depth of the burn.
- **Infection**: An infected surgical or wound site can result in pain, edema, cellulitis, drainage, erosion of the sutures and ulceration of the tissue. Surgical sites must be assessed carefully and laboratory findings reviewed.

ASSESSING OXYGENATION

Assessment of oxygenation includes:

- **Color**: Impaired oxygenation may cause a change in the color of the skin, including pallor and cyanosis, especially in the extremities and about the mouth and nose. Individuals with darker skin may take on a gray, ashy appearance.
- **Respiratory rate**: As oxygenation falls, air hunger may occur with the patient becoming increasingly dyspneic.
- **Oxygen saturation**: While normal oxygen saturation is greater than 95%, as oxygenation is impaired, the level may fall below 92%. Oxygen saturation loses accuracy if the level falls below 80%, so blood gas analysis should be done in those cases.
- **Blood gas analysis**: PO_2 should be greater than 80 mmHg but may fall below 60 mmHg (indicating hypoxemia).
- **Altered mental status**: As oxygen levels fall, the patient may exhibit confusion.
- **Blood lactate level**: Results higher than 2 mEq/L indicate impaired tissue oxygenation.

NEUROLOGICAL/NEUROVASCULAR ASSESSMENT

Neurological/neurovascular assessment includes:

- **Cranial nerve assessment**: Assess cranial nerves I through VII.
- **Inspection of muscles**: Determine if they are of normal size, strength, and tone and equal bilaterally. Note any involuntary movements (twitches, tremors).
- **Balance assessment**: Assess gait, Romberg test (feet together, eyes closed for 20 seconds), rapid alternating movements, finger-to-finger or finger-to-nose, and heel-to-shin test.
- **Sensory assessment**: Assess spinothalamic tracts for perception of pain, temperature, and light touch. Assess posterior column tract with vibration, position, fine touch, stereognosis, graphesthesia, two-point discrimination, extinction, and point location testing.
- **Reflexes**: Assess deep tendon reflexes (biceps reflex, triceps reflex, brachioradialis reflex, quadriceps reflex, Achilles reflex, and clonus) and superficial cutaneous reflexes (abdominal reflexes, cremasteric reflex, and plantar reflex).
- **Developmental status**: An age-appropriate assessment should determine if the patient's development is within normal parameters. Older adults may exhibit slower response times than younger adults and may exhibit tremors and unsteady gait related to age changes.

ELEMENTS OF WOUND ASSESSMENT

LOCATION AND SIZE

Wound location should be described in terms of anatomic position using landmarks (such as sternal notch, umbilicus, lateral malleolus), correct medical terminology, and directional terms:

- Anterior (in front)
- Posterior (behind)
- Superior (above)
- Inferior (below)

Wound size should be carefully described through actual measurement rather than association (the size of a dime). Measurements should be done with a disposable ruler in millimeters or centimeters. The current standard for measurement:

$$\text{length} \times \text{width} \times \text{depth} = \text{dimension}$$

However, a clear description requires more detail. The measurement should be done at the greatest width and greatest length. More than two measurements may be needed if the wound is very irregularly shaped. The depth of the wound should be measured by inserting a sterile applicator and grasping or marking the applicator at skin level and then measuring the length below. Ideally, the wound should be photographed as well, following protocols for photography.

WOUND BED TISSUE

Wound bed tissue should be described as completely as possible, including color and general appearance:

- **Granulation tissue** is slightly granular in appearance and deep pink to bright red and moist, bleeding easily if disturbed.
- **Clean non-granular tissue** is smooth and deep pink or red and is not healing.
- **Hypergranulation** is excessive, soft, flaccid granulating tissue that is raised above the level of the periwound tissue, preventing proper epithelization, and may reflect excess moisture in the wound.
- **Epithelization** should appear at wound edges first and then eventually cover the wound. It is dry and light pink or violet in color.
- **Slough** is necrotic tissue that is viscous, soft, and yellow-gray in appearance and adheres to the wound.
- **Eschar** is hard dark brown or black leathery necrotic tissue that accumulates with death of the tissue.

WOUND MARGINS

Wound margins and the tissue surrounding the wound should be described carefully and with correct terminology:

- **Color** should be described using color descriptions and such terms as blanched, erythematous (red), or ecchymosed (purple, green, yellow).
- **Skin texture** may be normal, indurated (hardened), or edematous (swollen). Note if there is cellulitis or maceration evident.
- **Wound edges** may be diffuse (without clear margins), well defined, or rolled. A healing ridge may be evident if granulation has begun. Note if the wound is closed (as with a surgical incision) or open (as with dehiscence or ulcerations). Note if wound edges are attached or unattached (indicating undermining or tunneling).
- **Tunneling or undermining** should be assessed by probing the wound margins with a moist sterile cotton applicator, using clock face locators (toward the head is 12 o'clock, for example). Tunneling may be described as extending from 3 o'clock to 4 o'clock. A large area is usually described as undermining. The size should be measured or estimated as closely as possible.

DISTRIBUTION, DRAINAGE, AND ODOR

Distribution of lesions should be clearly delineated if there is more than one lesion over an area. The arrangement of the lesions can be helpful for diagnosis and treatments.

- Linear (in a line)
- Satellites (small lesions around a larger one)
- Diffuse (scattered freely over an area)

Drainage may vary considerably from nothing at all to copious outpourings of discharge.

- Serous drainage is usually clear to slightly yellow.
- Serosanguineous drainage is a combination of serous drainage and blood.
- Sanguineous drainage is bloody.
- Purulent discharge may be thick and milky, yellow, brownish, or green, depending upon the infective agent.

Odor requires more subjective assessment, but the odor and type of discharge together can provide useful information. Some infective agents, such as *Pseudomonas*, produce distinctive odors, which may be described in various ways: musty, foul, sweet.

WOUND EXUDATE

Wound exudate is fluid found in the wound, consisting of blood serum, debris from cells, bacteria, and white blood cells (leukocytes). **Wound exudate** can occur in small to large amounts and, depending on the presence of an organism, may be colored clear or pale yellow (serous), pink or blood tinged (serosanguineous), red (sanguineous), or white/yellow (purulent pus). Consistency can range from thin to milky to thick, and odor may occur. When fluid covers less than one-third of the dressing, it is termed small in amount. Fluid covering one-third to two-thirds of the dressing is considered moderate, and fluid covering over two-thirds of the surface of the dressing is considered large. The presence of exudate can occur when the wound is left untreated or when venous insufficiency, congestive heart failure, malnutrition, kidney or liver disease, or infection is present. One must remember that some odors may be caused by the reaction of the wound fluid on the dressing. Odor can also be caused when the dressing is not changed often enough.

WOUND MEASUREMENT

Wound measurement determines the progress of healing and must be done accurately and consistently each time. When the wound is a surgical one, it is sufficient to measure length and width, but depth is important for pressure injuries:

- One should use millimeters or centimeters, not inches, in measurement.
- Linear measurement utilizes a plastic or paper ruler marked in centimeters, measuring the greatest length and the greatest width or making the measurements perpendicular to each other. This is the most common method, but it doesn't take into account the shape of the wound and can overestimate the surface area involved when the measurement is multiplied length by width.
- The outline of the wound may also be traced onto an acetate sheet marked in centimeters and the surface area determined by counting the squares.
- Depth is then determined by inserting a sterile moist cotton applicator into the deepest part of the wound.
- Undermining and tunneling tracts are measured in the same manner.

DIGITAL METHODS OF WOUND MEASUREMENT

A number of different tools are available for measuring and monitoring wounds using digital equipment. These tools are often more accurate than manual measurements and maintain a historical record that can be easily accessed to track changes. Most tools are software applications that can be loaded onto a smartphone (camera-enabled) or iPad, requiring only that the healthcare provider position the device and take photos. Some programs, such as WoundDesk (Digital MedLab) are primarily management software to improve documentation, but others, such as Scout (WoundVision) provide visual and infrared imaging and both physical and physiological (blood flow, metabolic activity) monitoring. Another program, WoundZoom, contains a 3D sensor and can provide an image of the wound that includes the length, depth, and breadth. Swift Skin and Wound, a widely-used program, offers a wound management system (Swift App for measurement, Swift HealX to calibrate size, color, lighting, and Swift dashboard to display data) that includes wound measurement, imaging, and tracking.

ASSESSMENT OF PERIWOUND ENVIRONMENT

The periwound environment includes the area around the wound and is an important part of wound assessment:

- Note signs of inflammation such as warmth, erythema, and edema.
- Palpate the skin for firmness and fluctuation that may indicate a subcutaneous abscess.
- Look for signs of breakdown from tape.
- Observe for signs of pale, moist, soft skin that may be maceration caused by exudate from the wound.
- Check the skin for flakiness or evidence of dryness, as the surrounding skin may be too dry if the dressing wicks the moisture out of the skin.
- Examine the skin for signs of circulatory impairment, such as abnormal hair distribution, rubor, or pallor.
- Note evidence of undermining or tunneling that extends under the tissue.

DOCUMENTATION OF THE WOUND ASSESSMENT

The care provider can use the acronym **ASSESSMENT** to help document the thorough assessment of a wound:

- **A**natomically locate the wound on the body and include the age of the wound
- **S**ize of the wound in centimeters: length, width, and depth, including shape and stage of the wound
- **S**inus tracts, tunneling, fistulas, and undermining at the edges
- **E**xudate color, amount, and consistency
- **S**epsis present in the wound or systemically
- **S**urrounding skin color, edema, status

Wound Care: Assessment

- **M**argins of the wound, attachment to the wound bed, rolling, presence of maceration
- **E**rythema, presence of epithelialization or eschar
- **N**ecrotic tissue presence, odor of wound, visible blood vessels
- **T**issue of wound bed, amount of granulation present, wound tenderness, tension, and temperature

ASSESSMENT CHARACTERISTICS OF ARTERIAL, NEUROPATHIC, AND VENOUS ULCERS

The assessment process is important in delineating between the arterial, neuropathic, or venous origin of the ulcer. Characteristics of each must be known and closely examined:

Location

- **Arterial**: Ends of toes, pressure points, traumatic nonhealing wounds
- **Neuropathic**: Plantar surface, metatarsal heads, toes, and sides of feet
- **Venous**: Between knees and ankles, medial malleolus

Wound Bed

- **Arterial**: Pale, necrotic
- **Neuropathic**: Red (or ischemic)
- **Venous**: Dark red, fibrinous slough

Exudate

- **Arterial**: Slight amount, infection common
- **Neuropathic**: Moderate to large amounts, infection common
- **Venous**: Moderate to large amounts

Wound Perimeter

- **Arterial**: Circular, well-defined
- **Neuropathic**: Circular, well-defined, often with callous formation
- **Venous**: Irregular, poorly-defined

Pain

- **Arterial**: Very painful
- **Neuropathic**: Pain often absent because of reduced sensation
- **Venous**: Pain varies

Skin

- **Arterial**: Pale, friable, shiny, and hairless, with dependent rubor and elevational pallor
- **Neuropathic**: Ischemic signs (as in arterial) may be evident with co-morbidity
- **Venous**: Brownish discoloration of ankles and shin, edema common

Pulses

- **Arterial**: Weak or absent
- **Neuropathic**: Present and palpable, diminished in neuroischemic ulcers
- **Venous**: Present and palpable

ASSESSING FOR WOUND COMPLICATIONS

CHRONIC INFLAMMATION

Chronic inflammation of a wound can last for months, delaying wound healing. The immune system may fail to adequately phagocytose debris and dead tissue in the wound and fight infection, and wound care may be inadequate, such as failure to debride the wound or clear infection. Chronic inflammation is caused by debris, necrotic tissue, repeated injury to the wound, and continued effects of histamine release from mast cells. The blood vessels stay dilated, causing warmth, redness, and swelling. The wound-encircling erythema is a ring of redness in light skin or a ring of darkness in dark skin. Pain may be absent or intense if there is infection or arterial vascular disease present. Necrotic tissue may extend over all or part of the wound bed and may be light or dark in color and hard, soft, or stringy. Exudate may be thick, yellow, brown, or green with an odor. The exudate should be cleansed from the wound so that the odor of the wound bed itself can be determined.

UNDERMINING

Undermining occurs at the edges of a wound and may result from shear injuries. The tissues pull away from the base of the wound and a cavity occurs under the intact skin of the wound periphery. The opening of the wound is thus smaller than the area of tissue damage beneath the surface of the skin surrounding the wound. The degree of undermining should be documented by using the face of the clock to describe the location of the undermining in relation to the opening and by recording the depth of the undermining into surrounding tissues by gently probing with a moist sterile cotton applicator. There are two basic **types of undermining**:

- **Initial**: This is related to discharge of liquefied necrotic tissue, leaving undermining that circles the wound. The wound usually lacks signs of epithelialization.
- **Late**: This is related to external pressure (after discharge undermining), and leaves more localized undermining, often in the direction of a bony prominence. The wound shows signs of epithelialization in non-undermined areas.

WOUND TUNNELING

Wound tunneling is a form of undermining that creates a tract that leads away from the wound through subcutaneous tissues between muscles. Tunneling occurs when the fascia that holds muscles together in bundles is cut. Tunneling must be measured with a sterile moist cotton applicator and documented as to depth and width, using the clock face to describe location (3 to 4 o'clock) and then packed loosely to stimulate the healing process. If tunneling ends in a dead space, infection of the wound can progress through the tunnel to cause development of abscess. Tunneling may be caused by infection, pressure that causes tissue necrosis (over bony prominences), or foreign bodies, such as a suture or dressing material left in the wound. It is important for tunnels to heal prior to wound closure to prevent abscess formation, necessitating surgical drainage later. Tunnels are common in surgical wounds in which dehiscence occurs, and the tunnels can join together to form sinus tracts.

ASSESSMENT OF LOWER EXTREMITIES

Assessment of lower extremities includes a number of different elements:

- **Appearance** includes comparing limbs for obvious differences or changes in skin or nails as well as evaluating for edema and color changes in skin, such as pallor or rubor.
- **Perfusion** should be assessed by checking venous filling time, capillary refill, skin temperature (noting changes in one limb or between limbs), bruits (indicating arterial narrowing), pulses (comparing both sides in a proximal to distal progression), ankle-brachial index, and toe-brachial index.
- **Sensory function** includes the ability to feel pain, temperature, and touch.
- **Range of motion** of the ankle must be assessed to determine if the joint flexes past 90° because this is necessary for unimpaired walking and aids venous return in the calf.
- **Pain** is an important diagnostic feature of peripheral arterial disease, so the location, intensity, duration, and characteristics of pain are important.

PULSE

Evaluation of the pulses of the lower extremities is an important part of assessment for peripheral arterial disease. Pulses should be first evaluated with the patient in supine position and then again with the legs dependent, checking bilaterally and proximally to distally to determine if intensity of pulse decreases distally. The pulse should be evaluated as to rate, rhythm, and intensity, which is usually graded on a 0-4 scale:

0 = pulse absent
1 = weak, difficult to palpate
2 = normal as expected
3 = full
4 = strong and bounding

Pulses may be palpable or absent with peripheral arterial disease. Absence of pulse on both palpation and Doppler probe does indicate peripheral arterial disease.

PROCEDURE AND SITES FOR PULSE CHECKS

Pulses can be assessed in the following order at the following sites:

- Beginning with the **dorsalis pedis** (on the top of the foot), palpate above the toes between the great and second toe and move upward until the pulse is palpable.
- Next, assess the **posterior tibial pulse**, which is located on the medial side of the ankle behind and slightly below the malleolus.
- Moving up the leg, the **popliteal pulse** should be assessed:
  o Ask the patient to place the leg straight and relax the leg.
  o Grasp the knee with both hands with thumbs on the sides of the knees, feeling for the pulse in the popliteal fossa.
- The **femoral pulse** is often difficult to assess in adults because the artery lies deep:
  o Apply deep pressure midway between the symphysis pubis and the anterior superior iliac spine.

BRUIT

Bruits (a sound indicating turbulent blood flow through a vessel) may be noted by auscultating over major arteries, such as femoral, popliteal, peroneal, and dorsalis pedis. Bruits often indicate peripheral arterial disease.

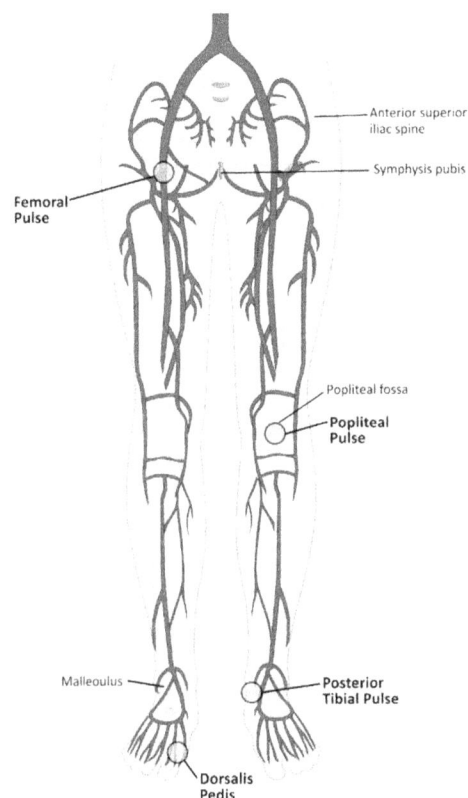

Anterior superior iliac spine

Symphysis pubis

Femoral Pulse

Popliteal fossa

Popliteal Pulse

Malleolus

Posterior Tibial Pulse

Dorsalis Pedis

PERFUSION

Assessment of perfusion can indicate venous or arterial abnormalities:

- **Venous refill time**: Begin with the patient lying supine for a few moments and then have the patient sit with the feet dependent. Observe the veins on the dorsum of the foot and count the seconds before normal filling. Venous occlusion or arterial supply inadequacy is indicated with times >20 seconds.
- **Capillary refill**: Grasp the toenail bed between the thumb and index finger and apply pressure for several seconds to cause blanching. Release the nail and count the seconds until the nail regains normal color. Arterial occlusion/insufficiency is indicated with times >2-3 seconds. Checks both feet and more than one nail bed.
- **Skin temperature**: Using the palm of the hand and fingers, gently palpate the skin, moving distally to proximally and comparing both legs. Arterial disease is indicated by decreased temperature (coolness) or a marked change from proximal to distal. Venous disease is indicated by increased temperature about the ankle.

ABI

The ankle-brachial index (ABI) examination is done to evaluate peripheral arterial disease of the lower extremities.

1. Apply a blood pressure cuff to one arm, palpate brachial pulse, and place conductivity gel over the artery.
2. Place the tip of a Doppler device at a 45-degree angle into the gel at the brachial artery and listen for the pulse sound.
3. Inflate the cuff until the pulse sound ceases and then inflate 20 mmHg above that point.
4. Release air and listen for the return of the pulse sound. This reading is the brachial systolic pressure.
5. Repeat the procedure on the other arm, and use the higher reading for calculations.
6. Repeat the same procedure on each ankle with the cuff applied above the malleoli and the gel over the posterior tibial pulse to obtain the ankle systolic pressure.
7. Divide the ankle systolic pressure by the brachial systolic pressure to obtain the ABI.

Sometimes, readings are taken both before and after 5 minutes of walking on a treadmill.

INTERPRETING RESULTS

Once the ankle-brachial index (ABI) examination is completed, the ankle systolic pressure must be divided by the brachial systolic pressure. Ideally, the blood pressure at the ankle should be equal to that of the arm or be slightly higher. With peripheral arterial disease, the ankle pressure falls, lowering the ABI. Additionally, some conditions that cause calcification of arteries, such as diabetes, can cause a false elevation. Calculation of the ABI ratio is simple: divide the ankle systolic BP by brachial systolic BP. For example, if the ankle BP is 90 and the brachial BP is 120, the ABI ratio is:

$$90 \div 120 = 0.75$$

The degree of disease relates to the ABI ratio as follows:

- >1.4 Abnormally high, may indicate calcification of vessel wall
- 1.0-1.4: Normal reading, asymptomatic
- 0.9-1.0: Low, but acceptable unless there are other indications of PAD
- 0.8-0.9: Likely some arterial disease is present
- 0.4-0.7 Moderate arterial disease
- <0.4 Severe arterial disease

TOE-BRACHIAL INDEX

The procedure for toe-brachial index (TBI) is as follows:

1. Apply blood pressure cuff to one arm, palpate brachial pulse, and place conductivity gel over the artery.
2. Place the tip of a Doppler device at a 45-degree angle into the gel at the brachial artery and listen for the pulse sound.
3. Inflate the cuff until the pulse sound ceases and then inflate 20 mmHg above that point.
4. Release air and listen for the return of the pulse sound. This reading is the brachial systolic pressure.
5. Repeat the procedure on the other arm and use the higher reading for calculations.
6. Repeat the same procedure on the great or second toe with the cuff applied around the base of the toes and the gel over the pulse to obtain the toe systolic pressure.
7. Divide the toe systolic pressure by the brachial systolic pressure to obtain the TBI (same calculations as for ABI). Normal values are >0.6.

ASSESSING THE GAITER AREA AND FOR HEMOSIDERIN STAINING

Two common signs of venous insufficiency that must be assessed in the lower extremities include:

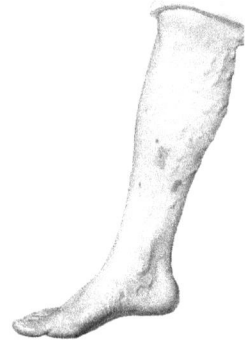

- **Gaiter area:** The region of the leg between the knee and ankle. This is the area in which most venous ulcers occur. Venous ulcers are commonly found around the medial or lateral malleoli within this region and tend to be large, shallow, and not painful. The wound bed is usually filled with irregular granulation tissue. Within this area, it is also common to see varicose veins and stasis dermatitis changes, as shown here.
- **Hemosiderin staining:** When a patient has a venous ulcer, there is frequently bleeding into the surrounding tissues. The blood cells break down in the tissues and their contents are absorbed by macrophages. The hemoglobin within red blood cells is broken down, and the iron within this is combined with proteins and changed into a stored form of iron. This stored form of iron contains a dark pigment called hemosiderin, which will give the patient a hyperpigmented area of skin. Patients frequently confuse this for a bruised area, though it may take years for the body to absorb this stored form of iron.

ASSESSING FOR PERIPHERAL NEUROPATHY

NYLON MONOFILAMENT TEST

A simple test for peripheral neuropathy, commonly used to determine risk of ulcers in diabetic patients, is the nylon monofilament test, which is available in kits:

1. Describe the procedure to the patient and ask the patient to indicate when the pressure of the monofilament is felt.
2. Grasp a length of #10 monofilament in the instrument provided.
3. Touch the monofilament against the bottom of the foot, and then press the monofilament into the foot until the line buckles.
4. Test the great, 3rd, and 5th toes.
5. Test the left, medial, and right areas of the ball of the foot.
6. Test the right and left of the arch.
7. Test the middle of the heel.

The test is evaluated according to how many of the 10 test sites the patient is able to detect. If the patient fails to detect the monofilament at fewer than 4 sites, this is indicative of decreased sensation and increased risk.

SENSORY VIBRATION TESTING

Sensory vibration testing is done with a tuning fork when a patient has a normal monofilament exam of the foot but still may be at risk for foot problems because of reduced sensation, especially patients with diabetes. To carry out the exam, the patient is placed in supine position with the feet exposed. Tap the tuning fork against the ball of the hand and then place the tip of the tuning fork against the bone near the end of the big toe, below the nail, or on top of the great toe joint. Ask the patient to indicate when the feeling of vibration stops. Both the examiner and the patient should feel the vibration stop at the same time if the patient has normal sensation. If the patient doesn't feel the vibration or feels it stop before the examiner, calculate the difference in seconds. Test both feet and note any differences.

ASSESSMENT OF LEND LEADING TO NEUROPATHIC/DIABETIC WOUNDS

The assessment for lower extremity neuropathic disease (LEND) and neuropathic/diabetic wounds includes:

- **History**: A history of general health and record of diabetes control and complications is critical. Risk factors should be identified and risks classified according to severity.
- **Physical examination**: The examination must identify any co-morbid conditions, such as heart disease, arthritis, and peripheral arterial or venous insufficiency.
- **Lower extremity/foot examination**: A thorough examination of the lower extremity and foot should include screening for neuropathy and sensory loss, pain, musculoskeletal changes or abnormalities, and vascular status. The skin should be carefully assessed for corns, calluses, pre-ulcerative lesions (such as blisters or cracks). Nails should be checked for fungus infections and thickening, which is common, and discolorations, such as red, black, or brown that may indicate trauma. Footwear should be examined for support and fit.
- **Evaluation and classification of the diabetic foot ulcer (DFU):** Ulcers should be measured and classified according to standard classification systems, observing for signs of infection.

ASSESSING ADEQUACY OF FOOTWEAR FOR THOSE WITH LEND

Examining footwear to determine if the fit is correct and if they are appropriate:

- **Examine shoes and slippers** for bulges on the side that may indicate the shoes are too tight, wear patterns on the shoes or heels that may indicate uneven gait or weight distribution. Check inside the shoes to see if there is worn or torn lining that could irritate the skin. Make sure that there is adequate cushioning. Sandals and open-toed shoes should be avoided because of the potential for foot injury.
- **Foot imprints**: Using the Harris Mat, the patient steps down barefoot on the mat that creates a visual (inked) image of the foot, showing pressure areas with darker images. It shows areas of the foot at greatest risk.
- **Forefoot test**: An outline of both bare feet is traced on paper while the patient is standing if possible. Then the shoes are placed over this and another outline drawn. The entire foot outline should be inside the shoe outline.

ASSESSMENT FOR FOOT DEFORMITIES RELATED TO DIABETIC ULCERS

The assessment for foot deformities related to diabetic ulcers is described below:

- Inflammation of connective tissue from the heel to ball of foot:
  - Plantar fasciitis—causes severe heel pain
- Bony heel growths:
  - Heel spurs—abnormal protruding growths of bone on the calcaneus, leading to plantar fasciitis.
- Distal muscle atrophy:
  - Hammer toe (contracture of proximal joint of toe)
  - Mallet toe (contracture of distal joint of toe)
  - Claw toe (contracture of both joints of toe)
- Changes in metatarsal bones:
  - Metatarsal bones lower or longer than adjoining bones uneven weight distribution, resulting in pain and ulceration
  - Bunion (enlargement of first metatarsal bone below first toe)
- Arch changes:
  - High cramped instep (*pes cavus*)
  - Flat foot (*pes planus*)
- Weakening of dorsum/plantar surfaces:
  - Charcot's arthropathy—involves weakened bones fracturing and the foot changing shape and becoming inflamed as the arch collapses, causing the foot to have a convex shape
- Nerve irritation:
  - Neuromas between toes

ASSESSMENT OF EDEMA

Edema is usually assessed by pressing the index finger into the tissue on top of each foot, behind the medial malleolus, and over the shin, starting distally and moving proximally to the highest level of edema, comparing both legs: Edema is rated on a 1- to 4-point scale:

- 1+ Slight pitting to about 2 mm; rebounds immediately.
- 2+ Moderate pitting to about 4 mm; rebounds in less than 15 seconds.
- 3+ Moderate-severe pitting to about 6 mm; rebounds in 15-30 seconds.
- 4+ Severe pitting to 8 mm or more; rebounds in greater than 30 seconds.

Types of edema:

- **Venous edema**: Edema from ankle to knee and may involve some limitation in ankle movement. Dependent pitting edema occurs, but may become non-pitting in chronic disease.
- **Lymphedema**: Usually unilateral non-pitting hard edema from toes to groin or fingers to axilla. In advanced disease, elephantiasis with huge enlargement of extremity may occur.
- **Lipedema**: Symmetrical bilateral soft rubbery tissue from ankle to groin and sometimes hips with pain on palpation and frequent bruising.

LIMB VOLUME MEASUREMENTS

Limb volume measurements are used primarily to assess muscle mass growth, assess peripheral edema, and evaluate lymphedema. Comparison is often done with an opposite limb. Methods utilized for limb volume measurements include:

- **Water displacement**: This method (inserting the limb into a container with a measured volume of water and then measuring the overflow water) enables a more accurate volume measurement of hands and feet but cannot be used with open wounds. It provides volume but no information about shape or condition. Additionally, it is difficult to do with full limbs.
- **Circumferential**: Skin markings are placed distally to proximally every 4 cm for the hand and arm and every 10 cm for the foot and leg. Foot should be in dorsiflexion position and hand flat. Measurements are taken and recorded at each mark, avoiding tension on the measuring tape. Tables are available to help calculate the volume based on the tape measurements.
- **Perometer**: Equipment that uses an infrared laser system to read limb measurements and software to calculate limb volume.

MANAGEMENT OF EDEMA

Chronic venous insufficiency (CVI) results in edema of the lower extremities, causing both discomfort and increased risk of ulcers. Treatment includes:

- **Leg elevation** when sitting to avoid dependency. Therapy may include lying down and elevating the affected limb above the heart for 1-2 hours two times daily and during the night. This is important for all patients with CVI, but especially for those unable to comply with compression therapy.
- **Compression therapy** can be used to suit the patient's specific clinical needs, based on mobility status, exercise needs, optimal pressure, and the available assistance they have to help with changing bandages or stockings. Common compression methods include elastic bandages, non-elastic bandages, multicomponent bandage systems, compression stockings, and intermittent pneumatic compression devices.
- **Surgical intervention** is indicated if more conservative treatment is unsuccessful in managing CVI.
- **Ligation and stripping** removes a vein or section of a vein that is damaged or has damaged valves. An incision below the vein allows an endoscope to be threaded into the vein to grasp and remove (strip) it. The vein is tied (ligated). Sometimes only ligation of a faulty valve is done and the vein is left in place.
- **Deep vein reconstruction** may be considered if other approaches fail.
- **Physical therapy** is important because effective calf muscle pumping requires ankle mobility with dorsiflexion over 90°. Some patients may benefit from gait training and exercises to improve the range of motion and strength of the ankle. Calf muscle exercises may include isotonic exercises. Patients need to alternate sitting and standing with walking on a regular schedule throughout the day.
- **Control of weight** often improves circulation and reduces edema, as obesity may be the primary cause of the circulatory impairment. Patients may need education and referral to a bariatric treatment center.
- **Medications** cannot correct venous insufficiency but some can help to control symptoms:
  - Pentoxifylline (Trental) enhances blood flow in capillaries.
  - Horse chestnut seed extract (HCSE) results in reduced pain and edema. It is widely used in Europe and has been studied in the United States. One problem is that it can cause low blood glucose levels in children and those with diabetes.

LYMPHEDEMA

Lymphedema is a dysfunction of the lymphatic system, resulting in a debilitating progressive disease. The healthy lymphatic system returns proteins, lipids, and fluids to the circulatory system from the interstitial spaces, but with lymphedema this accumulates, causing pronounced induration, edema, and fibrosis of tissues. As the fluid builds up, it causes distention, and the skin becomes thick and fibrotic with dimpling similar to that of an orange peel (peau d'orange). Scaly keratinous debris collects, and the skin develops cracks and leakage of lymphatic fluid. Lymphedema may be primary (developmental abnormality) or secondary. It can occur after mastectomy, radiation, infection, cancer, or surgery, such as joint replacements and vascular procedures. Patients are at risk of infection, cellulitis, and lymphangitis, as well as pain and limited mobility. Lymphedema has three **stages**:

- Stage 1 is reversible pitting edema distally with no fibrosis.
- Stage 2 is pitting or non-pitting edema with fibrosis and papillomatosis.
- Stage 3 is elephantiasis with massive enlargement and distortion of limb, fibrosis, and ulcerations.

MEDICAL MANAGEMENT

Medical management of lymphedema is intended to reduce the protein accumulation in the tissues and restore lymphatic circulation, but treatment needs to begin before extensive fibrosis occurs. Diuretics do not help and the treatments must be continued lifelong in order to be successful:

- Skin must be kept clean and dry and inspected for open areas or signs of infection. Mild emollients may improve skin barrier.
- Antimicrobial or antifungal topical agents are used for infections. About 15-25% requires long-term antibiotic prophylaxis.
- Limbs need to be elevated when possible during the day and always at night.
- Complex decongestive therapy with massage helps improve lymphatic drainage.
- Static compression bandaging during the day, providing 40-60 mmHg pressure. The bandaging may be removed at night if the limb is elevated.
- Dynamic compression (intermittent dynamic compression) may be used but can displace fluid or further damage lymphatics if not monitored carefully.
- Weight loss may be advised because obesity further compromises lymphatic circulation.

PATIENT MANAGEMENT

Because management of lymphedema is a lifelong process, compliance on the part of the patient is critical to controlling lymphedema and preventing further deterioration and complications. The patient must take an active role:

- Avoid excessive heat, such as sun exposure, saunas, and hot tubs.
- Use an electric razor instead of a straight razor or chemicals for hair removal to prevent injury to skin.
- Prevent trauma to limb. Wear protective gloves and clothing to prevent trauma to affected limb. Avoid blood tests or blood pressure readings in an affected arm.
- Observe skin carefully for signs of cellulitis or infection and follow prescribed protocols for treatment.
- Maintain good hygiene.
- Wear closed-toe shoes if lower limb is affected.
- Use sunscreen and bug repellent on affected limb.
- Avoid lifting and limit use of affected arm.

NUTRITIONAL FACTORS THAT AFFECT THE SKIN

Nutritional status is very important for maintaining the integrity of the skin:

- People who are on restrictive diets or do not have adequate protein in their diets will lack the amino acids for protein synthesis.
- A diet too low in fats can be deficient in essential fatty acids, which the skin cells need for the lipid barrier.
- Carbohydrates are necessary for the cell to carry out basic metabolic functions.
- Vitamin A helps to repair skin tissue.
- Vitamin B complex, especially biotin, is critical for skin formation and prevents dryness and itching.
- Vitamins C and E have been shown to reduce and counter the negative effects of ultraviolet radiation caused by exposure to the sun. Since Vitamin C is utilized for collagen formation, it is essential that intake is adequate.
- Minerals, such as iron, selenium, zinc, and copper are important also.

INITIAL NUTRITIONAL ASSESSMENT

Nutritional assessment should be done within the first 24 hours of care to ensure that nutritional requirements of the patient are met. The history and physical exam should include the following information about the **previous three months**:

- Changes in food intake, including number of meals eaten daily
- Weight loss (or gain)
- Episodes of depression or stress that may relate to dietary intake
- A sample of a usual daily menu

Additional screening should include:

- Daily number of proteins, fruit, grain, and vegetable servings
- Usual fluid intake, including type, amount, and frequency
- Method of feeding, independent or assisted
- Mobility
- Mental status
- Body mass index (BMI), mid-arm circumference, and calf circumference
- Living status (independent or dependent)
- Prescription and non-prescription drugs
- Pressure sores or other wounds or skin problems

NUTRITIONAL ASSESSMENT TOOLS

Standardized nutritional assessment tools include the following:

- **The MNA (Mini-Nutritional Assessment)** by Nestle Nutrition is designed for nutritional assessment of those over age 65 and is only valid for that population. It is a screening and assessment tool to determine the risk for malnutrition and comprises 15 questions about dietary habits and 4 measurements, including BMI using height and weight, and mid-arm and calf circumference.
- **The Nutritional Screening Initiative** is another tool for geriatric patients and screens for dietary information as well as social and environmental factors, such as whether the person eats alone, prepares meals, drinks alcohol, and has sufficient income.
- **The Subjective Global Assessment** assesses nutritional status by a thorough history and physical examination. The history assesses weight change, dietary intake, gastrointestinal symptoms, and functional impairment. The results of this assessment tool are evaluated subjectively and scores assigned to determine if malnutrition risks are normal to severe.

PHYSICAL ASSESSMENT OF NUTRITION
INDICATIONS OF NUTRITIONAL DEFICIENCY

The physical assessment is an important part of nutritional assessment to determine **malnutrition** or problems with **self-feeding**.

- **Hair** may be dry and brittle or thinning.
- **Skin** may show poor turgor, ecchymosis, tears, pressure areas, ulcerations, abrasions, or other compromises.
- The **mouth** may show dry mucous membranes. Lips may be scaly (riboflavin deficiency), have cheilosis, and be cracking at the corners. Gums may be swollen or bleeding, teeth loose or needing care, or dentures poorly fitting. The tongue may be inflamed, dry, cracked, or have sores.
- **Nails** may become brittle. Spoon-shaped or pale nail bed indicates low iron.
- **Hands** may be crippled or arthritic, making eating difficult.
- **Vision** may be compromised so that people can't see to prepare food or have difficulty feeding themselves.
- **Mental status** may be impaired to the point that people can't understand diet instructions or prepare or eat meals.
- **Motor skills** may decrease, including hand-mouth coordination or the ability to hold utensils.

TRICEPS SKINFOLD THICKNESS, MID-ARM CIRCUMFERENCE, AND MID-ARM MUSCLE CIRCUMFERENCE

Certain measurements aid in the diagnosis of weight- and nutrition-related disorders:

- **Triceps skinfold thickness (TST)** is measured using special calipers. The midpoint between the axilla and elbow of the non-dominant arm is measured and located, and then the skin is grasped between the thumb and index finger about 1 cm above the midpoint at the edges of the arm. The finger and thumb are moved inward until a firm fold of tissue is observed. The calipers are placed about this fold at the midpoint (right below the fingers) and squeezed for 3 seconds, and then a measurement is taken to the nearest millimeter. Three readings are taken with the average of the three used as the measurement.
- **Mid-arm circumference (MAC)** measurement is obtained by measuring in centimeters at the midpoint between the axilla and elbow.
- **Mid-arm muscle circumference (MAMC)** is calculated by multiplying the triceps skinfold thickness (in millimeters) by pi (3.14), and subtracting the result from the mid-arm circumference with results in centimeters.

Triceps skinfold thickness (TST) evaluates fat stores, which often change slowly, so this is not a sensitive test for malnutrition, but it can be used to determine if fat is increasing while muscle mass is decreasing. Mid-arm circumference (MAC) measures muscles, bones, and skin, and mid-arm muscle circumference (MAMC) measures lean body mass. These vary considerably from person to person so they are more useful for tracking muscle wasting over time than for comparisons between different individuals. The TST, MAC, and MAMC are recorded as a percentage of standard measurements, which are quantified for males and females.

- Males
  - TST: 12.5 mm
  - MAC: 29.9 cm
  - MAMC: 25.3 cm
- Females
  - TST: 16.5 mm
  - MAC: 28.5 cm
  - MAMC: 23.3 cm

In order to reach the percentage, the actual measurement for each test is divided by the standard measurement, and that result is multiplied by 100. Thus, if a male's TST measured 11.8:

$$11.8 \div 12.5 = 0.944 \times 100 = 94.4\%$$

BMI

The body mass index (BMI) formula is a measurement that uses height and weight as an indicator of obesity/malnutrition. This cannot be used alone to diagnose obesity as body types differ considerably. Women often have more body fat than men. Tables are available to make calculations simple, but the BMI can be calculated manually:

BMI formula using pounds and inches:

$$\text{BMI} = \frac{\text{weight in pounds} \times 703}{(\text{height in inches})^2}$$

BMI formula using kilograms and meters:

$$\text{BMI} = \frac{\text{weight in kilograms}}{(\text{height in meters})^2}$$

Resulting scores for adults age 20 and over are interpreted according to this chart:

- Below 18.5: Underweight
- 18.5-24.9: Normal weight
- 25.0-29.9: Overweight
- 30 and above: Obese

BMI for those under age 20 uses age-gender specific charts provided by the CDC, containing a curved line that indicates percentiles. The criteria for obesity based on these charts and BMI for age are as follows:

- <5th percentile: Underweight
- 85th-<95 percentile: At risk for overweight
- >95th percentile: Overweight

WAIST HIP RATIO

The Waist Hip Ratio (WHR) is the ratio of fat stored about the abdomen and the fat stored around the hips. This ratio is considered of increasing import because an increase in this ratio is associated with increased risk of heart disease, brain attacks, and diabetes mellitus. The formula:

$$\text{WHR} = \frac{\text{waist circumference in centimeters}}{\text{hip circumference in centimeters}}$$

The waist measurement is taken at the smallest circumference, usually slightly above the umbilicus, and the hip measurement at the widest part of the hips, usually about 7 inches below the waist.

The results of the calculation provide a score with risks according to gender:

- Males: WHR >1 means increased risk
- Females: WHR >0.85 means increased risk

Studies have indicated that people who carry more weight around their waists relative to their hips (apple-shaped) are more at risk for complications related to weight than those that carry more weight in their hips (pear-shaped).

MEASURING HEAD CIRCUMFERENCE TO ASSESS NUTRITION

Head circumference measurements are taken for children during the first 3 years. While there can be non-nutritional reasons for decreased growth of the head, it can also be a sign of a severe lack of nutrition and may be associated with decreased linear growth as well. The measurement is obtained through the following steps:

1. Use non-stretchable measuring tape.
2. Child should be standing or held in sitting position with head upright.
3. Place tape around head just above the eyebrows in the font and around the occipital area in the back.
4. Take at least 3 readings or more until 2 measurements are within 0.1 cm.
5. Use growth chart to determine if measurement is within normal limits.

The CDC provides growth charts for both head circumference and linear growth that are specific for gender, showing the percentile ranking of measurements. Evaluation depends upon various factors, including results of height and weight measurement, to determine if a child is undernourished. Findings below the 5th percentile are usually cause for concern.

MALNUTRITION

RISK FACTORS AND INDICATORS FOR MALNUTRITION

There are a number of risk factors for malnutrition:

- **Hypermetabolism** resulting from various diseases such as AIDS, as well as trauma, stress, or infection
- **Weight loss**, especially sudden or loss of 10% of normal weight over a 3-month period
- **Low body weight** of <90% of ideal body weight for age or **low body mass index** (BMI) <18.5
- **Immunosuppressive drugs** that interfere with absorption of nutrients
- **Malabsorption** of nutrients caused by diseases, such as chronic failure of kidneys or liver
- **Changes in appetite** that decrease intake of nutrients
- **Food intolerances**, such as lactose intolerance, resulting from lack of enzymes needed to completely digest food so it can be absorbed into the blood stream from the small intestine
- **Dietary restrictions**, such as the limiting of protein with kidney failure
- **Functional limitations**, such as an inability to feed oneself
- Lack of teeth or dentures, limiting intake
- **Alterations of taste or smell** that render food unpalatable

TYPES OF MALNUTRITION AND SYMPTOMS

Protein malnutrition (kwashiorkor or hypoalbuminemia) is characterized by inadequate protein but adequate fats and carbohydrates. It can result from chronic diarrhea, renal disease, infection, hemorrhage, burns, traumatic injuries, or other illnesses. Onset is usually rapid with loss of visceral protein while skeletal muscle mass is retained, so it may be difficult to detect on a physical exam. Symptoms include:

- Hypoalbuminemia and anemia
- Edema
- Delayed healing of wound
- Immuno-incompetence

Protein-calorie malnutrition (marasmus), inadequate protein and calories, is usually more obvious. Visceral protein is usually intact, as is immune function, because weight loss is gradual. However, patients are often very thin or emaciated from loss of skeletal muscle mass. Many are elderly and have chronic illnesses. Symptoms include:

- Decreased basal metabolism
- Lack of subcutaneous fat
- Tissue turgor
- Bradycardia
- Hypothermia

Mixed protein-calorie malnutrition (combination) is common in hospitalized patients and has an acute onset with low visceral protein as well as rapid loss of weight, skeletal muscle mass, and fat.

STARVATION AND EXCESSIVE INTAKE

In response wounds, the stress response causes a hypermetabolic state, and caloric and protein needs increase markedly at the same time intake decreases, leading to periods of **starvation**:

- A **short period** can result in increased nitrogen in urine and increased output with a rapid loss of muscle and weight.
- A **prolonged period** results in slower weight and muscle loss but can lead to metabolic acidosis with increased ammonia in urine and decreased nitrogen.
- An **extended period** becomes premorbid with obvious cachexia and weight loss. The mid-arm muscle circumference decreases and there is increase in creatinine/height index and urinary urea as well as decrease in serum albumin, transferrin, and lymphocytes.

Excessive intake may cause obesity, which delays wound healing, but it does not necessarily mean nutrition is adequate. Overweight people can still have inadequate protein, vitamins, and minerals. Because protein and caloric requirements for healing are tied to weight, nutritional needs are high, but fat stores help people to tolerate prolonged periods of starvation.

NOCICEPTIVE PAIN

There are two primary types of pain: nociceptive (acute) pain and neuropathic (chronic) pain although some people may have a combination.

Nociceptive or acute pain is the normal nerve response to a painful stimulus. Trauma that results in nociceptive pain can cause severe inflammation and damage to nerve endings. Nociceptive pain usually correlates with extent and type of injury: the greater the injury, the greater the pain. It may be procedural pain (related to wound manipulation and dressing changes) or surgical pain (related to cutting of tissue). It may also be continuous or cyclic, depending upon the type of injury. This type of pain is usually localized to the area of injury and resolves over time as healing takes place. This type of pain is often described as aching or throbbing, but generally responds to analgesia. Uncontrolled, this type of pain can result in changes in the nervous system that lead to chronic neuropathic pain.

NEUROPATHIC PAIN

Neuropathic or chronic pain occurs when there is a primary lesion in the nervous system or dysfunction related to damaged nerve fibers. Neuropathic pain may be associated with conditions such as diabetes, cancer, or traumatic injury to the nervous system. This type of pain is common in chronic wounds and is more often described as burning, stabbing, electric, or shooting pains. Often the underlying pathology causing the pain is not reversible. Pain may be **visceral** (diffuse or cramping pain of internal organs) caused by injuries to internal organs. It is also often diffuse rather than localized. It may also be **somatic pain** (involving muscles, skin, bones, and joints). Neuropathic pain is often more difficult to assess that nociceptive pain because the damage may alter normal pain responses. Neuropathic pain often responds better to antidepressants and anti-seizure medications than analgesics.

CONSEQUENCES OF PAIN

Part of managing pain is understanding patients' perceptions regarding pain and its consequences. Some expect and accept pain, and some lack the cognizant awareness to express that they are in pain. Pain, however, is very debilitating and limits quality of life for many patients:

- **Limited activity**: Patients may be unable to stand, walk, or do their jobs, resulting in their being more sedentary, impairing circulation.
- **Frustration**: Acute or chronic pain can lead to depression and anger, as well as withdrawal from activities or lack of desire to try new activities. Patients may withdraw from friends and family.

Additionally, pain has **physiological consequences**:

- **Wound care**: Adequate care of the wound may be limited by pain during treatment. Patients may not carry out prescribed treatments or may refuse treatments.
- **Perfusion**: Pain can result in peripheral vasoconstriction, decreasing perfusion of tissue and impairing leukocyte activity. This depresses angiogenesis, further impairing healing of the wound and continuing the cycle of pain.

PAIN ASSESSMENT METHODS

Pain is subjective and may be influenced by the individual's pain threshold (the smallest stimulus that produces the sensation of pain) and pain tolerance (the maximum degree of pain that a person can tolerate). The most common current **pain assessment tool** is the 1-10 scale:

- 0 = no pain
- 1-2 = mild pain
- 3-5 = moderate pain
- 6-7 = severe pain
- 8-9 = very severe pain
- 10 = excruciating pain

However, there is more to pain assessment than a number on a scale. Assessment includes information about **onset, duration, and intensity**. Identifying what **triggers** pain and what **relieves** it can be very useful when developing a plan for pain management. Patients may show very different **behavior** when they are in pain. Some may cry and moan with minor pain, and others may exhibit seemingly normal behavior even when truly suffering; thus, judging pain by behavior can lead to the wrong conclusions.

Assessing Activities in Relation to Pain

Assessment of pain must include determining those factors or activities that increase pain:

- **Site of pain**: While pain is often focused on the wound site, it may extend to the surrounding tissues, especially in chronic wounds, making application and removal of dressings especially painful.
- **Movement**: Pressure and touch caused by changes of position can increase pain, limiting mobility.
- **Time**: Pain often increases at night, making sleep difficult.
- **Dressings**: Dressings that are too tight or the wrong choice for a wound may cause intense site pain. Allowing the wound to become dry can also increase pain.
- **Personal/cultural**: Some people have difficulty expressing the degree of pain. Others react to the expectation of the medical personnel or family. Some believe that they should remain stoic or are afraid of becoming "addicted," so they resist taking pain medications until pain is severe.

Assessment of Pain for Those Who Are Cognitively Impaired or Cannot Verbalize Pain

Patients with cognitive impairment or an inability to verbalize pain may not be able to indicate the degree of pain, even by using a face scale with pictures of smiling to crying faces. The **Pain Assessment in Advanced Dementia (PAINAD) scale** may be helpful. Careful observation of nonverbal behavior can indicate that the patient is in pain:

- **Respirations**: Patients often have more rapid and labored breathing as pain increases, with short periods of hyperventilation or Cheyne-Stokes respirations.
- **Vocalization**: Patients may remain negative in speech or speak quietly and reluctantly. They may moan or groan. As pain increases, they may call out, moan or groan loudly, or cry.
- **Facial expression**: Patients may appear sad or frightened, may frown or grimace, especially on activities that increase pain.
- **Body language**: Patients may be tense, fidgeting, or pacing, and they may become rigid, clench fists, or lie in fetal position as pain increases. They may become increasingly combative as well.
- **Consolability**: Patients are less distractible or consolable with increased pain.

Wound Etiology

ETIOLOGY OF CHRONIC WOUNDS

Acute wounds heal fairly quickly, moving through stages of healing in a predictable manner; however, chronic wounds behave much differently and outcomes are less predictable. There are a number of factors related to chronic wounds:

- **Wound nature**: Chronic wounds are often related to underlying pathology, such as arterial insufficiency, rather than acute injury. Also, the lack of initial bleeding may impair fibrin production and release of growth factors.
- **Difference in healing**: The initial inflammatory stage of healing is often prolonged because of vascular insufficiency, necrosis, or bacteria.
- **Insufficient growth factors**: Growth factors are necessary to repair tissue, but there are insufficient numbers or they break down quickly, resulting in cellular senescence (inability of cells to proliferate or respond to growth factors).
- **Host factors**: Many factors, such as malnutrition and smoking, may interfere with healing.
- **Denervation**: Lack of adequate innervation impairs the inflammatory response and interferes with healing.

CHARCOT'S ARTHROPATHY

Charcot's arthropathy (Charcot's foot) is the direct result of neuropathy that weakens the muscles of the foot and reduces sensations. The neuropathy weakens the muscles supporting the bones, which in turn become weak and fracture easily. Because of the lack of sensation, the patient may be unaware of the fracture and continue to walk, causing further deformity. The foot becomes inflamed and swollen with increased temperature in foot, but usually there is no pain. In time, the joint dislocation causes the arch to collapse. Treatment includes:

- Compression bandages for 2-3 weeks to reduce edema and inflammation
- Total contact or non-weight-bearing cast applied for up to 9 months
- Gradual weight bearing after skin has resumed normal temperature
- Electrostimulation of the bone may improve healing
- Medications, such as Fosamax and Aredia may be used to decrease bone destruction
- Gradual weight bearing is resumed as foot temperature improves

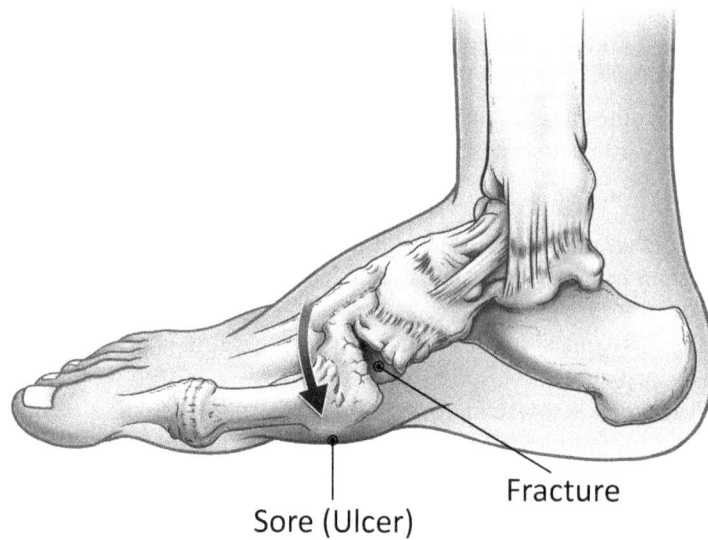

Fracture

Sore (Ulcer)

VENOUS INSUFFICIENCY
VENOUS ULCERS

Venous ulcers were once thought to be caused by venous stasis. Now it is thought that venous hypertension is the cause and the underlying reason that healing doesn't occur. Incompetent valves cause a backup of blood that distends the veins and increases intracapillary pressure. This results in leakage of fluid into the tissues and edema around the ankle areas. Red blood cells leak as well, depositing hemosiderin into the tissues. Hemosiderin is seen as a brownish stain in the lower leg in both Caucasian and black skin. The edematous skin becomes shiny and taut and is extremely itchy. Excoriation and ulceration with infection often occur. The skin may weep or be dry and scaly. Varicose veins and telangiectasia (spider veins) may be seen. The legs feel heavy and ache. A typical venous ulcer has exudate and may have a yellow fibrous film over the wound bed. The shape is irregular and surrounding skin is indurated with a brownish rust color. Scars from previous ulcers are often seen.

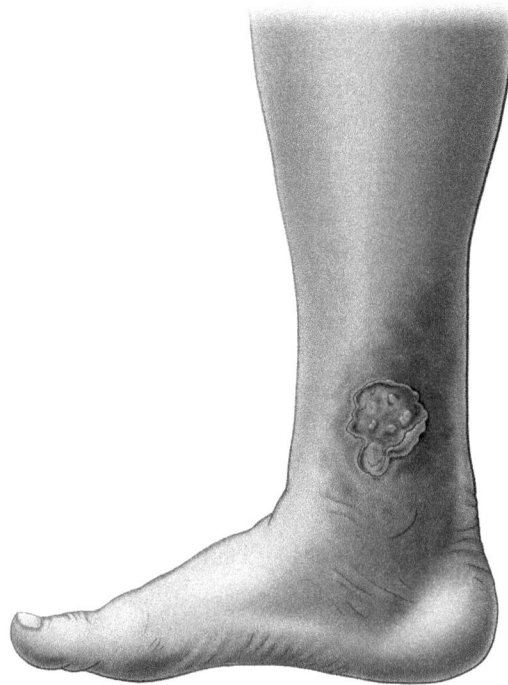

Risk Factors for Chronic Venous Insufficiency

There are a number of risk factors for chronic venous insufficiency (CVI) also known as lower-extremity venous disease (LEVD), primarily those that result in valvular dysfunction or calf-muscle dysfunction:

- **Obesity** with BMI >25 causes patients to be more likely to have pressure on pelvic veins, causing valvular dysfunction.
- **Intravenous drug use** into lower extremities may damage vessels.
- **Thrombosis/leg trauma** may damage vessels and valves.
- **Thrombophlebitis** may cause direct damage to valves.
- **Thrombophilic conditions**, such as protein C deficiency, decrease clotting time of venous blood, increasing risk of thrombosis.
- **Varicose veins** slow venous return.
- **Pregnancy**, especially multiple or close pregnancies increase pressure on pelvic veins.
- **Lack of exercise/sedentary lifestyle** with prolonged periods of sitting result in calf muscle dysfunction.
- **Smoking** causes vascular changes.
- **Age and gender** studies show that older women most commonly develop CVI.
- **Co-morbid conditions**, such as arthritis or those that limit mobility, affect calf-muscle function.

Skin Changes and Abnormalities Related to LEVD

Skin changes and abnormalities, in addition to edema, related to lower-extremity venous disease (LEVD) include:

- **Hemosiderin staining** occurs when hemosiderin, a brownish granular iron-containing pigment resulting from breakdown of hemoglobin, builds up in the interstitial fluid as a result of venous hypertension, causing the erythrocytes to seep into the tissues. As the cells break down, the deposits along with melanin remain in the tissue. This causes a brownish, splotchy discoloration of the skin from the ankle to the anterior tibial area.

- **Lipodermatosclerosis** occurs in the lower leg area as the tissue becomes fibrotic from fibrin and protein (collagen) deposits, causing the skin to feel waxy and the tissue to harden with narrowing of the tissue around the ankle compared to proximal tissue above.
- **Venous (stasis) dermatitis** is inflammation of the epidermis and dermis resulting in scaly, erythematous, crusty, weepy, itchy skin, usually in the lower leg (ankle and tibia). It is progressive with redness and itching appearing before other symptoms.
- **Malleolar flare** is caused by capillaries in a sunburst pattern inferior and distal to the medial malleolus.
- **Atrophie blanche lesions** are smooth white avascular sclerotic skin plaques that occur in about one-third of patients with LEVD. They are usually associated with torturous vessels and hemosiderin staining on the ankles or foot. They may appear similar to scarring from healed ulcers but actually have a high risk for deteriorating into ulcer formation.
- **Varicosities** (varicose veins) are veins where blood has pooled, causing them to become distended, twisted, and palpable, often appearing as blue rope-like vessels on back of the knee and calf or inside of the leg. They are the result of venous reflux and venous hypertension.

VENOUS DERMATITIS

Venous dermatitis appears on the ankles and lower legs and can cause severe itching and pain. Without treatment to control the dermatitis, it may deteriorate, causing ulcers to form, so treatment is needed to alleviate the symptoms:

- Topical antihistamines are used to decrease itching and prevent excoriation from scratching. Low dose topical steroids should be used only for short periods (2 weeks) to reduce inflammation and itching only because of danger of increasing ulceration.
- Compression therapy, usually with compression stockings, is used on affected legs to improve overall venous return.
- Leg elevation when sitting helps to avoid dependency.
- Topical antibiotics, such as bacitracin, should be administered as indicated to reduce danger of infection. Oral antibiotics as indicated for systemic infection.
- Hypoallergenic emollients (without perfume), such as petrolatum jelly, can improve the skin's barrier function and is a preventive measure that should be used when the acute inflammation has subsided.

ARTERIAL INSUFFICIENCY
RISK FACTORS FOR LOWER EXTREMITY ARTERIAL DISEASE (LEAD)

There are a number of risk factors for lower extremity arterial disease (LEAD):

- **Smoking** is a primary cause of LEAD, with diagnosis of disease 10 years before non-smokers. It increases the rate of atherosclerosis, decreases HDL, increases blood pressure, and decreases clotting time.
- **Obesity** raises blood pressure, decreases HDL in cholesterol while raising cholesterol and triglycerides, and increases risk of circulatory disease, including heart attack.
- **Lack of exercise** decreases pain-free walking distance.
- **Hypertension** correlates with changes in the vessel walls that result in narrowing of blood vessels and decreased circulation.
- **Diabetes mellitus** causes increased plaque formation, decreased clotting time, increased blood viscosity, and hypertrophy of vasculature. Insulin resistance, related to Type II diabetes, increases atherosclerosis. Arterial disease typically progresses faster with diabetes.
- **High blood cholesterol**, especially LDLs, increases atherosclerosis and circulatory impairment.

SUBTLE INDICATIONS OF INFECTION WITH ARTERIAL INSUFFICIENCY

Because of the lack of circulation, the normal signs of inflammation and infection may be evident with arterial insufficiency, so observing for subtle signs of infection is critically important. Prompt identification and treatment is necessary to prevent cellulitis and/or osteomyelitis that may result in amputation. Dry necrotic wounds should be painted with 10% povidone-iodine and covered with dry gauze, but the ulcer and the skin around should be inspected daily. **Indications of infection** include:

- Increased pain in the ischemic limb or ulcer and/or increased edema.
- Increase in necrotic area of ulcer.
- Periwound tissue has fluctuance evident on palpation (soft wave-like texture) that may indicate infection in the tissue.
- Erythema about the perimeter of the wound may be very slight.

At any indication of infection, culture and sensitivities should be done so that appropriate therapy can begin.

DIABETIC WOUNDS

DIABETIC FOOT ULCERS

Most diabetic ulcers are on the foot, ranging from the toes to the heels. Ulcers may first appear as laceration, blisters, or punctures, and the wound is usually circular with well-defined edges. There is often callus in the periwound tissue. The following are common sites:

- **Toes**: The toes are frequent sites for ulcers because of the potential for trauma. The interphalangeal joints often have limited flexibility that causes pressure and friction. The dorsal toes may have hammertoes from injuries or improperly fitted shoes that are easily injured. Distal toes may suffer injury from poor perfusion, heat, or short footwear.
- **Metatarsal heads** may have poor flexibility, increasing pressure.
- **Bunions** may erode because of deformities or narrow footwear.
- **Midfoot** may suffer injury from trauma or Charcot's fracture.
- **Heels** are susceptible to unrelieved pressure, often related to prolonged periods of bed rest.

RISK FACTORS

There are a number of risk factors for the development of neuropathic/diabetic ulcers:

- **Sensory loss** can cause sores and ulcers to go undetected in early stages.
- **Vascular insufficiency**, especially peripheral artery disease, occurs four times more frequently in diabetics.
- **Autonomic neuropathy** decreases sweating, leaving feet dry and more prone to cracks and sores.
- Long-term diabetes mellitus with poor glucose control causes severe damage to the circulatory system.
- **Smoking** increases vascular damage and arterial insufficiency.
- **Deformities or lack of mobility** may increase risk of developing ulcers or having ulcers be undetected.
- **Obesity** decreases circulation and interferes with control of diabetes. Between 80% and 90% of diabetics are overweight.
- **Male gender** increases risk.
- **Poor vision** may cause people to overlook dangers or prevent them from examining feet and skin.
- **Age** is associated with an increased danger of ulcers.
- **Ethnic background** can determine genetic risks: Native Americans, Hispanic Americans, African Americans, and Pacific Islanders have higher risk for diabetes, and therefore diabetic neuropathy and ulcers.
- Improperly fitted and supportive footwear can cause ulcerations.

Wound Issues Specific to the Pediatric Population

Pediatric patients, especially infants and young children, have skin that is more fragile and easily injured than that of adults. Incontinence increases risks of tissue breakdown. The incidence of pressure injuries in pediatric and neonatal intensive care units is high with the greatest risk of pressure injuries in children under three being the occiput (because the head is proportionately larger in children). Older children are at increased risk of pressure injuries in the sacral area and heels. Children with intellectual disabilities, spinal cord injuries, and myelomeningocele are especially at risk because of decreased mobility, awareness, and sensation. Risk factors include prolonged immobilization (such as with premature infants), medical equipment/devices that apply pressure to the tissue (such as NG and IV tubing and arm boards). Pressure redistribution devices intended for adults are not always effective with children because of their smaller size and weight, so products intended for pediatric patients should be utilized. Appropriate pain assessment tools, such as NIPS, CHEOPS, and NCCPC, should be utilized as children may express pain differently from adults.

Contact Dermatitis

Contact dermatitis is a localized response to contact with an allergen, resulting in a rash that may blister and itch. Common allergens include poison oak, poison ivy, latex, benzocaine, nickel, and preservatives, but there is a wide range of items, elements, and products to which people may react.

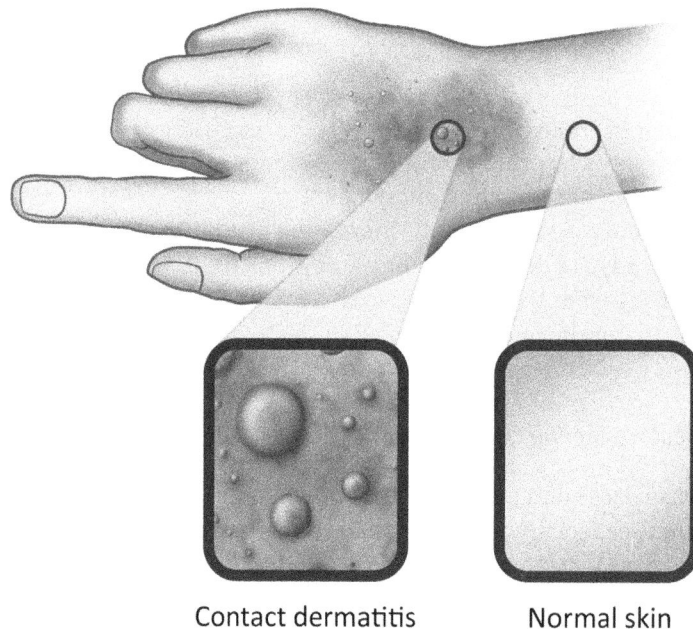

Contact dermatitis   Normal skin

Treatment includes:

- Identifying the causative agent through evaluating the area of the body affected, careful history, or skin patch testing to determine allergic responses.
- Corticosteroids to control inflammation and itching.
- Soothing oatmeal baths.
- Caladryl lotion to relieve itching.
- Antihistamines to reduce allergic response.
- Lesions should be gently cleansed and observed for signs of secondary infection.
- Antibiotics are used only for secondary infections as indicated.
- Rash is usually left open to dry.
- Avoidance of allergen will prevent recurrence.

CANDIDIASIS

Candidiasis, infection of the epidermis with *Candida* spp. (commonly referred to as "yeast" or "thrush"), causes a pustular erythematous papular rash that is commonly scaly, crusty, and macerated with a white cheese-like exudate. It may burn, is usually extremely pruritic, and grows in warm moist areas of the skin, such as under breasts, in abdominal folds, and in the perineal area. Antibiotic use, immunocompromised status, and diabetes mellitus may predispose people to fungal infections, so candidiasis must be differentiated from bacterial infections because antibiotic treatment will worsen the condition. Treatment includes:

- Preventing humid, moist conditions of skin
- Controlling hyperglycemia
- Burow's solution soaks with air drying to relieve itching
- Topical antifungal creams (clotrimazole, nystatin, fluconazole, and ketoconazole) twice daily
- Topical antifungal powders for mild cases
- Oral antifungal medications for severe cases

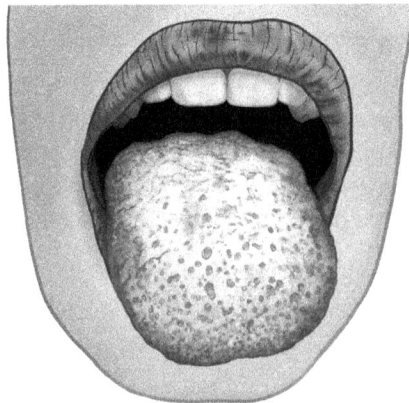

MANAGEMENT OF BACTERIAL INFECTIONS

FOLLICULITIS AND IMPETIGO

Folliculitis is a bacterial infection of the hair follicles, often on the face, resulting in pustules, erythema, and crusts that are painful and itchy. Recently, there has been an increase in cases of community-acquired methicillin-resistant *Staphylococcus aureus* folliculitis infections. Folliculitis may occur as a primary or secondary infection and may result from chronic nasal colonization of *MRSA*.

Treatment includes:

- Antibacterial soaps
- Topical or oral antibiotics

Impetigo is a contagious itchy bacterial infection of the skin, commonly on the face or hands, causing clusters of blisters or sores, especially in children. Group A *Streptococcus* usually causes small blisters that crust over. *Staphylococcus aureus* usually causes larger blisters that may be bullous and cause lesions 2-8cm in size that persist for months. Treatment includes:

- Avoid itching
- Gently cleanse area with soap and water
- Topical Bactroban 3 times daily until healed

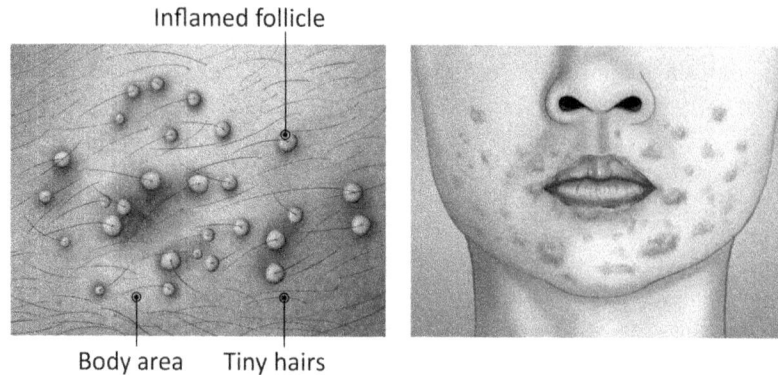

Inflamed follicle

Body area   Tiny hairs

Folliculitis   Impetigo

STAPHYLOCOCCAL SCALDED SKIN SYNDROME

Staphylococcal scalded skin syndrome (SSSS) is a superficial partial-thickness infection of the skin caused by toxins produced by a localized *Staphylococcus aureus* infection, resulting in generalized erythema followed in 24-48 hours by blisters that rupture and peel off, leaving large areas of superficial necrosis and denuded skin, giving the skin a burned or "scalded" appearance. It is most common in neonates and children under 5 but can affect adults who are immunocompromised or in renal failure. Pain is usually mild unless the infection is very widespread. Treatment includes:

- IV antibiotics (such as flucloxacillin) are usually needed initially, followed by a course of oral antibiotics.
- Maintenance of fluids and electrolytes.
- Debridement of skin.
- Moisture-retentive dressings, such as foam dressings, sheet hydrogels, and alginates, avoiding adhesives.
- Excessive tissue loss may be treated the same as partial-thickness burns.

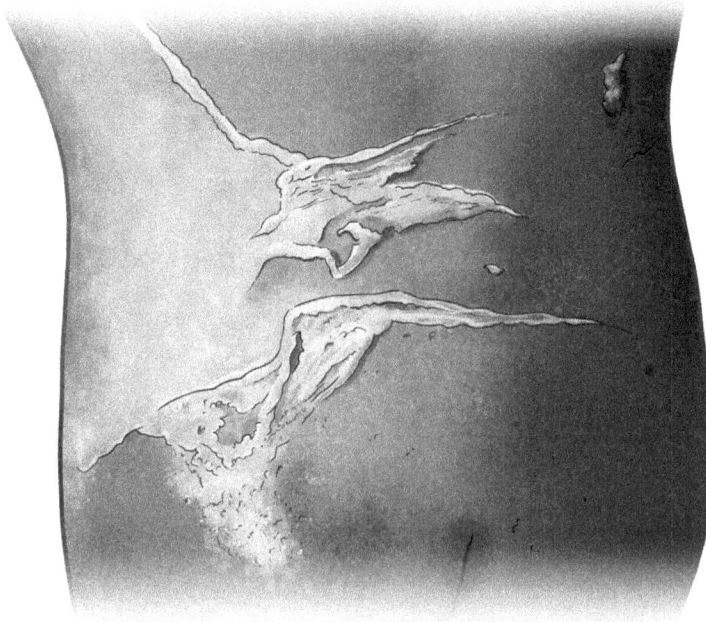

ERYSIPELAS

Erysipelas is a superficial bacterial infection, primarily of the face or legs, involving the cutaneous lymphatic system and invading the skin in areas of trauma. Facial erysipelas is usually caused by group A *Streptococcus* following a nasopharyngeal infection. Infections on the legs are more often related to non-group A *Streptococcus*. The infection spreads rapidly with streaking and clearly demarcated erythema and cellulitis. Local lymph nodes become inflamed, sometimes resulting in lymphedema because of damage to lymph nodes. Erysipelas most commonly affects children and the elderly. Treatment includes:

- Bed rest with elevation of affected limb and warm saline packs to improve circulation.
- Oral antibiotic (usually penicillin G and penicillin VK). IV antibiotics may be indicated for severe cases.

- Hospitalization is recommended for severe cases or those who are very young, elderly, or immunocompromised.
- Analgesics to control pain.

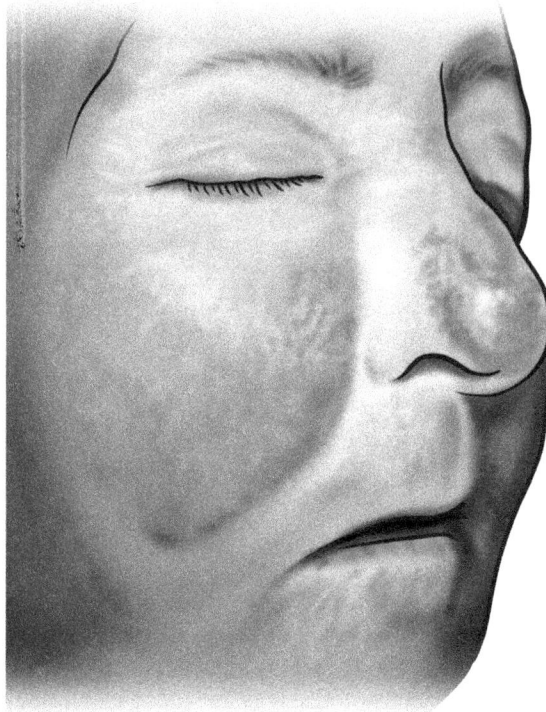

TOXIC SHOCK SYNDROME

Toxic shock syndrome (TSS) is an acute, severe life-threatening bacterial infection that causes a systemic infection with high fever, hypotension, myalgia, diarrhea, and widespread erythematous rash that has the appearance of bad sunburn, with subsequent desquamation (peeling). The original causative agent was *Staphylococcus aureus* and infections were related to the use of tampons, but the infection can occur with wounds or surgical sites where the bacteria can find entry. There are now 2 forms: *Staphylococcus aureus* (TSS) and *Streptococcal* toxic shock syndrome (STSS). *STSS* occurs secondary to an infection in the body, often an infected wound, causing severe hypotension, dyspnea, tachycardia, liver and kidney failure, and a splotchy rash that may peel. Treatment includes:

- Hospitalization for aggressive antibiotic therapy
- Intravenous fluids to treat hypotension
- Topical non-adhesive, non-occlusive dressings with absorbent materials as indicated

HERPES ZOSTER

Herpes zoster ("shingles") is caused by varicella zoster virus retained in the nerve cells after childhood chickenpox. The virus remains dormant until it is reactivated, often in older adults who are immunocompromised. Initial symptoms include pain (often severe burning) and redness. Painful blistering lesions then occur along sensory nerves, usually in a line from the spine around to the chest, although sometimes the head and face are involved. Facial nerve involvement can cause loss of taste and hearing. Eye involvement can cause blindness. The lesions eventually crust over and heal in 2-4 weeks, although some have persistent post-herpetic neuralgia for 6-12 months or longer. The lesions are contagious to those who contact them and have not been immunized or had chickenpox.

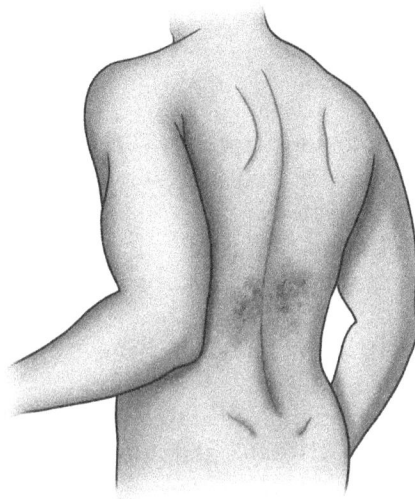

NECROTIZING FASCIITIS

Necrotizing fasciitis is a rapidly spreading infection of the soft tissues involving extensive necrosis of the fascia and subcutaneous tissue as well as destruction of the vasculature with thrombosis. It most often occurs in the extremities after a minor infection. The most common organisms are group A β-hemolytic *Streptococci*, but there may be polymicrobial infections or other causative agents. It may result from surgical procedures, including cardiac catheterization. The infection begins with pain, edema, fever, toxemia, and cellulitis that spreads rapidly, becoming increasingly cyanotic as tissue and perfusion is impaired. Bullae form and progress to necrosis, gangrene, and sepsis within 3-5 days. Mortality rates are 25%. Treatment includes:

- Aggressive extensive surgical debridement of all non-viable tissue. Repeat surgical debridement may be necessary.
- Antibiotic therapy.
- Wound care as indicated by the extent of the wound with careful monitoring to determine if the wound is deteriorating.
- IV immunoglobulin may be used.

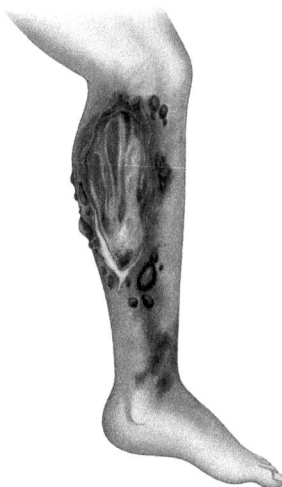

PEMPHIGUS VULGARIS

Pemphigus vulgaris (PV), an autoimmune disorder causing blistering of both the skin and the mucous membranes (presenting symptoms in 50-70% of patients), creates burn-like wounds, which may heal slowly or not at all, often starting in the mouth and genital areas. Untreated the disorder can lead to death. Blisters on skin rupture, causing ulcerations, and those in folds may develop hypergranulation and crusting. Treatment includes:

- Corticosteroids (Prednisone) and immunosuppressive drugs (Imuran).
- Nutritional assessment: vitamin D and calcium supplement may be needed.
- Careful observation for secondary infections.
- Protective clothing and minimize trauma to skin.
- Rituxan, a drug used for lymphoma and leukemia, has helped patients go into remission when used with other drugs.
- Sheets should be kept clean and dry at all times, and changed immediately when soiled.
- Good oral care with soft toothbrush.
- Plasmapheresis with plasma removed to reduce antibodies and donated plasma infused.
- Potassium permanganate lotion bath (1:10000) and chlorhexidine tulle gauze dressing of the denuded areas.

FUNGATING NEOPLASTIC WOUNDS

Fungating neoplastic wounds occur in up to 10% of those with metastasis, especially involving oral or breast cancer. Fungating wounds are ulcerating with necrosis and slough and may have a foul odor and small to copious amount of drainage. Infection is common and the periwound tissue may become inflamed, macerated, or tender. The prognosis is very poor and treatment may be primarily palliative, depending upon the condition of the patient:

- **Control bleeding**: The ulcers bleed as the vasculature erodes, so hemostatic dressings (Gel foam, alginates) and cauterization with silver nitrate may be necessary. Use non-adherent dressings or long-term dressings to reduce trauma.
- **Manage exudate**: Foam, alginate, or hydrofiber dressings or wound pouch as indicated.
- **Control odor**: Use of charcoal dressing or Chloromycetin solution.
- **Protect periwound tissue**: Skin sealants, barrier ointments, and hydrocolloid waters to anchor tape.

- **Cleanse wound**: Use ionic cleansers or antiseptics.
- **Control pain**: Analgesia as indicated.

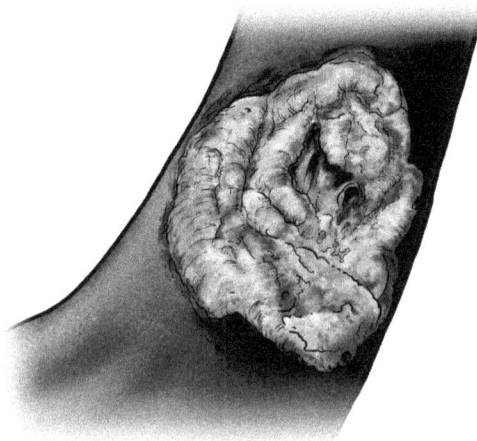

CALCIPHYLAXIS

Calciphylaxis is a rare fatal disease related to end-stage renal disease and uremia, resulting in vascular calcification of cutaneous blood vessels and necrotic lesions with typical violet discoloration. Mortality rates range from 60-80%, usually caused by sepsis. Patients present with painful discolored lesions that progress to nodules and ulcerations that become infected and gangrenous. Lesions are most common in areas with accumulation of fatty tissue. Blood flow distal to the ulcerations is usually intact. The etiology is unclear, but it is associated with hypercalcemia, hyperphosphatemia, and hyperparathyroidism. Treatment is often palliative as there is no successful standardized approach, although the disorder frequently results in amputation of the affected limb.

Treatment includes:

- Control of calcium and phosphorus levels
- Intravenous sodium thiosulfate to reduce calcium deposits
- Surgical or medical treatment of hyperparathyroidism
- Antibiotics as indicated for wound infections
- Aggressive debridement with absorbent moisture-retentive dressings
- Analgesia as indicated

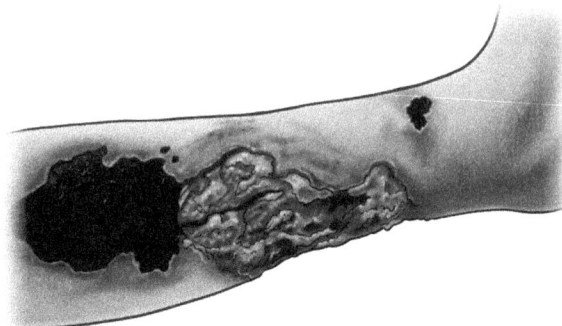

PYODERMA GRANULOSUM

Pyoderma granulosum is a painful ulcerative condition of the skin that is often associated with underlying systemic diseases (such as inflammatory bowel disease) and dysregulation of immunity involving neutrophils. There are two types:

- **Classical**: Deep ulcerations with border overhanging wound bed, most common on the legs but may be around stomas.
- **Atypical**: Vesiculopustular draining lesions, usually on the tops of the hands, the forearms, or face.

Treatment includes:

- Topical and systemic corticosteroids and systemic immunosuppressive drugs
- Local wound care and dressings as indicated for the type and degree of wound, includes moisture-retentive non-adherent dressings
- Autolysis is only debridement because of danger of extending the disease
- Topical antibiotics may be necessary to control infection
- Treating the underlying systemic cause, such as colectomy for ulcerative colitis, may reduce symptoms
- Surgical treatment of lesions is usually avoided

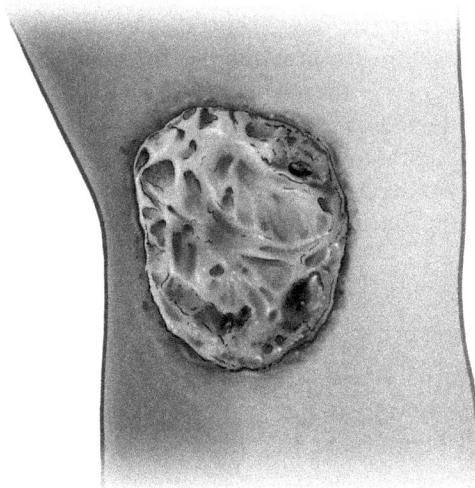

EPIDERMOLYSIS BULLOSA

Epidermolysis bullosa (EB) comprises a group of inherited and non-inherited bullous (blistering) disorders of different levels of the epithelial tissue, with even mild mechanical trauma resulting in blistering. Symptoms vary widely and may range from slight seasonal blistering to life-threatening erosions of skin. It may affect internal epithelial tissue in mucous membranes and organs as well as the external dermal layers. There are different **categories** of EB:

- **Simplex (EBS)**: Intraepidermal lesions.
- **Junctional (JEB)**: Blistering at lamina lucida (between epidermis and basement membrane).
- **Recessive dystrophic (RDEB)**: Separation at basement membrane. Excessive scarring and blistering from slight mechanical trauma, leading to hemorrhage and ulceration. Predisposes to squamous cell carcinoma.
- **Dominant dystrophic (DDEB)**: Blisters below basement membrane with scarring, less severe than RDEB.

Treatment includes:

- Nutritional assessment and supplements as needed
- Topical antibiotics or silver-impregnated dressings for infection
- Protection to avoid trauma
- Fenestrated non-adherent dressings, secured with stockinet, roll gauze, or tubular gauze

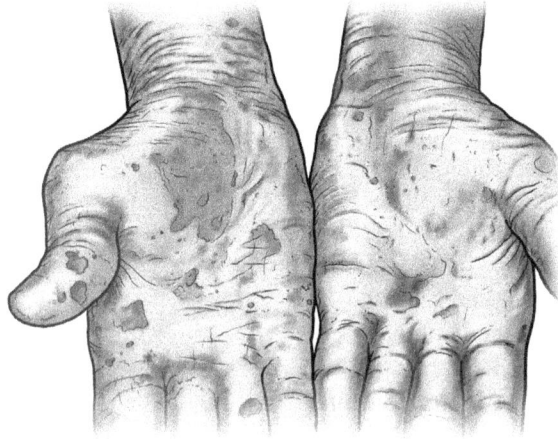

VASCULITIS

Vasculitis comprises a large number of disorders that result in inflammation of veins, arteries, and capillaries, causing changes in vessel walls. Symptoms vary widely, but frequently include fever, general malaise, myalgia, loss of appetite, and skin lesions. Skin lesions may range from macular rashes to large necrotic ulcerations. Lesions are commonly on the lower extremities and may be confused with venous lesions. Disorders that may cause vasculitis with hemorrhagic rash or ulcerations include Behcet's syndrome, Henoch-Schönlein purpura, rheumatoid vasculitis, systemic lupus erythematosus, polyarteritis nodosa, and Wegener's granulomatosis.

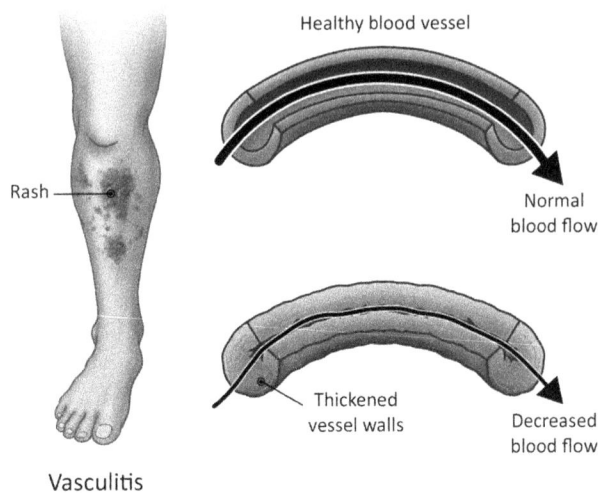

Vasculitis

Treatment includes:

- Medical control of underlying disease process
- Systemic corticosteroids, antihistamines, and immunosuppressants

- Debridement of necrosis
- Observation for infection and treatment with topical or systemic antibiotics as indicated
- Moisture retentive dressings with absorptive material if needed for exudate
- Skin sealants or barriers to protect periwound tissue from exudate
- Monitor nutrition and provide supplements as needed

TOXIC EPIDERMAL NECROLYSIS

Toxic epidermal necrolysis is a rare life-threatening condition of the epidermis caused by drug reactions to 3 types of drugs: antibiotics (sulfonamides, allopurinol, and ampicillin), anticonvulsants (phenytoin, carbamazepine, and phenobarbital), and analgesics (acetaminophen and NSAIDS). An initial maculopapular rash gives way to erythema and painful skin that sloughs with the slightest pressure, leaving >10% of the body denuded of epidermis. The skin, mucous membranes, eyes, and respiratory tract may be involved with mortality rates of 30-40%. Treatment includes:

- Surgical debridement of sloughing skin with saline-moistened cloth
- Porcine xenografts stapled into place
- Patient placed in air-fluidized bed in burn unit
- Fluid and electrolytes monitored and replaced
- NG feedings
- Systemic antibiotics and cessation of any corticosteroids
- Pain control with opioids
- Pulmonary and ophthalmic care
- Grafts trimmed as they desiccate and wounds heal

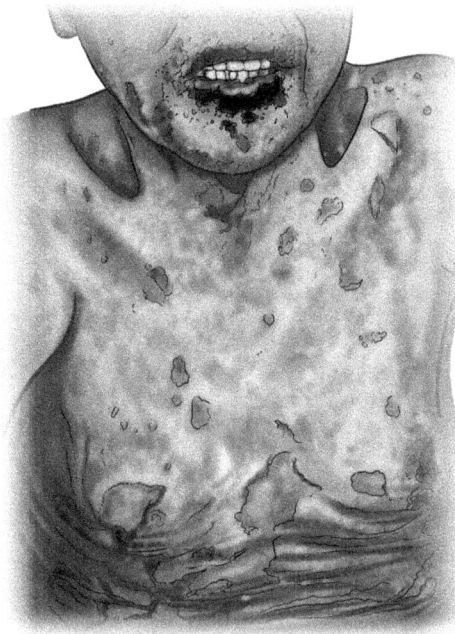

GRAFT-VERSUS-HOST DISEASE

Graft-versus-host disease (GVHD) is caused by a severe host reaction to bone marrow or stem cell transplantation. Acute GVHD occurs within 100 days after surgery, and chronic GVHD occurs after 100 days. The skin, liver (causing jaundice and pruritus), and large and small intestines (causing bleeding and diarrhea) may all be involved. A maculopapular (red to violet) rash usually begins on the hands, plantar area of the feet, face, and upper trunk, then spreads and may results in desquamation and formation of bullae. The disease is staged 1-4 depending on severity.

Treatment includes:

- Colony-stimulating factor (CSF) for 6 months and other appropriate immunosuppressive therapy.
- Topical corticosteroids may be used.
- Careful observation and cleansing of skin for signs of infection.
- Severe denudement requires debridement and transfer to the burn unit for treatment appropriate to the condition to prevent further deterioration.
- Adhesive occlusive dressings should be avoided.

CLASSIFICATION OF BURNS

Burn injuries may be chemical, electrical, or thermal and are assessed by the area affected, percentage of the body burned, and the depth of the burn, as follows:

- **First-degree burns** are superficial and affect the epidermis, causing erythema and pain.
- **Second-degree burns** extend through the dermis (partial thickness), resulting in blistering and sloughing of the epidermis and severe pain.
- **Third-degree burns** affect the underlying tissue, including the vasculature, muscles, and nerves (full thickness). Depending on the extent of the nerve damage, third-degree burns may present with less pain.

Burns are **classified** according to the American Burn Association's criteria as follows:

- **Minor**: <10% body surface area (BSA) in adults or <5% in children and elderly, or 2% BSA with third-degree burns without serious risk to the face, hands, feet, or perineum.
- **Moderate**: 10–20% BSA combined second- and third-degree burns in adults or 5-10% in children or elderly, or 2-5% third-degree burns without serious risk to the face, hands, feet, or perineum.
- **Major**: >20% BSA in adults or >10% in children/elderly; >5% third-degree burns; any burns that are to the face, hands, feet, perineum and will result in functional/cosmetic defect; or burns with inhalation or other major trauma.

Head and Neck 9%

Trunk
Anterior 18%
Posterior 18%

Arms
9% each

Genitalia and Perineum 1%

Legs
18% each

or

if IV

RULE OF NINES

The Rule of Nines is helpful when assessing burn patients to determine fluids (needed if ≥10% total BSA) or transfer to a burn unit is necessary (needed if >20% total BSA, 2nd degree >10% total BSA, 3rd degree >5% total BSA).

Note that the percentage calculations are modified for infants and children under 10 years old because of their larger head and smaller body size. The head is assigned 18%, and the legs are given 13.5% each.

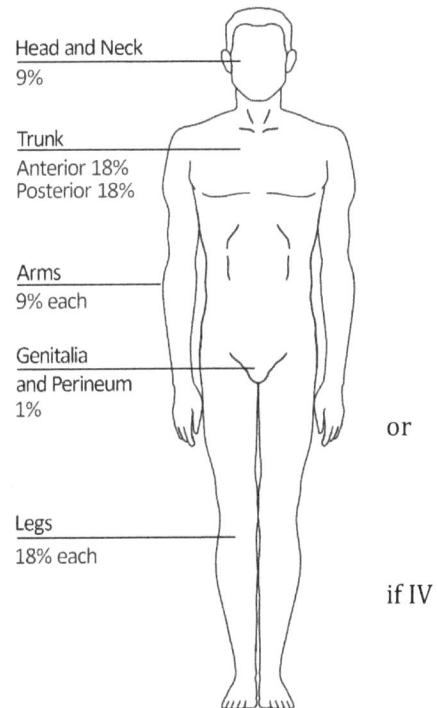

> **Review Video: Rule of Nines**
> Visit mometrix.com/academy and enter code: 846800

COMPLICATIONS ASSOCIATED WITH BURN INJURIES

Burn injuries begin with the skin but can affect all organs and body systems, especially with a major burn. Complications include the following:

- **Cardiovascular**: Cardiac output may fall by 50% as capillary permeability increases with vasodilation and fluid leaks from the tissues, resulting in hypovolemia and hypothermia. Vasoconstriction occurs as a compensatory mechanism, but it may impair circulation and result in further hypoxia.
- **Pulmonary**: Injury may result from smoke inhalation or (rarely) aspiration of hot liquid. Pulmonary injury is a leading cause of death from burns and is classified according to the degree of damage as follows:
  - **First**: Singed eyebrows and nasal hairs with possible soot in airways and slight edema, increasing hypoxia.
  - **Second**: Stridor, dyspnea, and tachypnea with edema and erythema of the upper airway, including the area of the vocal cords and epiglottis, resulting in severe hypoxia, sometimes with rapid onset.
- **Infection**: Open wounds are vulnerable to infection.
- **Circumferential burns**: Swelling beneath eschar can create a tourniquet effect, impairing distal circulation.

ELECTRICAL BURNS

Electricity injures the skin by heating tissues and destroying cellular membranes:

- **Flash burns** look the same as a thermal burn and any hair in the area will be singed. This is the type of burn that usually occurs when a person is struck by lightning. There may be entry and exit burns.
- **Arc burns,** in which the patient is part of a circuit of electricity (≤4000 °C) arcing through the air, have a dry parchment-like center with a surrounding circle of congestion.
- **Contact burns** may show a branding the size of the object touched. Hair is not usually burned in this case.

High-voltage burns of the extremities may require a fasciotomy to save the limb. Care at a specialized burn center is needed for those with moderate to severe burns or for those with electrical burns around the mouth. Disfigurement may be severe when nerves and muscles are destroyed.

LIGHTNING BURNS AND INJURIES

Lightning burns and injuries may occur with a direct strike (≤5%), side splash from a strike nearby, contact voltage when touching an item that has been struck, ground current (from a more distant strike), and blunt trauma from being too close to a strike (which often results in the patient being thrown). Symptoms may vary, but they can include external burns (Lichtenberg figures) in a fernlike pattern, acute pain, fixed and dilated pupils (temporary), eye injuries, confusion, headache, hearing loss, perforated eardrum, hypotension, paralysis/paresis, spinal cord injury, altered mental status, brain injury, fractures, and cardiac arrest. Patients may be responsive initially but lapse into unconsciousness as cerebral edema increases, resulting in secondary respiratory and/or cardiac arrest. Burns are usually mild because of the brief contact.

MANAGEMENT OF BURN INJURIES

Management of burn injuries must include both wound care and systemic care. Treatment includes establishment of airway, treatment for inhalation injury, and intravenous fluids and electrolytes, based on weight and extent of burn.

Parkland formula: 4 mL/kg/day × BSA%

The type of wound treatment depends upon the **severity** of the burn:

- **First-degree**: Superficial and affects the epidermis. Usually, only emollients are needed and symptoms recede within 3-4 days, usually with peeling skin.
- **Second-degree**: Superficial partial-thickness. The skin blisters and sloughs off, denuding the area. These burns may be very painful. Silvadene or other silver preparations are commonly applied to the burns in the initial stages. The skin is debrided and covered with dressings, which are changed every 1-3 days. Healing usually occurs within 2 weeks.
- **Third-degree**: Deep partial-thickness through the epidermis and the dermis. The wounds are painful and may be wet or dry and nonblanchable. The wound requires debridement and grafting as they rarely heal on their own.
- **Fourth-degree**: Full-thickness and may extend through muscle, vessels, and nerves. Third-degree burns require extensive debridement, grafting to prevent massive protein/fluid loss and infection, and application of topical antibiotics and compression dressings.

SKIN DAMAGE CAUSED BY RADIATION TREATMENT

Skin damage/burns caused by radiation treatment vary widely depending upon the dose, duration, fraction-size, treatment area, and type of equipment as well as the condition of the patient. Acute radiation dermatitis usually occurs when radiation is higher than 10 Gy. Patients vary in the progression of symptoms. There may be an initial inflammatory response in the tissue, with increased perfusion and WBCs to the area.

STAGING OF SKIN DAMAGE

Acute skin damage begins within 2-3 weeks of exposure to radiation with changes that are reversible. Because the cells in the skin are constantly going through mitotic division, they are vulnerable to the effects of irradiation. Most reactions subside 1-3 months after therapy ends. Damage is staged according to the type and degree of reaction, and staging determines treatment:

- **Stage I**: Slight edema and inflammation with erythema that may result in burning, itching, and discomfort, caused by dilation and increased permeability of capillaries.
- **Stage II**: Dry, itching, scaly skin with partial sloughing of epidermis, caused by inability of basal epidermal cells to adequately replace surface cells and decreased functioning of skin glands.
- **Stage III**: Moist blistering skin with loss of epidermal tissue, serous drainage, and increased pain with exposure of nerves, caused by continued deterioration of skin.
- **Stage IV**: Loss of body hair and sweat gland suppression resulting in permanent hair loss, atrophy, pigment changes, and ulcerations, caused by accumulation of radiation in the tissues.

TREATMENT FOR RADIATION DAMAGE

Management of tissue damage related to irradiation focuses on treating damage and preventing deterioration in order to relieve discomfort and promote healing. Patients must be educated about the need for skin care during therapy:

- **Protect skin** by maintaining cleanliness, avoiding irritants, using electric razors, protecting the skin from sunlight and extremes of heat and cold, applying appropriate emollients, using mild soaps, and wearing loose, protective clothing.
- **Relieve discomfort** by using cornstarch or powders (NOT talcum) in dry areas, applying topical corticosteroids sparingly to reduce itching.
- **Treat open areas** by using saline compresses, Sitz baths, and semi-occlusive dressings as indicated to protect nerve endings. Prevent damage to wounds by using non-adherent dressings and securing them with mesh or stockinet instead of tape. Culture wounds and treat bacterial or fungal infections as indicated. Use dressings appropriate for the amount and type of exudate to prevent further skin damage or irritation of periwound skin.

ASSESSMENT OF PRESSURE INJURIES

When assessing a tissue injury, it is necessary to determine whether it is a pressure injury or non-pressure injury because the treatment protocol may vary depending upon whether the injury is caused by pressure, venous or arterial insufficiency, or neuropathic disorders. The clinical basis for this determination should be clearly outlined.

- The pressure injury should be classified according to the stage and the characteristics, including size (length, width, and depth).
- Pain associated with the pressure injury should be described.
- Photographs should be taken if a protocol is in place.
- Pressure injuries should be monitored daily and any changes carefully documented.
- The injury should be evaluated for signs of infection.

It is important to differentiate between colonization, which is very common, and infection, which usually presents with symptoms such as periwound erythema, induration, and increased pain as well as delayed healing of the wound. Wound culture and blood tests should be done if there are indications of infection. Treatment should be determined according to the characteristics of the wound.

CAUSES OF PRESSURE INJURIES

PRESSURE INTENSITY, PRESSURE DURATION, AND TISSUE TOLERANCE

Pressure injuries are caused primarily by pressure, but there are numerous additional considerations:

- **Pressure intensity**: Capillary closing pressure (10–32 mmHg) is the minimal pressure needed to collapse capillaries, reducing tissue perfusion. This pressure can be easily exceeded in the sitting or supine position if weight is not shifted.
- **Duration of pressure**: Low pressure for long periods and high pressure for short periods can both result in pressure injuries.
- **Tissue tolerance**: The tissue tolerance is the ability of the skin to tolerate and redistribute pressure, preventing anoxia. Both extrinsic and intrinsic factors can affect tissue tolerance. Extrinsic factors include shear (the skin stays in place but the underlying tissue slides), friction (moving the skin against bedding or other objects), and moisture. Intrinsic factors include poor nutrition, advanced age, low blood pressure, stress, smoking, and low body temperature.

SHEAR AND FRICTION

Shear occurs when the skin stays in place and the underlying tissue in the deep fascia over the bony prominences stretches and slides, damaging vessels and tissue and often resulting in undermining. Shear is one of the most common causes of pressure injuries, which are often described as pressure ulcers but are technically somewhat different, although the effects of shearing are often combined with pressure. The most common cause of shear is elevation of the head of the bed over 30°. Friction against the sheets holds the skin in place while the body slides down the bed, resulting in pressure and damage in the sacrococcygeal area. The underlying vessels are damaged and thrombosed, leading to undermining and deep ulceration.

Friction is a significant cause of pressure injuries because it acts with gravity to cause shear. Friction by itself results only in damage to the epidermis and dermis, such as abrasions or denudement referred to as "sheet burn." Friction and pressure can combine, however, to form tissue injury.

Wound Care: Assessment

MEASURES TO CONTROL SHEAR AND FRICTION

Because **shear** and **friction** are primary factors in the development of pressure injuries, measures to reduce them are essential:

- The head of the bed should never be elevated more than 30°; however, bed-bound patients may not be able to feed themselves at this angle. If the bed is elevated higher, the patient should be carefully positioned, using a pull sheet or overhead trapeze to make sure the patient is at the right position. The bed should be lowered as soon as possible.

Note: Elevating the foot of the bed to prevent sliding and shear simply increases pressure to the sacrococcygeal area, solving one problem by creating another.

- Making sure that the skin is dry; using fine cornstarch-based powders may help prevent the skin from "sticking" to the sheets.
- Pull sheets or mechanical lifting devices should be used to lift, move, or transfer the patient.
- Medical treatments may reduce restlessness.
- Heel and elbow protectors provide protection.

MANAGEMENT OF PRESSURE INJURIES

MEASURES TO PROMOTE MOBILITY

Mobility is a problem for many patients with pressure injuries because their restricted mobility is often the cause of the injury in the first place. However, promoting mobility to the extent possible improves circulation, aids healing, and decreases risk of developing further pressure injury:

- Bed-bound patients must be repositioned on a scheduled basis and should receive passive ROM exercises and active bed exercises if tolerated daily. The patient's head should be elevated only to 30° for short periods of time.
- Patients with limited mobility should be evaluated by physical and occupational therapists in order to develop an individualized plan for activities. Patients may need assistive devices, such as walkers, canes, or wheelchairs. Because the wound must be protected without compromise to circulation, the amount and type of mobility or exercises must be designed with respect to the area and stage of the pressure injury as well as underlying pathology or co-morbid conditions.

MEASURES TO CONTROL FECAL INCONTINENCE

Control of fecal incontinence is necessary to prevent deterioration of tissue that can increase the risk of pressure injuries and to prevent contamination of existing pressure injuries:

- Assess incontinence to determine cause and whether it is temporary, related to health problems, or chronic.
- Determine the type of incontinence:
  - Passive, in which the person is unaware.
  - Urge, which is the inability to retain stool.
  - Seepage, after a bowel movement or around a blockage.
- Use medications as indicated to control diarrhea or constipation.
- Place on a bowel-training regimen with scheduled bowel movements, using suppositories, stool softeners, and bulk formers as indicated, according to cause of incontinence. Use skin moisture barriers and absorbent pads or adult briefs as needed.
- Modify diet as needed with foods to control diarrhea or constipation.
- Ensure adequate fluid intake.
- Consider fecal pouches or fecal containment devices if incontinence cannot be otherwise controlled.

MEASURES TO CONTROL URINARY INCONTINENCE

Control of urinary incontinence is necessary to prevent deterioration of the tissue that can increase the risk of pressure injuries:

- Assess incontinence to determine cause and whether it is temporary, related to health problems, or chronic.
- A temporary Foley catheter may be used in some cases while tissue heals, but long-term use is contraindicated because of the danger of infections.
- Medications may be indicated to treat urinary infections or frequency. Scheduled toileting with reinforcement may help to decrease incidence.
- Use absorbent pads or adult briefs that wick liquid away from the body, and establish a regular schedule for changing.
- Cleanse soiled skin with no-rinse wipes, as they are less drying to skin than soap and water.
- Use skin moisture barrier ointments to protect skin from urine.
- Use protective and support devices as needed.
- Avoid positioning on existing pressure injuries.

FACTORS INFLUENCING THE HEALING OF SURGICAL WOUNDS

There are a number of **factors that affect surgical wound healing**:

- Preoperative showering and skin preparation without shaving decreases incidence of infection.
- Patient condition prior to surgery, type of illness, and the procedure performed all affect healing.
- Breaks in sterile procedure, contamination of the wound by the GI tract, or encountering inflammation or necrotic tissues during the course of the surgery creates a "dirty" wound that has a greater chance of infection.
- Longer procedures increase infection risk.
- The amount of mechanical stress on tissues during the surgery affects inflammation.
- The wound must have a proper blood supply and be able to be closed without causing tension of the tissues.

TOPICAL THERAPY FOR SURGICAL WOUNDS

Topical therapy for surgical wounds is generally conservative, observing for signs of healing and infection. The standard use of antimicrobials and antiseptics is generally not indicated because of the danger of resistance and the cytotoxic properties of some that delay healing. Therapy includes:

- Initial dressing to provide protection, to absorb any exudate, and to provide thermal insulation to promote healing. Dressings should be lightly applied in order to prevent compression that may impede perfusion to the wound. These may be left in place for 48-72 hours to allow the wound to begin to seal.
- If there are signs of local infection, a topical antimicrobial (such as Neosporin) or antiseptic (such as povidone iodine) may be applied to the surgical incision site.
- Depending upon the site of the incision, after the initial healing has taken place, the wound may be left uncovered or a soft dressing may be kept in place to prevent local irritation.

WOUND DEHISCENCE

Wound sutures should be long lasting, at times permanent, as opposed to absorbable. They should be placed 1 cm from the wound edge and 1 cm apart. If sutures are too thin, they may stretch, break, or cut through tissues. Knots may become undone if there are too few sutures to hold tissues together adequately when the wound is under tension due to obesity or movement. Suture problems can cause wound dehiscence to occur. Wound dehiscence occurs more often in those older than 65. Other factors include obesity, cancer, emergency surgery situations, steroid use, hypoalbuminemia, and hypovolemia. Wound infections or intra-abdominal sepsis also predisposes the wound to dehiscence. Coughing, vomiting, and ascites put strain on the incision. The first indication of dehiscence is leakage of serosanguineous fluid. Evisceration can occur suddenly or gradually as the incision opens. The patient is taken to surgery and any necrotic tissues are removed to allow the wound to be resutured through healthy tissues. Hernias often form in these scars.

KELOID AND HYPERTROPHIC SCARS

Keloid scars are thick, rope-like, and extend over the borders of the wound, rarely regressing with healing. Keloids occur more frequently in African Americans and Asians. They occur due to excess collagen deposition, causing increased growth. Normal collagen degradation that occurs in wound remodeling is overtaken by the rate of deposition. Keloids respond to cutting or abrasion by growing even bigger. They are most common on the upper back, chest, earlobes, and deltoids. Keloids may be painful or itch. The tendency to form keloid scars should be assessed when treating a patient's wound so that precautions may be taken in the early stages of wound healing to try to prevent keloid formation.

Hypertrophic scars are also thick but they stay within the borders of the wound and occur most often over joints where there was tension on the wound. They may regress in time. They can also itch, cause pain, and decrease functional movement if they contract.

FACTORS TO CONSIDER ABOUT TRAUMATIC WOUNDS

There are many types of traumatic wounds: slashes, incisions, crush injuries, degloving, and penetrating. However, they hold the following elements in common:

- Traumatic wounds may not only have tissue trauma but also trauma to blood vessels, nerves, tendons, muscles, and bone.
- There may be extensive bleeding that must be stopped.
- The wound may be contaminated with bacteria, dirt, or foreign bodies that must be removed with irrigation or exploration. Wounds that are contaminated or missing significant tissue must remain open to heal by secondary intention.
- There may be nonviable tissue that must be removed, requiring skin grafts to cover the underlying tissue.
- Wounds involving joint capsules are at risk for septic arthritis, and those of the extremities may be at risk for compartment syndrome, requiring a fasciotomy to save the limb from ischemia due to edema.

TREATMENT OF TRAUMATIC BITE WOUNDS

ANIMAL BITES

There is no one topical therapy for traumatic wounds because they vary so widely in the type and degree of injury. A scrape on the knee is treated very differently from a car accident that involves massive tissue injury or tissue loss. Animal bites, including human, are frequent causes of traumatic injury. Treatment includes:

- Cleanse the wound by flushing it with 10-35 cc syringe with an 18-gauge angiocath to remove debris and bacteria using normal saline or dilute Betadine solution.
- Hand, puncture, and infected wounds or those more than 12 hours old may be closed by secondary intention.
- Use moisture-retentive dressings as indicated by the size and extent of wound left open. Dry dressings may be applied to injuries with closure by primary intention.
- Topical antibiotics may be indicated although systemic antibiotics are commonly prescribed for animal bites.
- Tetanus toxoid or immune globulin is routinely administered.

SPIDER BITES

Spider bites are frequently a misdiagnosis of a *Staphylococcus aureus* or MRSA infection, so unless the spider was observed, the wound should be cultured and antibiotics started. If the wound responds to the antibiotic, then it probably was not a spider bite. There are two main types of venomous spider bites:

- Producing neurological symptoms (Black widow)
- Producing local necrosis (brown recluse, yellow sac, and hobo spiders)

Treatment of spider bites universally includes first cleansing the wound and applying a cool compress. The body part should be elevated if possible.

Black widow bite treatment includes:

- Narcotic analgesics
- Nitroprusside to relieve hypertension
- Calcium gluconate 10% solution IV for abdominal cramps
- Latrodectus antivenin for those with severe reaction

Necrotic/ulcerated bites (brown recluse, etc.) treatment includes the following considerations:

- There is no consensus on the best treatment as ulceration caused by the venom may be extensive and surgical repair with grafts may be needed.
- Treatment as for other necrotic ulcers, with moisture retentive dressings as indicated.

SNAKE BITES

About 45,000 snake bites occur in the United States each year, about 8,000 of which are venomous. In the United States, about 25 species of snakes are venomous. There are 2 types of snakes that can cause serious injury, classified according to the type of fangs and venom.

CORAL SNAKES

Coral snakes have short fixed permanent fangs in the upper jaw and venom that is primarily neurotoxic, but may also have hemotoxic and cardiotoxic properties:

- Wounds show no fang marks but there may be scratches or semi-circular markings from teeth.
- There may be little local reaction, but neurological symptoms may range from mild to acute respiratory and cardiovascular failure.

Treatment includes:

- Cleanse the wound thoroughly of dirt and debris and leave it open or cover with dry dressing.
- Antibiotics are not usually needed.
- Administer antivenin immediately even without symptoms, which may be delayed.
- Administer tetanus toxoid or immune globulin.

PIT VIPERS

A second type of snake that can cause serious injury are pit vipers, including rattlesnakes, copperheads, and cottonmouths. These snakes have erectile fangs that fold until they are aroused, and their venom is primarily hemotoxic and cytotoxic but may have neurotoxic properties.

- Wounds usually show 1-2 fang marks.
- Edema may begin immediately or may be delayed up to 6 hours.
- Pain may be severe.

Wound Care: Assessment

- There may be a wide range of symptoms, including hypotension and coagulopathy with defibrination that can lead to excessive blood loss, depending upon the type and amount of venom.
- There may be local infection and necrosis.

Treatment includes:

- Cleanse the wound thoroughly and apply dressings as indicated.
- Administer tetanus toxoid or immune globulin.
- Administer analgesics, such as morphine sulphate.
- Avoid NSAIDs and aspirin because of anticoagulation properties.
- Mark edema every 15 minutes.
- Administer antivenin therapy if indicated (observation for serum sickness if horse serum used).
- Administer prophylactic antibiotics for severe tissue necrosis.
- Administer platelets, plasma, or packed RBCs for coagulopathy.

ALLIGATOR BITES

Alligators are found in 10 coastal states in the southeastern United States with the largest population in Florida, where most injuries are reported. Animals between 4-8 feet often bite once and release, but larger animals may bite repeatedly, engaging in typical biting and feeding activities, and resulting in severe injury, amputations, or death. Most wounds involve the limbs, with the hands and arms the most frequently bitten. Treatment includes:

- Treatment for shock and blood loss.
- Apply pressure to the wound.
- Retrieve the amputated limbs if possible.
- Flush the wound with copious amounts of normal saline to reduce contamination.
- Collect wound cultures.
- Administer prophylactic broad-spectrum antibiotics for Gram negative organisms, such as *Aeromonas hydrophila* and *Clostridium*.
- Observe for signs of infection, such as erythema, cellulitis, exudate, necrosis.
- Administer tetanus toxoid or immune globulin.
- Repair fractures.
- Surgical repair and debridement as indicated with wounds usually healing by secondary intention or delayed primary closure.

MANAGEMENT OF MECHANICAL TRAUMA

Mechanical trauma may result in stripping of the epidermis and sometimes the dermis of the skin or lacerations. Mechanical trauma may occur from tape removal or blunt trauma, such as colliding with furniture. Treatment includes:

- Recognize fragile skin and treat it carefully.
- Apply emollients, skin sealants, and skin barriers as indicated.
- Apply and remove tape appropriately.
- Avoid adhesives when possible.
- Use hydrocolloids, SteriStrips, and transparent dressings to stabilize flaps.

MANAGEMENT OF CHEMICAL TRAUMA

Chemical trauma may be caused by leakage or incontinence of body fluids, such as urine, feces, and exudate, or chemicals applied to the skin, such as lotions, iodine, soap, organic solvents, acids, and adhesives. Reactions to irritant contact dermatitis may vary widely, from an itching rash similar to allergic contact dermatitis to cracks and fissures in the skin, especially on the hands, or denudement of skin, often in the perineal area. The skin reaction may be rapid and extremely painful. Treatment includes:

- Identify the irritant and eliminate its contact with skin.
- Gently cleanse the skin to remove the irritant, avoiding further skin irritation.
- Use skin sealants or skin barriers as indicated to protect the skin and allow healing.
- Use appropriate skin care products and containment devices.
- Monitor dressings and peri-wound condition daily.

Wound Classification Systems

CLASSIFICATION OF WOUNDS BY CAUSE

Wounds can be classified in various ways. The most common classification of wounds is that according to cause:

- **Vascular wounds:** Vascular changes can result in wounds that occur most commonly in the lower extremities, such as those that result from arterial insufficiency and ischemia, those that relate to changes in the lymphatic system, and those related to venous insufficiency.
- **Neuropathic wounds:** Neuropathic changes that occur with chronic diseases, such as diabetes, and chronic alcoholism can decrease sensation and circulation, resulting in ulcerations.
- **Pressure injuries:** Shear friction and pressure, especially over bony prominences such as the sacral area and heels, causes erosion of the tissue.
- **Traumatic wounds:** Trauma often results in contaminated wounds.
- **Surgical wounds:** Surgery can result in wounds that are originally contaminated or originally clean, depending upon the type of surgery and the reason.
- **Infected wounds:** Inflammation and infection may result in deteriorating wounds or fistulas.
- **Self-inflicted wounds:** Vary widely, from minor cuts to traumatic gunshot wounds.
- **Dysfunctional healing wounds:** Hypergranulation/keloid formation can change the character of a wound and prevent adequate healing.

STAGING SYSTEM FOR PRESSURE INJURIES

Pressure-related injuries result from pressure with or without shear and/or friction over bony prominences. The National Pressure Injury Advisory Panel developed a staging system to ensure that definitions for pressure injuries were standardized:

- **Suspected deep tissue injury**: Skin discolored, intact or blood blister
- **Stage I**: Intact skin with non-blanching reddened area
- **Stage II**: Abrasion or blistered area without slough but with partial-thickness skin loss
- **Stage III**: Deep tissue injury with exposed subcutaneous tissue; tunneling or undermining may be evident with or without slough or epibole (rolling inward of wound edge)
- **Stage IV**: Deep tissue injury, full thickness, with necrosis into muscle, bone, tendons, and/or joints
- **Unstageable**: Eschar and/or slough prevents staging prior to debridement

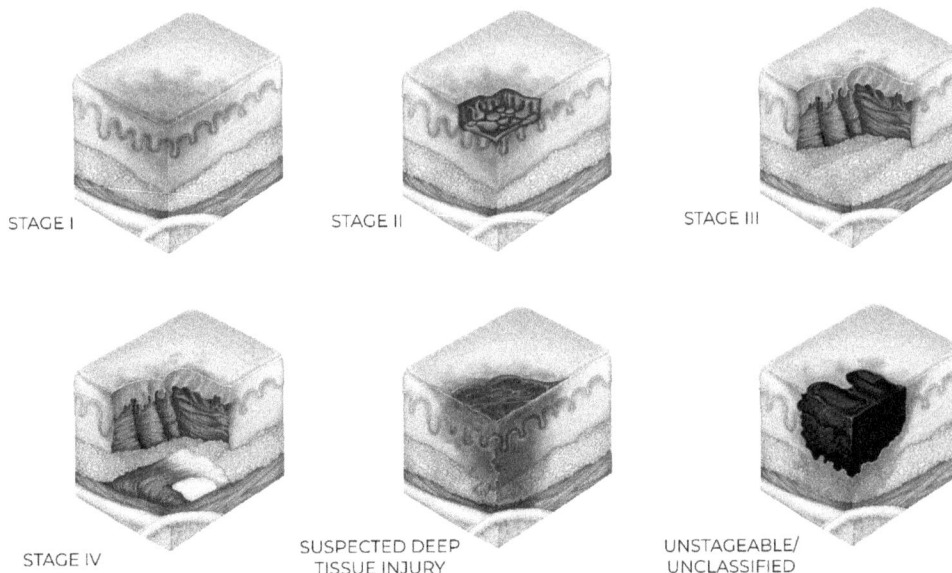

STAGE I

STAGE II

STAGE III

STAGE IV

SUSPECTED DEEP TISSUE INJURY

UNSTAGEABLE/ UNCLASSIFIED

MODIFIED WAGNER ULCER CLASSIFICATION SYSTEM FOR FOOT ULCERS

The modified Wagner Ulcer Classification System divides foot ulcers into six grades, based on lesion depth, osteomyelitis or gangrene, infection, ischemia, and neuropathy:

- **Grade 0**: At risk but no open ulcers
- **Grade 1**: Superficial ulcer, extending into subcutaneous tissue; superficial infection with or without cellulitis
- **Grade 2**: Full-thickness ulcer to tendon or joint with no abscess or osteomyelitis
- **Grade 3**: Full-thickness ulcer that may extend to bone with abscess, osteomyelitis, or sepsis of joint and may include deep plantar infections, abscesses, fasciitis, or infections of tendon sheath
- **Grade 4**: Gangrene in one area of foot, but the foot is salvageable
- **Grade 5**: Gangrene of entire foot, requiring amputation

While this classification system is useful in predicting outcomes, it does not contain information about the size of the ulcer or the type of infection, so it should be only one part of an assessment, as more detailed information is needed to fully evaluate an ulcer.

UNIVERSITY OF TEXAS DIABETIC FOOT WOUND CLASSIFICATION SYSTEM

The University of Texas created a wound classification system to account for the shortcomings of the Wagner classification system. Although the Wagner system is still used today, it has limitations at predicting outcome after grade 3 and lacks certain aspects of the wound assessment, making it less comprehensive in nature. The University of Texas wound classification system considers the wound's depth and infection status, as well as the presence of peripheral arterial occlusive disease, and evaluates the wound by both grade (0 through 3) and Stage (A, B, C, or D), which are defined as follows:

Stage	Grade 0	Grade 1	Grade 2	Grade 3
A	Lesion (pre- or post-ulcerative) is completely epithelialized	Ulcer is superficial and does not involve tendon or bone	Ulcer penetrates to the tendon	Ulcer penetrates to the bone/joint space
B	Infection present	Infection present	Infection present	Infection present
C	Ischemia present	Ischemia present	Ischemia present	Ischemia present
D	Both infection and ischemia present	Both infection and ischemia present	Both infection and ischemia present	Both infection and ischemia present

S(AD) SAD CLASSIFICATION SYSTEM

S(AD) SAD stands for Size (Area and Depth), Sepsis, Arteriopathy, and Denervation. The S(AD) SAD classification system for lower-extremity neuropathic disease is one of many that builds upon the original or modified Wagner classification system and assigns a 0-3 grade based on 5 categories: area, depth, sepsis, arteriopathy, and denervation.

- **Grade 0**: No pathology is evident.
- **Grade 1**: Ulcer is <10 mm^2, involving subcutaneous tissue with superficial slough or exudate, diminution or absence of pulses, and reduced sensation.
- **Grade 2**: Ulcer is 10-30 mm^2, extending to tendon, joint, capsule, or periosteum with cellulitis, absence of pulses except for neuropathy dominant ulcers that have palpable pedal pulses.
- **Grade 3**: Ulcer is >30 mm^2, extending to bones and/or joints; seen with osteomyelitis, gangrene, and Charcot's foot.

This grading system is useful, but as with most other classification systems, it doesn't provide a simple way to distinguish those wounds that follow an atypical pattern or may be consistent with the grade in some areas and inconsistent in others.

CEAP CLASSIFICATION FOR CHRONIC VENOUS DISORDERS

Clinical (C0-C6)

- 0: No apparent venous disease
- 1: Telangiectasia/reticular veins
- 2: Varicose veins
- 3: Edema
- 4: Skin changes
- 5: Healed ulcer
- 6: Active ulcer

Etiologic

- E_C: Congenital
- E_P: Primary
- E_S: Secondary
- E_N: No cause identified

Anatomic distribution

- A_S: Superficial veins
- A_D: Deep veins
- A_P: Perforating veins
- A_N: No location identified

Pathophysiological classification

- P_R: Reflux
- P_O: Obstruction
- $P_{R,O}$: Reflux and obstruction
- P_N: No pathophysiology identified

Wound Infections

STAGES OF WOUND INFECTION

The skin contains natural flora that cause no problem with intact skin, but if the skin barrier is breached, these microorganisms can migrate in to an open wound. Additionally, some pathogens, such as *Staphylococcus aureus,* are endemic to hospital environments and can contaminate wounds. Furthermore, **bioburden** (the presence of necrotic tissue and debris that prevent epithelialization from occurring) contributes to the development of infection in the wound.

There is a continuum to the **infectious process**:

- **Colonization** occurs when microorganisms replicate. There may be superficial signs of infection, but this phase is not pathogenic and should not be treated with antibiotics.
- **Critical colonization** occurs when the bioburden increases, arresting healing of the wound. Wounds may appear red and clean but lack granulation. The infection remains localized, and there is no systemic response. Topical antibiotics may be used at this phase.
- **Infection** occurs when the microorganisms invade the tissue and there is a systemic response. Acute wounds show signs of inflammation, but chronic wounds may only exhibit increased pain, exudate, or further delay in healing. Cultures and sensitivities should be done to ascertain the correct treatment.

ASSESSMENT OF WOUND INFECTION

There are a number of different aspects to the assessment for wound infection:

- **Patient history**: A complete history is critical. Any prior hospitalizations or recent surgeries should be noted as well as medication history. The history should show when and how the wound first occurred to help determine if the wound is acute or chronic. Co-morbidities should be noted as well as age and cognitive, functional, and nutritional status.
- **Examination**: A complete assessment of the wound, noting wound characteristics and drainage, should be done along with a careful and complete physical examination.
- **Laboratory testing**: Laboratory findings provide indications of the type and extent of infection and should include the complete blood count to determine if there is elevation of the white blood count. Wound cultures and sensitivities should be done to identify the microorganism and treatment. CT scans may be done to identify abscesses.

> **Review Video: Wound Infections**
> Visit mometrix.com/academy and enter code: 761736

SURGICAL SITE INFECTIONS
CDC CRITERIA FOR INCISIONAL AND ORGAN/SPACE SURGICAL SITE INFECTIONS

The CDC classifies surgical site infections as superficial incisional, deep incisional, or organ/space, depending on the severity of the infection:

- **Superficial incisional**:
  - Occurs within 30 days of surgery
  - Purulent discharge evident, organisms isolated, signs of infection and wound opened by surgeon, or diagnosis by physician

- **Deep incisional**:
  - o Occurs within 30 days of surgery if no implant is in place, or 1 year if an implant is in place
  - o Purulent discharge evident, signs of infections and incision dehisces or is deliberately opened by physician
  - o Abscess or other evidence of infection found on examination, radiology, or histopathology
  - o Diagnosis by physician
- **Organ/space**:
  - o Occurs within 30 days of surgery if no implant is in place, or 1 year if an implant is in place if infection appears related
  - o Infection involves any part of the body (organs, tissues) manipulated during surgery
  - o Purulent discharge evident from drain to organ/space, organisms isolated from fluids or tissue in organ space, abscess in area, or diagnosis by physician

RISK FACTORS FOR SURGICAL SITE INFECTIONS

Risk factors should be carefully assessed to determine the likelihood of surgical site infections:

- **Duration of surgery**: Surgeries more than 2 hours in length increase risk.
- **Co-morbidity**: Some conditions, such as diabetes mellitus or skin disease in surgical area, predispose patients to infection.
- **Steroids**: Immunosuppressive response allows infection.
- **Malnutrition**: Nutrients needed for healing are lacking.
- **Recent surgery**: Each procedure increases risk.
- **Extended hospitalization**: Risk increases with length of hospitalization prior to surgery.
- *Staphylococcus aureus*: Nasal colonization or presence on skin allows bacteria to migrate to wound.
- **Remote infection**: Infection anywhere else in the body poses risk.
- **Prior radiation**: Radiation therapy compromises tissue and delays healing, allowing for infection to occur more easily.
- **Old/young**: The very young and elderly are more easily infected.
- **Circulatory impairment**: Hypoxemia or localized impairment, such as with peripheral vascular disease, compromise tissue. Smoking interferes with circulation as well.

VITAL SIGNS INDICATING SYSTEMIC INFECTION LEADING TO SEPSIS

Infections caused by viruses, fungi, bacteria, and parasites can lead to sepsis, especially in the immunocompromised or those who have injuries that impair the body's defense, such as large contaminated wounds or burns. Signs of wound infection, such as warmth, pain, odorous exudate, and pus, or changes in condition should prompt one to check the patient's vital signs for typical **signs that may indicate sepsis**:

- Hyperthermia with temperature >38 °C OR hypothermia with temperature <35 °C
- Temperature changes possibly occurring with chills
- Increased respiratory rate (>20/min)
- Increased pulse rate
- Hypotension with falling blood pressure and <90 mmHg systolic or >40 mmHg decrease from normal reading

The symptoms indicating sepsis may relate to the underlying infection, such as pneumonia or meningitis, so symptoms may vary considerably, depending upon the causative agent and the site of infection. Some people may exhibit few symptoms while others may develop severe symptoms.

Risk Assessment

DETERMINING RISK FROM PATIENT'S MEDICAL HISTORY

A thorough medical history will uncover information about diseases that have an impact on the condition of the skin:

- Medication and supplements taken, allergies, and hygiene practices should be noted as well as soaps, lotions, and other skin care products used.
- Environmental conditions and exposure to agents that are harmful to the skin at home, at work, or during recreation are important.
- Previous skin problems, problems with wound healing, and hereditary conditions affecting the skin should be determined.
- Nutritional status and dietary habits should be discussed.
- Symptoms of vascular problems should be noted.
- The patient's support system is important if help is needed for ADLs.
- Past exposure to radiation is noted along with the location, duration, strength of radiation, and effects on the skin.
- Financial status and health care insurance status of those who require wound care must also be considered.

IMPACT OF SMOKING ON PERIPHERAL CIRCULATION

Smoking is a primary cause of lower extremity arterial disease, with diagnosis of disease 10 years before non-smokers. The effects of smoking on peripheral circulation include:

- Smoking decreases the blood flow to the extremities by causing arterial spasms that last 1 hour or longer.
- Carboxyhemoglobin from smoke is thought to harm the lining of the blood vessels, thus encouraging thrombus formation.
- Platelet function is also affected, increasing the formation of blood clots.
- Prostacyclin, a prostaglandin that inhibits platelet aggregation and causes vasodilation, is inhibited in production by smoking.
- Smoking increases the rate of atherosclerosis, decreases HDL, increases blood pressure, and decreases clotting time.
- The risk of claudication is nine times higher for smokers. Those with intermittent claudication who quit do not usually progress to having pain at rest.

RISK FACTORS FOR PRESSURE INJURIES

BRADEN SCALE FOR PRESSURE INJURY RISK ASSESSMENT

The Braden scale is a risk assessment tool that has been validated clinically as predictive of the risk of patient's developing pressure injuries. It was developed in 1988 by Barbara Braden and Nancy Bergstrom and is in wide use. The scale scores 6 different areas with 1-4 points.

- **Sensory perception**
  - 1. Completely limited (unresponsive to pain or limited ability to feel)
  - 2. Very limited (responds to painful stimuli and moans)
  - 3. Slightly limited (responds to verbal commands but limited communication)
  - 4. No impairment

- **Moisture**
  - 1. Moist constantly
  - 2. Very moist (linen change each shift)
  - 3. Occasionally moist (linen change each day)
  - 4. Rarely moist

- **Activity**
  - 1. Bed bound
  - 2. Chair bound
  - 3. Walks occasionally (short distances)
  - 4. Walks frequently

- **Mobility**
  - 1. Completely immobile
  - 2. Very limited (makes occasional slight position changes)
  - 3. Slightly limited (makes frequently slight position changes)
  - 4. No limitations

- **Usual nutrition pattern**
  - 1. Very poor (eats < half of meals and has inadequate protein intake, and hydration)
  - 2. Inadequate (eats about half of food with 3 protein servings or not enough liquid or tube feeding)
  - 3. Adequate (eats more than half of meals and 4 protein servings)
  - 4. Excellent

- **Friction and shear** (3 parameters only)
  - 1. Problem moving (skin frequently slides down sheets, needs help to move)
  - 2. Potential problem (moves weakly or needs some assistance, skin slides somewhat during moves)
  - 3. No apparent problem

The scores for all six items are totaled, and a risk is assigned according to the number:

- 23 (best score) excellent prognosis, very minimal risk.
- ≤16 break point for risk of pressure injury (will vary somewhat for different populations).
- 6 (worst score) prognosis is very poor, strong likelihood of developing pressure injury.

Braden Q and Braden QD Scales

The Braden Q scale is the pediatric version of the Braden scale, meant to rate risk for pediatric patients. This scale uses all six subscales from the original Braden scale, and adds a seventh for **tissue perfusion/oxygenation** which is broken down as follows:

- 1. Extremely compromised (hypotensive or unable to tolerate repositioning)
- 2. Compromised (normal blood pressure with oxygen saturation <95% OR hemoglobin <10 mg/dL OR capillary refill >2 seconds with a serum pH of <7.4)
- 3. Adequate (normal blood pressure with oxygen saturation <95% OR hemoglobin <10 mg/dL OR capillary refill >2 seconds with a serum pH that is normal)
- 4. Excellent (normal blood pressure, oxygen saturation, hemoglobin, and capillary refill)

In 2018, the Braden Q scale was updated to the Braden QD scale. The Braden QD scale has 7 subscales, each rated from 0 to 2 (except for the *number of medical devices* subscale, which is a total count of all medical devices, with a max of 8). 0 indicates no problem, 1 indicates potential problem, and 2 indicates a problem. The 7 subscales are as follows:

- Mobility
- Sensory perception
- Friction and shear
- Nutrition
- Tissue perfusion and oxygenation
- Number of medical devices
- Repositionability/skin protection

A score of 13 or higher places the patient at risk for a pressure injury.

Norton Scale

Often compared to the Braden Scale, the Norton Scale is another scale measuring risk for pressure injuries in the adult population. This scale was created in 1962, before the Braden Scale, and has been criticized for being less predictive of pressure injuries than the Braden Scale. Five categories are rated, with scores stratifying risk as low (>18), medium (14-18), high (10-14), and very high (<10). Categories are as follows:

- Physical Condition
  - Good (4)
  - Fair (3)
  - Poor (2)
  - Very Bad (1)
- Mental Condition
  - Alert (4)
  - Apathetic (3)
  - Confused (2)
  - Stuporous (1)
- Activity
  - Ambulatory (4)
  - Walks with help (3)
  - Chairbound (2)
  - Bedfast (1)

- Mobility
  - Full (4)
  - Slightly impaired (3)
  - Very limited (2)
  - Immobile (1)
- Incontinence
  - None (4)
  - Occasional (3)
  - Usually urinary (2)
  - Urinary and fecal (1)

COMMON RISK FACTORS FOR PRESSURE INJURIES

The Centers for Medicare and Medicaid Services (CMS) established a list of common risk factors for pressure injuries. Many people present with more than one risk factor. Assessment should include evaluation of risks for following:

- Impairment or decreased mobility or functional ability that prevents a person from changing position.
- Co-morbid conditions affecting circulation or metabolism, such as renal disease, diabetes, and thyroid disease.
- Drugs that interfere with healing, such as corticosteroids.
- Impaired circulation, such as generalized atherosclerosis or arterial insufficiency of lower extremity, reducing tissue perfusion.
- Patient refusal of care, increasing risk (positioning, hygiene, nutrition, hydration, skin care).
- Cognitive impairment that prevents the patient from reporting discomfort or cooperating with care.
- Fecal and/or urinary contamination of skin, usually related to incontinence.
- Under nutrition or frank malnutrition and/or dehydration.
- Previous healed pressure injuries. Healed pressure injuries that were Stage III or IV may deteriorate and breakdown again.

IMMOBILITY

Immobility increases the chance of pressure injury development by reducing the voluntary shifting of pressure off of bony prominences. The patient who is unable to move independently must rely on others to change position. Reduced sensory perception of pain adds to the risk. The patient who has restricted mobility may not be able to maintain posture when upright, allowing the body to slump and increasing the chance of shearing as the body succumbs to gravity causing the skeleton to slide downwards as the skin of the sacrum remains in place due to friction against the bed. When caregivers reposition the patient without the aid of a lifting sheet friction against bed linens occurs and increases the chance of skin breakdown. Turning and repositioning plans must be developed for patients who are unable to change position voluntarily. Reconditioning exercises are needed for those who are debilitated but have intact muscular and sensory capabilities.

IMPAIRED COGNITION

The patient with impaired cognition is unable to translate sensory input that warns them of impending problems. They are not alert enough to shift position or signal the need for help from others to do so. They may not recognize sensations of pain, the location of the pain, or the connection between pain and the need to reposition. They do not associate the need for proper fluid and nutritional intake with their health status. They are dependent upon others for all activities of daily living and are often unable to recognize or stop harmful activity. They may engage in activities, such as picking or scratching the skin, without realizing that they are causing damage. They may be incontinent of stool and feces, and the added risk factor of moisture adds to the risk of skin breakdown.

POPULATIONS AT RISK FOR PRESSURE INJURIES

Populations at risk for pressure injuries include the following;

- The **elderly**, especially those with impairment of mobility or changes to the skin, experience the most pressure injuries, often associated with hospitalization or long-term care. For those admitted to long-term care facilities, 10-18% have at least one pressure injury on admission.
- People with **spinal cord injuries** are at risk because of loss of sensation. Studies have shown that approximately one-third of patients with spinal cord injuries will develop a pressure injury at some time.
- **Children** who are hospitalized are also at risk, but rates vary widely depending upon the child's condition and the setting. Rates may be as high as 27% in pediatric care units and as high as 20% in neonatal intensive care units. Pressure injuries usually occur within the first 2 days after admission.
- **Surgical patients** have pressure injury rates of 4-45%, depending on age, nutrition, and co-morbidities. Tissue damage may not be evident for up to 3 days after injury.

RISK FACTORS FROM LOWER EXTREMITY WOUNDS

A lower extremity wound can impact the person's ability to function physically, and put the patient at risk for additional wounds:

- Pain and discomfort may limit the amount of standing and ambulation.
- Enforced immobility, such as being on bed rest with leg elevated, severely constrains physical functioning, leading to pressure injuries.
- Bowel function may be compromised, and constipation from decreased activity is common. Antibiotic therapy associated with the wound may cause diarrhea, which leads to skin breakdown.
- The person's quality of sleep and energy level may be decreased, causing fatigue at home and at work.
- Side effects from antibiotics and other medications also may impair the ability to function.
- The ability to perform ADLS can also be affected by pain, limited mobility, bulky dressings, and fatigue or other symptoms and side effects.

The care provider should assess the patient for these problems and help to find solutions. The care provider should also assess this patient for new wounds. Many of these patients will need help with ADLs at home.

RISKS FACTORS FOR MEDICAL ADHESIVE-RELATED SKIN INJURY AND SKIN TEARS

Medical adhesive-related skin injury (MARSI) occurs when the superficial layers of the skin are peeled away when adhesive is removed. Other evidence of MARSI may include skin tears, erythema, itching, and vesicular lesions. MARSI persists more than 30 minutes after the adhesive is removed and may result from traumatic injury to the tissue (such as epidermal stripping or tension injury), contact dermatitis, or allergic dermatitis. Risk factors include age (those of older age and neonates are at higher risk), and history of dermatologic disorders, malnutrition, dehydration, and underlying medical conditions.

Skin tears occur when layers of the skin are peeled away or separate from underlying tissue. Risk factors include older age, corticosteroid therapy, impaired mobility, and cognitive impairment. Skin tears are categorized with the **Payne-Martin Classification System**:

1. Skin tear (linear full thickness or flap partial thickness) leaves avulsed skin adequate to cover wound. Tears may be linear or flap-type.
2. Skin tear with loss of partial thickness, involving either scant (<25% of epidermal flap over tear is lost) to moderate-large (>25% of dermis in tear is lost).
3. Skin tear with complete loss of tissue, involving a partial-thickness wound with no epidermal flap.

Documenting on Wound Assessment

PATIENT CARE DOCUMENTATION

Patient documentation provides a legal record of patient status and care given. It acts as a communication tool between healthcare providers in their efforts to meet patient needs and ensure the best outcome. It serves as a record of services ordered and services given for billing purposes. Documentation also provides history of previous disease and treatments for reference. Allergies or sensitivities that may impact the patient's condition or treatments are recorded through documentation as well. Entries must always be precise, thorough, factual, and legible. Information must be updated as needed so that the record reflects the current status of the patient during the hospital stay. These principles also apply to care given in clinics, the doctor's office, or during a home health visit.

DOCUMENTATION OF ADMISSION SKIN ASSESSMENT

A pressure injury that develops after 24 hours in a facility is generally considered to be acquired at that facility. Therefore, it is crucial to conduct a thorough skin assessment documentation at the time of admission. The problem comes when an innocent looking bruise present on admission develops into a full-blown pressure injury. Therefore, one should utilize the new definition of deep tissue injury in the guidelines by the National Pressure Injury Advisory Panel (NPIAP) when assessing skin status on admission and designate any area with maroon or purple skin or a blood-filled blister as a suspected deep tissue injury on admission. This designation should also be given to any areas of skin that are painful to the patient, appear changed in texture and firmness from the surrounding skin, or are warmer and cooler. A good-quality photograph of these areas may be included, according to facility policy, with written documentation.

ONGOING WOUND OR TISSUE INJURY DOCUMENTATION

The primary documentation of the wound or injury at the time of presentation for care must be as thorough as possible to establish the baseline to measure the success or failure of healing interventions. The size (length, width, depth), extent (tunneled, undermined), character (granulation, slough, eschar), color (red, pink, black), odor (none, slight, foul), and degree and type of drainage should be initially documented for baseline measurement and then regularly documented to show changes. Photographs should be taken. Consistent photography is valid documentation, but sporadic photography is not. Each photo must be dated and matched with a written description of the wound at the time of the photo. Documentation on wound progress should occur daily with a thorough assessment at least weekly. Documentation should be done in a consistent manner to indicate that care is consistent.

TOOLS TO MONITOR AND DOCUMENT WOUND HEALING

There are three tools used to help monitor wound healing. They all assess the wound, and two also assess the peri-wound areas. The tools all differ in the manner that they are set up. They allow the person doing the assessment to assign a numerical score to the wound:

- **The Sussman Wound Healing Tool (SWHT***)* is used by physical therapists to measure the results of various PT treatments on pressure injuries. Changes in the wound are classified as "good" or "not good" for healing.
- **The Pressure Ulcer Scale for Healing (PUSH)** was developed by the National Pressure Injury Advisory Panel (NPIAP) and measures the surface area of the wound, the amount of exudate, and the wound appearance.
- **Bates-Jensen Wound Assessment Tool (BWAT)**, formerly known as Pressure Sore Status Tool (PSST), assesses 13 wound characteristics and grades them from best to worst.

DOCUMENTATION OF WOUND CARE PROCESS

Documentation of the wound care process should include the following elements:

- **Medication Administration**: Document the name of the medication, the dosage and the route of administration, site of administration (such as for IM injections) as well as the time of administration and follow-up response (such as relief of pain after analgesia) and times of monitoring.
- **Wound Progression (Healing)**: The description must be accurate, including the location, size, depth, stage, and character of the wound, supplemented with photographs (especially at the beginning of treatment and after debridement) or drawings. Changes should be noted at each dressing change and physician visit or intervention, such as debridement. Any complicating factors, such as PAD, and interventions to alleviate them should be documented. The plan of care with expected outcomes should be included.
- **Billing**: Documentation requirements must be met, including the reason for treatment. Documentation must support the service that is billed, and the correct ICD and CPT codes must be utilized for the institution.

USING PHOTOGRAPHS TO DOCUMENT WOUND CHANGES

Documenting wound changes with photographs is an issue of risk management, so facility-wide procedures must be in place regarding the use of photographs. Guidelines must specify:

- The type of camera and film that can be used. Some facilities mandate only Polaroid pictures because digital images can be manipulated. Others use digital cameras because of ease of entering pictures into computerized systems.
- Specific guidelines as to distance requirements indicating how many inches the camera should be from the wound
- Guidelines for including the date in the photograph and using measures (such as disposable rulers)
- Designation of staff allowed to photograph and training required
- Types of wounds/conditions that may be photographed
- Consent form

A wound photo may be taken by any type of camera. Low-cost instant cameras may not deliver the close-up, clear, true color photo that is desired. Moderately priced digital cameras with as high a resolution as possible deliver the best quality photo and provide instant feedback.

TIPS FOR TAKING PHOTOS OF WOUNDS

Tips for taking photos of wounds:

- The correct distance from the wound should be verified using a measuring device, such as a length of string attached to the front of the camera (changed between patients).
- Lighting will affect the colors of the wound. A flash camera will give a blue color and incandescent light will give a yellow cast to the photo. Good ambient light is helpful.
- The patient should be positioned so only the wound is shown in the photo. Other parts of the body should be screened off with drapes. The patient's face should not be shown unless the wound is on the face.
- A ruler should be placed next to the wound to indicate wound size.
- A sign with patient identification and the date may be included in the photo.
- The patient position at the time of the photo should be documented for future reference.
- A written description of the wound must be included in the record with the photograph.

PHOTOGRAPHIC WOUND ASSESSMENT TOOL

The **Photographic Wound Assessment Tool (PWAT)** is a modification of the Bates-Jenson Wound Assessment Tool (BWAT). The tool contains 6 domains (areas) of information that can be determined from the photo:

- Edges of the wound
- Type of necrotic tissue
- Amount/degree of necrotic tissue
- Periwound color
- Evidence of granulation
- Evidence of epithelialization

Each domain is scored from 0 to 4, with a total resulting score that can range from 0 (healed) to 24. Serial photographs are taken on a regular schedule. Studies have shown that this photographic method of assessment is as accurate as bedside assessment of the wound, especially for pressure wounds as the BWAT is designed for pressure wounds rather than other types. PWAT provides a tool for telemedicine use when a clinician cannot be at the patient's bedside to evaluate a wound.

Wound Care: Assessment

Wound Care: Intervention and Treatment

Pressure Redistribution

TISSUE INTERFACE PRESSURES

Tissue interface pressure is the amount of pressure exerted on the body by a surface that the body is lying or sitting on. Small sensors are placed between the patient and the surface to measure pressures in localized areas. The measurement is important to assess whether the pressure is great enough to occlude the capillaries in the area, increasing the risk of tissue ischemia and injury formation. The force that closes capillaries is 12-32 mmHg. This range is used as a comparison along with patient condition, skin condition, nutrition, and other factors to decide whether a support surface relieves enough pressure in a specific location on that particular patient. However, research has not demonstrated that there is a specific threshold at which pressure will cause harm, so the tissue interface pressure should only be used as a guide and not a substitute for observation.

PRESSURE INJURY PREVENTION

Every patient should be assessed for **risk factors** for pressure injuries. These include immobility, inactivity, moisture and incontinence, poor nutritional state and intake, friction and shear, decreased sensation, mental status changes, fragile skin condition, and certain medications. Tools are available for assessing patient risk for pressure injuries, including the Gosnell Scale and the Braden Scale. Use of these scales provides consistency in assessment from patient to patient and can be used to assess changes in risk level as a result of interventions. Once the risk factors are defined, prevention can concentrate on alleviating these factors. Interventions are designed, and patient and family teaching is performed. Interventions are specific for each patient, disease status, and individual situation. Several solutions for risk factors are possible, and solutions must be individualized for the patient.

TURNING AND REPOSITIONING TO REDUCE PRESSURE

Measures to reduce pressure include turning and repositioning.

- Goals for repositioning and a turning schedule of at least every 2 hours should be established for each individual, with documentation required.
- Devices, such as pillows or foam, should be used to correctly position patients so that bony prominences are protected and not in direct contact with each other.
- Re-position patients carefully to avoid friction or shear.
- Assistive devices should be used if necessary to move patients.
- Use chairs of correct size and height and use pressure relieving devices for the seats.
- Limit chair time for those who are acutely ill to no more than 2 hours.
- Patients should be taught or reminded to redistribute weight every 15 minutes. A timer may be used to remind patients.
- Use the 30° lateral position rather than the 90° side-lying position.

POSITIONING STRATEGIES IN THE BED AND CHAIR

Passive repositioning should be performed on the patient in both the bed and the chair:

- **Bed**: When positioned on his or her side, the patient should be turned to a 30° laterally-inclined position rather than a 90° side-lying position, which puts pressure on the trochanter. Two people should use a turn sheet, draw sheet, and pillows to pull up in bed, turn, and position the patient. Pillows should be placed under the head, under the legs to keep heels off the bed, behind the back, and between the ankles and knees.
- **Chair**: Patients in chairs need repositioning hourly as well. The patient should be assisted to stand and sit down again. Small changes in seated patients include changing leg position from dependent to elevated. The body should be in proper alignment, using pillows or cushions if needed. Patients who are cognizant and able to shift position should be instructed to do so every 15 minutes while seated.

USE OF SUPPORT SURFACES TO PREVENT PRESSURE INJURIES

A support surface redistributes pressure to prevent pressure injuries and reduce shear and friction. There are various types of support surfaces for beds, examining tables, operating tables, and chairs. General use guidelines include:

- Pressure redistribution support surfaces should be used in beds, operating tables, and examining tables for at-risk individuals.
- Patients with multiple injuries or with stage II to stage IV injuries require support surfaces.
- Chairs should have gel or air support surfaces to redistribute pressure for chair bound patients, critically ill patients, and those who cannot move independently.
- Support surface material should provide at least an inch of support under areas to be protected when in use to prevent bottoming out. (Check by placing hand palm-up under overlay below the pressure point.)
- Static support surfaces are appropriate for patients who can change position without increasing pressure to an injury.
- Dynamic support surfaces are needed for those who need assistance to move or when static pressure devices provide less than an inch of support.

CATEGORIES OF SUPPORT SURFACES

There are five elements that are used to categorize support surfaces:

- **Pressure redistribution** may be preventive (≤32 mmHg, but not consistently) or therapeutic (≤32 mmHg, consistently). Preventive devices are used for those at risk or with stage I or II injuries. Therapeutic devices are used for those with stage III and IV pressure injuries.
- **Device forms** are varied and may supplement or replace existing equipment. Devices include chair cushions, mattress overlays, pressure-reducing mattresses, and specialty bed systems used in place of traditional hospital beds.
- **Active support surfaces** are powered, requiring attachment to an electrical motor for utilization, (dynamic) or non-powered (static).
- **Medium** may be different types of foam, water, gels, or air.
- **Medicare reimbursement group**:
  - Group 1: Used as a preventive measure and includes overlays and mattresses.
  - Group 2: Used as a therapeutic measure and includes non-powered and powered overlays and mattresses.
  - Group 3: Used as a therapeutic measure and includes air-fluidized beds.

Wound Care: Intervention and Treatment

93

FUNCTIONS OF SUPPORT SURFACES

Support surfaces are designed for a number of functions:

- **Pressure redistribution** occurs through *immersion* (spreading the pressure out) and *envelopment* (conforming to shape without increasing pressure). The aim is to reduce pressure on the skin to less than the capillary closing pressure (<32 mmHg), but lower pressures may be necessary for elderly patients. *Interface pressure measurement* is measurement of the pressure exerted between the body and the support surface. This measurement is currently used to evaluate the pressure redistribution efficiency of devices although it has not been demonstrated through research that this measurement can predict clinical performance. Thin, flexible sensors are placed under the support surface and the patient and computerized readings indicate if the support surface is adequate. A number of new measurement devices are now marketed that show colored-coded computerized pictures demonstrating different levels of pressure.
- **Temperature control** is important because temperature increases can lead to skin breakdown. Skin temperature relates to the specific heat of the material in the support surface. Specific heat (the ability to conduct heat) varies considerably from one type of material to another. Air has a low specific heat, and water has a high specific heat. Material with high specific heat may conduct heat away from the body, decreasing skin temperature.
- **Moisture control** prevents moisture damage to skin, but there are wide ranges of materials in use in support surfaces. Some materials, such as rubber or plastic, may increase perspiration and moisture, while some porous materials, such as some foams, may reduce perspiration.
- **Friction/shear control** is more difficult to achieve although some surface coverings, such as those with Gortex, are purposely slick to decrease friction. However, proper positioning, lifting, and repositioning still must be done.

REDISTRIBUTION MEDIA

WATER

Water in overlays or mattresses is a common redistribution medium. The water may flow between cells or may be in one large space. Weight floating on water is evenly distributed, so waterbeds provide good weight distribution, and they have good immersion qualities, so the patient's body sinks into the surface, which then molds to their body shape. While these devices are popular in the home, there are a number of disadvantages to their use in healthcare facilities:

- They require electricity and a heater to keep the correct temperature.
- Water is very heavy, so they are difficult to move and maneuver.
- Draining and filling is messy and time-consuming.
- They may leak if punctured or around connections.
- Water is pulled by gravity, so if the head of the bed is elevated, the water flows downward, leaving uneven distribution.
- Moving or repositioning patients on a water support surface can be difficult because of the constant movement of the water.

FOAM

Foam varies considerably according to density and indentation load definition (ILD). Foam can be closed-cell (resistant) or open cell (viscoelastic). The number of chemicals used in the manufacturing of polyurethane foam determines the weight and viscoelasticity. Higher densities have higher viscoelastic (molding) properties. Open-cell foam is temperature-sensitive, helping it to mold to the body as it reaches the patient's body temperature. The density number of foam indicates the weight per cubic foot. Firmness is determined by the ILD, which is the number of pounds of pressure needed to indent a 4-inch foam 25% of its thickness using an indentation of 50 square inches. (Body weight and pounds of pressure should not be confused.) Foam is relatively inexpensive and was one of the first support surfaces used. Overlays should be 3-4 inches thick with densities of 1.3-1.6, and ILD of about 30.

Foam also has some **disadvantages**:

- Increases skin temperature
- Has a short lifespan
- Loses fire-retardance if it gets wet

AIR

Non-powered (static) air redistribution devices are manufactured in various forms: cushions, pads, overlays, and mattresses. The **air-filled overlays** may have a single bladder or the multi-cells/cylinders, with multi-cell forms providing the most pressure redistribution. Most forms are reusable and are filled with pumps to levels prescribed by the manufacturer according to the size and weight of the individual. The air moves with the individual, and the degree of immersion determines the effectives of the device.

Powered (dynamic) alternating pressure overlays have cells or cylinders that are alternately inflated and deflated at prescribed intervals by way of a pump that is attached to the overlay. Air overlays must be checked frequently to ensure that there is adequate air filling. Disadvantages include susceptibility to shear when the bed is elevated and bottoming out. Air overlays are recommended only for those <250 pounds. The degree of temperature and moisture control depends on the covering.

Air-fluidized (high air loss) beds are special bed systems that have a high flow of air through silicon beads, originally designed for treatment of burn patients. As the air flows through the beads, it fluidizes them so that they move and provide support and redistribution of pressure in much the way water does. The beads are contained in a bathtub-like frame. The lower part of the body becomes immersed in the beads so that the person appears to be floating as the beads move about because of the air. The air-fluidized bed is most commonly used for patients with multiple pressure injuries, making positioning to avoid pressure on sores very difficult, or who have had surgery for myocutaneous flaps. These expensive beds provide a warm alkaline environment and a bactericidal effect. There is some indication that capillary perfusion may become occluded, resulting in pressure injuries, although existing injuries heal faster.

Low air loss beds, overlays, and cushions have porous surfaces that allow air that is pumped in the support surface to leak, so there is a continuous flow of air through the air pillows in the device. The air pressure in the pillows in the devices can be adjusted according to the individual needs. The low air loss bed systems provide better immersion than air overlays and the patient cannot bottom out if the device is properly maintained. The covers for the devices are usually made of nylon or polytetrafluoroethylene fabric, both of which minimize friction. Only linen coverings or special pads that are air-permeable should be used with low air loss devices so that the air can flow beneath the skin. Disadvantages are that the equipment is expensive and contraindicated for those with an unstable spine. The airflow in beds must be maintained properly or there is a danger of entrapment in the bed. Hypothermia sometimes occurs.

Wound Care: Intervention and Treatment

GELS

Gels, which consist of silicone elastomer, silicone, or polyvinyl chloride, are fluid emulsions used in the manufacture of numerous devices, such as chair cushions and other types of flotation pads, such as overlays for beds, operating tables, and exam tables. There are also gel mattress replacements. Gel flotation pads usually have covers that can be disinfected so they can be used by multiple patients, a factor in their versatility. They are relatively inexpensive and require no electricity. Gels provide protection against shear and have good immersion properties, molding well to the body shape and providing good pressure redistribution. There are, however, some **disadvantages**:

- They are heavy.
- The gel filling may break up over time, leading to uneven distribution.
- They are difficult to repair.
- They may increase body temperature.
- They are not suitable for moisture control.

OFF-LOADING

Off-loading is relief of pressure on an ulcerated area of the foot while walking. Meticulous effective wound care plus off-loading promotes rapid healing of foot ulcers or other pressure injuries. Any material used must be able to be compressed to half of its thickness to be effective. Pressure testing of the standing foot or insoles that conform to the patient's foot is used to identify areas needing off-loading. Temperature testing reveals areas with increased temperature indicating tissue trauma:

- Specialized inserts may be used inside a shoe, tailored to relieve pressure in areas as needed.
- Special shoes are designed for some patients to relieve pressure.
- Crepe soles may provide relief.
- The heel of a shoe may be modified to compensate for limited toe motion, a varus deformity, or a decreased arch.
- A wide shoe that allows 0.5-0.75 in above the toes is needed for neuropathic feet.
- Cast shoes, wedged shoes, healing sandals, and half shoes are all alternative shoes that may provide the proper off-loading for the patient's needs.

TOTAL CONTACT CASTS

Total contact casts (TCCs) are the most successful way to off-load a foot ulcer/pressure injury to promote healing. A TCC is like a fracture cast but differs in that more padding is used and the toes are covered. The cast is applied by a skilled person and molded closely to the foot and leg below the knee. This prevents any movement of the foot or leg within the cast. An ambulation platform is added to the cast to force the patient to off-load the injury while walking. The cast is confining, hot, and must be kept dry during bathing. It is very effective in healing wounds when combined with good wound care. It is changed every 1-2 weeks or more often for wound care or when edema is present.

INDICATIONS AND CONTRAINDICATIONS

Total contact casts (TCCs) are indicated for uninfected, debrided ulcers on the bottom of the foot when associated with neuropathy. TCC also is used to treat Charcot neuroarthropathy by reducing the stress of weight bearing.

TCC must not be used if infection or arterial insufficiency is present. Wounds with necrotic material can hide an abscess or osteomyelitis, so ulcers must undergo total debriding prior to TCC application. Open exposure of tendons, bones, or joint capsules is a contraindication to the use of a TCC. The skin must be free of active problems, and the patient must be free of allergies to cast materials. A TCC is contraindicated for obese patients or those who can't tolerate total enclosure of the foot and lower leg. It should not be used for those who are blind or who have an unsteady gait.

REMOVABLE CAST WALKER TO OFF-LOAD A FOOT ULCER/PRESSURE INJURY

A removable cast walker is a good alternative to a total contact cast (TCC) for the patient who can't tolerate the TCC or when it is contraindicated. It is easy to apply and removable for hygiene and more frequent wound care. It can be used to control edema in combination with compression therapy. There are several available for use that can be modified for the patient's particular needs. They are often made of plastic with foam inserts and padding and are secured with Velcro straps. Patient compliance is important when a removable cast-walking boot is used. An expensive custom-built ankle foot orthotic is sometimes used for difficult foot pathology. It consists of a molded polypropylene shell and acts as a splint. Another method is to mold a TCC and then cut a hinged opening to make it removable. It is then customized to off-load pressure. A cast shoe is placed over this splint for ambulation.

WALKING AIDES USED BY PATIENTS WITH FOOT ULCERS

Patients with an unsteady gait and the elderly may need to have a walking aid when they use special shoes, a TCC and cast shoe, or an orthotic splint to heal an ulcer. Walking aides should be chosen with individual needs in mind. They must be customized to the person's height:

- A conventional walker with or without wheels may suffice.
- A 2-, 3-, or 4-wheeled walker with brakes may be more useful. They are available for use by both hands or just one hand. Some have seats so people can rest, but people must be cautioned to keep the walker braked when they are sitting.
- Quad canes are safer to use than a single-leg cane.
- Crutches may be suitable for younger patients with good upper body strength, but they must be fitted properly.

CONSIDERATIONS WHEN PATIENT NEEDS WHEELCHAIR DUE TO FOOT ULCERS

The patient who needs to be totally non-weight bearing may need a wheelchair to allow mobility instead of being confined to bed with the attendant problems caused by immobility. The chair should be fitted by measuring the patient's seat depth, seat width, seat-to-foot support height, seat to top of sacrum for lumbar support, and height of backrest. The height of armrests must also be determined. Seat back height may need to be increased to accommodate special seat padding to reduce pressure on the ischial tuberosities. The leg rests may need to be elevated so they must be of the proper height and length and padded. The patient may need upper body strength training and must have training for proper wheelchair mobility and safe transfers into and out of the wheelchair.

Wound Care: Intervention and Treatment

Wound Preparation

CLOSURE OF DEAD SPACE

Dead space is the defect of soft tissue left behind after debridement or excision of a space-occupying lesion. Dead space may also occur if portions of the wound separate beneath the skin after primary closure, leaving an open pocket if air/fluid becomes trapped between tissue layers. Closure of the dead space is essential because it promotes healing and decreases the risk of infection. Treatment options vary depending on the location, extent of the dead space, and the cause, but may include application of a compression bandage (using care not to apply excessive pressure that may impair oxygenation), insertion of a drain (open or closed, active or passive), and/or aspiration of fluid contents (seroma) of the dead space. Negative pressure wound therapy may be utilized for large wounds. Dead spaces open to the surface should be completely filled with suitable wound packing material (depending on the extent of drainage) but should be lightly packed so as to avoid pressure on healthy tissue. Patients may need to restrict activity during treatment for dead space.

WOUND EDGE OPTIMIZATION

Chronic wounds may take weeks or months to heal, so wound edge optimization is essential to healing. If the wound edges are not advancing or there are indications of undermining or deterioration, this may indicate that the wound cells are nonresponsive and that there are abnormalities of protease activities. Wound optimization methods include careful wound assessment and adequate debridement of the wound to remove necrotic tissue through sharp excision or enzymatic debridement, such as with collagenase, which debrides and promotes epithelialization. Maintaining appropriate moisture balance is also important as excessive moisture may cause maceration and deterioration of the wound, while inadequate moisture may result in desiccation of the wound and slowed epithelialization. The choice of dressing, therefore, may affect the healing process. If infection occurs appropriate antimicrobials (systemic or topical) may be necessary. In some cases, bioengineered skin or skin grafts may be appropriate. Additionally, edema slows healing, increases the risk of bacterial colonization, and must be controlled, such as through compression therapy. Wound exudate should be controlled because exudate, especially with chronic wounds, depresses cell proliferation (fibroblasts, keratinocytes).

MAINTAINING A WARM AND MOIST WOUND ENVIRONMENT

One of the basic principles of current wound care is the use of occlusive dressings that keep the wound warm and moist. There are a number of reasons for keeping a healing wound warm and moist:

- **Reduction in dehydration** allows cells such as neutrophils and fibroblasts to carry out their functions in wound repair, as they require a moist environment. This also results in less cell death.
- **Angiogenesis** requires a moist environment and low oxygen tension, which is found in occlusive dressings.
- **Autolytic debridement** with proteolytic enzymes is enhanced in a moist environment.
- **Re-epithelization** of tissue occurs because the epidermal cells are able to spread across the surface of the wound.
- **Reduction in microorganisms, facilitated by the seal provided by occlusive dressings, decreases infection.**
- **Pain reduction** results from the protection of the nerve endings and the need for fewer dressing changes.

PERIWOUND SKIN PROTECTION

The area extending about 4 cm from the wound edges is the periwound tissue, and it is especially vulnerable to irritation from drainage and adhesive. The periwound tissue should be evaluated for increased warmth and erythema as well as signs of maceration from exposure to exudate. Moisture-associated and adhesive associated skin damage can be prevented and treated by gentle cleansing of the periwound tissue with NS or water and application of a skin barrier. Moisture-retentive dressings help to keep the wound surface moist while avoiding excessive wetness and can wick fluid away from the periwound tissue. Dressing changes should be minimized to prevent stripping of periwound skin. Barriers may include:

- **Alcohol-based skin sealants**: Provide a sticky surface to help adhesives adhere and provide some skin protection. Available in wipes and spray.
- **Creams/Ointments**: May contain petrolatum, zinc oxide, or dimethicone and are applied in a thin layer to the skin and covered with absorptive dressings or applied in the perineal area to prevent skin irritation from incontinence.
- **Topical corticosteroids**: Used for allergic reactions, such as to adhesives.

Wound Care: Intervention and Treatment

Wound Cleansing

WOUND CLEANSING WITH EACH DRESSING CHANGE

Microorganisms, contaminants, and cellular debris in a wound can significantly delay healing and increase inflammation. Antiseptics such as hydrogen peroxide, acetic acid, povidone-iodine, or sodium hypochlorite (Dakin solution) are toxic to developing fibroblasts and interfere with healing over time. They are sometimes used and rinsed with saline for a short period of time to control heavily infected wounds. The current standard is to use irrigation to deliver normal saline in a manner forceful enough to break the adhesion of debris to the wound bed yet gentle enough to prevent injury to developing cells. Pressures of at least 5-15 psi delivered by mechanical irrigators are needed for effective cleansing. Higher pressures can cause penetration of the fluid into tissues. Irrigation using a 12 mL syringe and a 22 G needle will deliver a force of 13 psi. The use of a 35 mL syringe and a 19 G needle will deliver 8 psi and is more effective than using a bulb syringe when mechanical irrigation is not available.

CLEANSING A WOUND BY SOAKING

Soaking is a beneficial way to cleanse a wound that has a large amount of necrotic debris or contamination. Contamination must be removed from new wounds to avoid excess inflammation that will delay wound healing. Soaking softens any necrotic tissue and helps to ease it away from the healthy tissue at the bottom of the wound bed. It also helps to loosen contaminants that are embedded in the wound. Antiseptic agents should not be used in the soaking solution. Soaking may be accomplished using any container that will hold the wound area, or by whirlpool. The container must be disinfected well prior to and after the soaking. It may take several soaks to remove tough, dry eschar, and once the necrotic material has been removed, soaking should be discontinued, as it will then delay healing.

IRRIGATING A WOUND FOR CLEANSING PURPOSES

When **irrigating a wound** for cleansing purposes, the area beneath the wound should be covered to prevent contamination of the bed linens:

1. Place a basin beneath the wound to catch the returned solution.
2. Wash hands and wear gloves.
3. Use pulsatile lavage or a syringe to deliver water or saline with a force of 5-15 psi to the wound bed. Using pressure >15 psi forcefully injects irrigating fluid into newly formed tissues and risks inoculating microorganisms into deeper tissues. Highly contaminated or infected wounds may require pressure at the higher range of 15 psi to cleanse. Use low pressure (5-8 psi) to cleanse healthy wounds so new capillaries are not damaged.
4. Flush undermined, tunneled areas well, and then massage over the area of tunneling or undermining to dislodge debris and encourage the fluid to return.
5. Repeat as needed until the return fluid is free of debris.
6. Finish by packing these areas as ordered.

CLEANSING A SHALLOW WOUND BY SCRUBBING

Scrubbing is sometimes combined with a cleansing solution to initially cleanse a wound to remove debris. It is best performed using a very porous, soft sponge and a nonionic surfactant cleansing solution to avoid damaging the wound bed as much as possible. Even so, damage to the wound bed is often unavoidable, so scrubbing may be done initially to a traumatic wound, but the practice should not be continued after the wound is clean and beginning to heal because it can disrupt the development of granulation tissue and damage areas of epithelialization. When scrubbing, one should begin cleansing in the center of the wound and work in a circle toward the edges of the wound, avoiding recleansing an area to prevent recontamination of the center of the wound.

PULSED LAVAGE

Pulsed lavage (pulsatile high-pressure lavage) is irrigation of an infected or necrotic wound under pressure, using an electrically powered device. Normal saline is commonly used for lavage treatments, with the amount varying according to the size and amount of exudate on the wound. It is recommended that the pressure be 8-15 psi. The pressure can be varied as needed. While there is concern that higher pressure may inoculate tissue with bacteria, studies have not indicated this. Exposed blood vessels, graft sites, and muscle tissue should be avoided with the lavage treatments, and treatments should be discontinued if bleeding occurs with patients taking anticoagulants. Treatment is usually done 1-2 times daily. Both the hose and irrigating nozzle are intended for one-time use, so treatments can be expensive.

WOUNDS REQUIRING PULSED LAVAGE

Pulsatile lavage can be used on almost any type of wound but is particularly indicated for the following:

- Clean wounds to encourage granulation and healing
- Wounds with delayed healing to encourage granulation and stimulate epithelialization
- Severely contaminated or infected wounds to reduce microorganisms in the wound bed
- Pre-graft wound preparation to remove any contamination, foreign material, or necrosis and provide an optimal graft surface
- Diabetic neuropathic ulcers to treat without damaging callus or fragile areas
- Sacral wounds to allow easy access and comfort (as opposed to sitting in whirlpool)
- Wounds with undermining and tunneling to effectively irrigate (using smaller, flexible irrigation wands)

Patients who have cardiac monitoring, urinary catheters, IV lines, or other invasive monitoring avoid compromise to these areas when they have bedside irrigation of wounds. Febrile patients do not experience core warming as they do in whirlpools.

PRECAUTIONS

Aerosolization of microorganisms is possible during the use of pulsatile lavage with suction to cleanse wounds. The patient should wear a facemask, and all areas of the body, except for the wound, should be covered. The cleansing should be done in a ventilated private room with cupboards, drawers, and doors closed with no one else present. Waterproof mattresses or pads without surface tears should be used. Unnecessary equipment in the room should be stowed during irrigation since all exposed areas of the room must be disinfected after irrigation is done. Wheelchairs or transport stretchers should be removed from the room. The person performing pulsatile lavage should have full personal protective gear on, including hair and shoe coverings, face shields, mask, gown, and gloves. Suctioned fluids should be emptied into a toilet or designated commode. Disposable equipment should be disposed of as hazardous waste. Suction canisters should be disposable or sterilized after use if made of glass. Bed linens and towels used during lavage should be double bagged and laundered.

HYDROTHERAPY

Hydrotherapy, often in the form of whirlpool treatments to a limb or the whole body, is used to cleanse and debride wounds that are large with significant necrosis. Hydrotherapy is frequently used to treat burn injuries. Water is used at a temperature of 37 °C. Antiseptics are sometimes added to the water but can interfere with healing. Hydrotherapy has been implicated in a number of outbreaks of wound infections caused by cross-contamination; so many facilities have discontinued the use of whirlpools. Additionally, they are contraindicated for venous ulcers because vasodilation can increase edema. Diabetic patients may be insensitive to temperature, so therapy must be used cautiously. Wounds related to arterial insufficiency may not benefit. Whirlpool treatments do not appear to reduce surface bacteria of wounds, but rinsing the tissue after the treatment does. Equipment must be thoroughly disinfected between patients to prevent spread of infection.

PATIENT SAFETY MEASURES DURING WHIRLPOOL TREATMENTS

Whirlpools are used to cleanse wounds with a large amount of contamination or necrotic tissue. Small whirlpools are best for extremity wounds so the entire body does not need to be immersed. Water used in whirlpools should first be tested for the presence of microorganisms. If antiseptics are used in the water, the patient should wear a mask to avoid allergic reactions to aerosolized antiseptic or pneumonia from water vapor droplets. Additional **patient safety measures** include:

- Transfer the patient into and out of the whirlpool cautiously if a large whirlpool is used.
- Monitor vital signs before, during, and after whirlpool treatments and observe for fainting, dizziness, or altered mental status.
- Position the patient away from the jets to avoid damage to the wound or other tissues from the high pressure.
- Adjust or discontinue agitation if tissues are fragile.
- Rinse all body surfaces and the wound after whirlpool to remove antiseptics, contamination, and cellular debris. This is best done by a vigorous warm water rinsing or by showering.

PERIWOUND CLEANSING

The stratum corneum of the **periwound skin** is not as stable as normal skin. Periwound skin has more skin debris, such as water-insoluble proteins, amino acids, urea, ammonia, microorganisms, and cholesterol, than other tissue. Microorganisms up to 10 cm away from the wound edge can be more numerous and differ from those found in the wound bed, so cleansing prevents wound contamination. The microorganism level increases when the amount of protein on the periwound surface is increased. This area must be cleansed along with the wound when dressing changes are done. Cleansing reduces bacterial counts within and around the wound for about 24 hours. Normal saline may not remove these substances adequately. A skin cleanser that is mild and will not harm skin or strip away intercellular lipids may be used on the periwound area.

Compression Therapy

INDICATIONS FOR COMPRESSION THERAPY

When edema is present, wounds are unable to receive adequate nutrients, immune defenses are decreased, and epithelialization is poor or nonexistent. Compression therapy is used to control edema when there are lymphatic or venous insufficiencies. Compression must be used consistently to improve these conditions. It increases venous return by compressing superficial venous capillaries and forcing the blood into deeper veins for transport back to the heart. This minimizes venous hypertension and superficial capillary leakage. Arterial studies must be performed prior to compression therapy to ensure an adequate arterial blood supply. Pulses are assessed and Doppler studies are performed if pulses are weak. The Doppler ankle arterial pressure is divided by the Doppler brachial arterial pressure to determine the Ankle/Brachial Index to assess peripheral arterial disease. Baseline measurements are done prior to beginning therapy to establish the circumference of the extremity at several points. Serial measurements then demonstrate the effectiveness of the compression therapy. Ambulation and exercise are combined with compression to maximize the removal of edema.

STATIC COMPRESSION THERAPY

Static compression therapy is applying external graduated pressure to a lower extremity, from the ankle to the knee, to support the calf muscle and increase venous flow. Compression therapy is not curative, but is used as a preventive and therapeutic treatment to eliminate edema. It is contraindicated in those with heart failure or peripheral arterial disease as it may further impair compromised arterial circulation. Compression should not be used if the ankle brachial index (ABI) is <0.5. There are many different types of static compression products, and they should be chosen according to individual needs. They are graded according to the level of compression:

- **High level** provides therapeutic compression at 30-40 mmHg at the ankle. Some may provide pressure at 40-50 mmHg. ABI should be >0.8.
- **Low level** provides modified pressure up to 23 mmHg at the ankle. ABI must be >0.5 to <0.8. While this level is less than therapeutic, some authorities believe that even low levels of pressure provide some therapeutic benefit.

Wound Care: Intervention and Treatment

ELASTIC

There are many products and different types of elastic static compression therapy:

- **Layered wraps** (Profore, ProGuide, and Dynapress) combine both elastic and non-elastic layers in 2-4 layers with the inner layers providing protection to bony prominences and absorbing drainage. Different products require different wrapping methods, spiral or figure-8. The skin is usually lubricated to prevent drying. These are used for both ambulatory and non-ambulatory patients. The dressing must be applied by a professional and changed 1-2 times weekly. Layered wraps are frequently used for early treatments. Some wraps have visual pressure indicators.
- **Single-layer wraps** (SurePress) are long reusable elastic wraps that are used for early treatment or maintenance and can be used by both ambulatory and non-ambulatory patients. Competent caregivers can be taught to apply these dressings, especially those with visual pressure indicators. Because they are reusable, they are more cost effective than single-use dressings.
- **Therapeutic compression stockings** (Jobst, Juzo, Sig-Varis, Medi-Strumpf, Therapress Duo) are used to prevent ulceration in those with varicose veins and stable venous insufficiency after edema is controlled or with existing ulcers when edema recedes. They are contraindicated with lipodermatosclerosis because of the difficulty fitting the stocking. They may be used for both ambulatory and non-ambulatory patients who are able to apply the stockings. The stockings come in many sizes and colors and may extend from the foot to the knee or the groin. The stockings must be fitted properly and have the correct level of compression:
  - **Class 1**: 20-30 mmHg (varicose veins)
  - **Class 2**: 30-40 mmHg (venous ulcers and prevention)
  - **Class 3**: 40-50 mmHg (refractory venous ulcers & lymphedema)
  - **Class 4**: 50-60 mmHg (lymphedema)

APPLYING 4-LAYER PRESSURE BANDAGES

The following is the technique for applying a 4-layer pressure bandage:

- Wounds present on the limb are dressed and padded. The limb is then covered with stockinet. Foam padding is applied to bony prominences over the stockinette.
- The first elastic bandage is applied from the base of the toes or fingers up the limb, overlapping the previous turn by 50%, in a clockwise fashion.
- The next layer of elastic bandage is applied over top of the first, with the same 50% overlap, but in a counterclockwise fashion.

The application of the two elastic bandages in the opposite direction to each other ensures smooth even pressure up the limb. Care is taken with both layers not to exert pressure over the bony prominences to minimize damage to the delicate thin layer of skin in these areas. Short or long stretch bandages are used, depending on the amount of exercise and resting pressure desired.

Mometrix

NON-ELASTIC

There are many products and different types of non-elastic static compression therapy:

- **Unna's boot** (ViscoPaste) is a gauze wrap impregnated with zinc oxide, glycerin, or gelatin to provide a supporting compression "boot" to provide support to the calf muscle pump during ambulation, so they are not suitable for non-ambulatory patients. They can be used for those with peripheral arterial disease. The bandage must be applied carefully without tension. It may be left open to dry or covered with an elastic or self-adherent wrap. The dressings are changed according to the individual needs, determined by a decrease in edema, the amount of exudate, and hygiene with dressing changes ranging from 2 times weekly to every other week.
- **Short-stretch wrap** (Comprilan) is reusable and indicated for ambulatory patients and those with borderline ABIs (0.5-0.8). It is used for both initial and maintenance therapy. Caregivers can be taught to apply, but dressings slip out of place easily.

SHORT STRETCH AND LONG STRETCH BANDAGES

Differences between short and long stretch bandages:

- Short stretch bandages have less elasticity than long stretch. They stretch to 90% of their length whereas long stretch bandages stretch to about 140% of their length.
- Short stretch bandaging exerts more pressure on the limb during ambulation or exercise and low pressure when the limb is at rest. Long stretch bandages exert a higher pressure than short stretch. Since they stretch more, there is less pressure on the limb during exercise than with short stretch. There is more pressure on the limb when at rest, however. This makes it more likely that the long stretch bandage will exert too much pressure during rest, reducing perfusion to tissues and increasing the risk of tissue ischemia.
- Both short and long stretch bandages are applied by exerting tension on the bandage. The amount of tension determines the amount of pressure of the wrapped bandage. Bandaging should never cause numbness or tingling of the distal extremity and circulation, motion, and sensation (CMS) should be frequently monitored while bandages are worn.

NON-ELASTIC ORTHOTICS

Non-elastic orthotics, such as The CircAid Thera-Boot, are stockings with multiple Velcro straps that can be adjusted to fit each patient. The straps make adjusting easy for patients or caregivers. The ankle-foot wrap is attached to cover the foot and ankle but is thin enough to fit into a standard shoe. The orthotic provides continuous compression as well as supporting the calf muscle pump function. The orthotic comes in three sizes (small, medium, and large) according to ankle and calf measurement. It is washable, reusable, and can adjust to changes in limb size, so it is more cost-effective than some other devices. Also, it can be adjusted as needed during activities. The CircAid Thera-Boot was designed specifically for treatment of venous ulcers, but should not be used until edema has subsided. It can be used initially for treatment as well as for maintenance.

INTERMITTENT PNEUMATIC COMPRESSION THERAPY

Intermittent pneumatic compression (IPC) therapy is indicated if static compression therapy is ineffective or if the patient is immobile. (Medicare reimbursement requires a six-month trial of static compression therapy.) IPC devices are used on the lower leg or plantar area of the foot. IPC devices have a garment and a pneumatic pump that inflates the garment. The device for the leg typically has a double-lined stocking that fits over the leg. One lining contains an air bladder with segments so that the intermittent inflations occur segmentally up the leg, increasing venous return. The foot pump takes advantage of the physiologic pumping function in the sole of the foot to stimulate blood flow. The Circulator Boot is an end-diastolic IPC that is timed to the end of diastole to improve arterial flow while improving venous return. Treatments are usually 1-2 times daily for 1-2 hours and decrease edema and promote healing of ulcers. IPC therapy is contraindicated for those with uncompensated heart failure and for those with an active thrombus.

Dressings

BASIC DRESSING REQUIREMENTS

The **basic dressing requirements**, regardless of the type, are the following:

- Maintain a moist environment in order to promote healing.
- Absorb wound drainage and prevent leakage.
- Increase wound temperature to promote healing.
- Provide a protective barrier to prevent mechanical injury to the wound.
- Provide a protective barrier to prevent colonization and infection with microorganisms.
- Allow exchange of gases and fluids.
- Retain and absorb odor of the wound or drainage.
- Remove easily without causing additional trauma to the wound or disrupting the healing process.
- Debride wound of dead tissue and exudate.
- Provide protection without toxicity or causing sensitivity reactions.
- Provide a sterile protective covering for the wound.

The dressing that directly covers the wound may be inadequate to absorb large amounts of drainage, so sometimes additional secondary dressings are needed.

WOUND DRESSING SELECTION

The proper **dressing** for a wound may change over time depending on wound characteristics:

- The wound environment's moisture content may call for a dressing that either wicks away too much moisture or provides moisture to a dry wound to enhance epithelialization.
- Slough and dry eschar calls for a dressing that will enhance debriding.
- The presence of tunneling or undermining will require a packing material.
- Some wounds need dressings that are absorbent and deodorizing to control exudate.
- Control and prevention of infection is important in some wounds.
- Dressings must allow oxygen, water, and carbon dioxide to be exchanged between the environment and the wound.
- Dressings need to provide warmth as well.
- Dressings must not adhere to or harm the wound tissues but must be kept in place reliably without harming the skin around the wound.

CATEGORIES OF DRESSINGS AND METHODS OF SECURING DRESSINGS

Dressings are considered primary if they are next to the wound surface and secondary if they are used to cover the primary or to secure the dressing. There are **three main types of dressings** to consider when determining which will be the most effective for a particular type of wound:

- **Traditional topical dressings** are used primarily to cover the wound, such as gauze and tulle.
- **Interactive dressings**, such as polymeric films, are generally transparent so that the wound can be observed and are permeable to water vapor and oxygen but provide an effective barrier for microorganisms, such as hyaluronic acid, hydrogel, and foam dressings.
- **Bioactive dressings** provide substances that directly promote wound healing, such as hydrocolloids, alginates, collagens, and chitosan.

Securing a dressing depends on the health of the surrounding skin and the type of dressing. Skin protection and tape may be appropriate. Some are self-adherent. Tubular dressings or wraps can help to secure dressings with fragile skin.

GAUZE DRESSINGS

Gauze dressings are made from cotton, rayon, or polyester, and are frequently used with primary closure where there is little or no exudate. The purpose of these dressings is to provide protection of the partial or full-thickness wounds or those with cavities or tracts. They may be sterile or non-sterile. In the past they were used for wet to dry dressings. Wet-to-dry dressings have little use in current wound care unless the wound is very small because the gauze adheres to the wound and can disrupt granulation or epithelization. Wet to moist saline gauze dressings are sometimes used to treat wounds but are less effective than hydrocolloid dressings. Gauze dressings may be used as secondary dressings with another type of dressing in direct contact with the wound or as packing to fill dead space in combination with amorphous hydrogel or other dressings. When used to fill space, the gauze should be fluffed to avoid causing excess pressure.

TULLE OR IMPREGNATED GAUZE DRESSINGS

Tulle dressings, also known as paraffin gauze, (Jelonet, Paranet) are open weave gauze that are coated with paraffin so they do not adhere to the wound. They are suitable only for flat or shallow wounds. They may be useful for people with sensitive skin. When these are placed in contact with the wound, secondary dressings may be used to absorb exudate.

Impregnated gauze may contain antimicrobials, medications, nutrients, and moisture (such as normal saline). Commonly used gauzes are impregnated with petrolatum, zinc oxide, and iodoform. They are used for partial or full-thickness wounds or those with cavities, tracts, or infection. The choice of gauze depends upon the needs of the wound. They should be loosely packed into cavities and avoid contact with intact skin as they may cause maceration because of the moisture content of the dressing. Exudate should be carefully monitored so dressings can be changed as needed.

FOAM DRESSINGS

Foam dressings are made of semi-permeable hydrophilic foam, and sheet forms may have an impermeable barrier. They come in a wide variety of sizes and shapes (wafers, rolls, pillows, films) depending upon the manufacturer. Some types have a charcoal layer to control odor. Foam dressings provide a warm, moist environment and provide cushioning. Foam dressings may be used for partial and full-thickness wounds. Non-sheet forms are used as packing and are appropriate for minimal to heavy exudate. When used as packing, a secondary non-occlusive dressing is secured over the foam. They are used for leg ulcers as well as pressure injuries. Because they are intended for wounds with exudate in order to provide the appropriate environment for healing, they are not suitable for dry epithelializing wounds or those with eschar. Sheet forms can be used as secondary dressings with alginates, pastes, or powders. Some have adhesive borders. Foam dressings are changed every 2-7 days, depending on the dressing type and the wound.

SEMI-PERMEABLE FILM DRESSINGS

Semi-permeable film (OpSite, Tegaderm, Polyskin II) dressings are composed of polyurethane with a coating of acrylic adhesive so the dressing will adhere to the skin. These types of dressings are frequently used over intravenous sites to allow observation of tissue. They are suitable only for shallow partial-thickness wounds that have little or no exudate because they are not able to absorb; therefore, they are not suitable for infected wounds. They are permeable to air and water vapor but provide a barrier to pathogenic agents and liquid. The tissue under the dressing is maintained in a warm moist environment, encouraging autolysis. The dressings are comfortable and may be left in place for up to 1 week although some people may develop local irritation from the adhesive. Semi-permeable film may be used as a protective dressing and is often used for stage I and II pressure injuries.

Wound Care: Intervention and Treatment

ALGINATES OR OTHER FIBER GELLING DRESSINGS

Alginates (AlgiSite M, Sorbsan, Aquacel, Hydrofiber) are very absorbent dressings made from brown seaweed. Through ion exchange, they absorb drainage and form a hydrophilic gel that conforms to the size and shape of the wound. They are useful for full-thickness wounds with moderate to heavy exudate or slough, such as pressure injuries and cavity wounds, especially if there is undermining or tunneling. They are effective for infected and foul-smelling wounds. Alginates are sold in sheet form or fibers for packing. Alginate dressings or packing fibers are loosely packed into the wound to allow for swelling and then secured with a secondary dressing. They are usually changed once daily. Alginates serve to cushion and protect the wound as well as contain exudate. They are easier to remove than gauze dressings used for packing and cause less discomfort. Alginates need differing times to gel with some requiring 24 hours, so they are not interchangeable.

HYDROCOLLOID DRESSINGS

Hydrocolloids (DuoDerm, Restore, Tegasorb) are sheets or wafers of absorbent adherent material with an occlusive coating so that they provide a barrier to moisture. They are used for clean granulating wounds that are partial and full thickness with minimal to moderate amounts of drainage. They may be used with pastes or alginates. Hydrocolloids come in various sizes and shapes and can be cut to fit, overlapping the wound by 2-3 cm. They are usually changed about every 2-5 days. Hydrocolloid material may be stiff and should be warmed between the hands to soften before application. Some hydrocolloids emit an unpleasant odor when active. Because the dressings are occlusive, infected wounds should be observed carefully for signs of infection with anaerobic bacteria. They may be used with compression for venous ulcers but are not recommended for third degree burns. Hydrocolloids may cause hypergranulation tissue to form.

HYDROGEL DRESSINGS

Hydrogel dressings (AquaForm, Curasol, Hypergel, Elastogel, Vigilon, Intrasite gel) are produced in amorphous form, supplied in tubes, or impregnated in packing strip materials. They are also produced in sheet form, with or without an adhesive border. They have a high moisture content with water or glycerin with hydrophilic sites allowing them to absorb exudate and provide a warm, moist wound environment. Hydrogels are used for partial and full-thickness wounds, dry to small amounts of exudate, necrotic wounds, and infected wounds. They are applied directly to the wound and provide rehydration and autolysis, effectively and quickly debriding the wound. They are usually used with a secondary dressing, such as gauze or films. Dressings may be changed every 1-3 days, depending upon the type of product used. Hydrogels are contraindicated for wounds with heavy exudate, as the leakage may cause maceration of periwound tissue or candidiasis.

CONTACT LAYER DRESSINGS

Contact layers (Dermanet, Mepitel, Tegapore) are composed of woven polyamide net and may be coated with silicone (Mepitel). They adhere lightly to the wound but have pores that allow exudate to pass through to absorbent secondary dressings. They are particularly useful in wounds in which adherence of dressings to the tissue may pose problems, such as with abrasions, second degree burns, grafts, full-thickness granular wounds, and skin damaged by radiotherapy or steroids. They may be used with negative pressure wound therapy. They protect the wound base but are not recommended for shallow or dry wounds. Usually, the contact layer stays in place for up to a week while the secondary absorbent dressings are changed more often. If exudate is extremely viscous, it may not penetrate the net and can build up beneath the contact layer. Some types of contact layers may need to be kept moistened with normal saline so they don't adhere to the wound base.

COMPOSITE DRESSINGS

Composites are combination dressings that are frequently used to secure primary dressings or with other dressings, such as alginates. The material in composites varies from one dressing to another, but usually consists of some type of impermeable exterior barrier to prevent leakage of exudate, an absorptive layer (*not* alginate, foam, hydrocolloid, or hydrogel), a semi-adherent or non-adherent surface for covering the wound, and an adhesive rim to secure the dressing to the periwound tissue. Used alone, they are most suitable for partial or shallow full-thickness wounds but used with other dressings they are suitable for larger wounds with minimal to large amounts of exudate. A paper backing must be removed prior to application. They are usually changed about 3 times a week or more often if needed for wounds with larger amount of exudate.

ABSORPTIVE DRESSINGS AND WOUND FILLERS

Absorptive dressings (Surgipad, Tendersorb, ABD pad, Exu-dry) are composed of cellulose, cotton, or rayon fibers. Some have adhesive borders. They are highly absorptive and are intended for wounds that have moderate to heavy drainage. They are changed every 1-2 days.

Wound fillers (Biafine WDE, DuoDerm Sterile Hydroactive Paste, Multidex Maltodextrin Wound Dressing) are composed of starch copolymers in numerous different forms, such as pastes, granules, beads, gels, and powders. They fill dead space in shallow wounds, hydrate, provide a warm, moist environment, and absorb exudate. They soften necrotic tissue and aid debridement. Wound fillers are indicated for partial and shallow full-thickness wounds with minimal to moderate exudate and can be used for both infected wounds and uninfected wounds. They are used with secondary dressings, such as films and hydrocolloids. Wound fillers are not recommended for use in dry, eschar-covered, or tunneled wounds. Dressings are usually changed daily.

WOUND POUCHES

Wound pouches (Convatec Wound Manager, Hollister Wound Manager) are adapted from ostomy appliances and work in a similar way to contain heavy exudate from fistulas, wounds, drains, and tubes. The pouches provide a skin barrier to protect the skin and a drainage spout so that the pouch can be attached to straight drainage and a bedside bag. The pouch provides odor control as well. The opening in the pouch is cut to fit around the wound and paste, such as Stomahesive, is applied about the cut opening to ensure seal. The skin is usually wiped with a skin barrier prior to application, and any skin crevices are filled with paste. Forceps are used to feed drains or tubes through the opening of the pouch. Pouches are usually changed about every 4-7 days or when there is leakage or drainage under appliance.

Wound Care: Intervention and Treatment

Wound Debridement

AUTOLYTIC DEBRIDEMENT

Autolysis takes advantage of the body's enzymes and white blood cells to debride the wound by using proteolytic, fibrinolytic, and collagenolytic enzymes to soften and liquefy slough and eschar. Autolysis takes place in a warm, moist environment with adequate vasculature to provide white blood cells and neutrophils, so the neutrophil count must be adequate (>500 mm³) or sepsis can occur. Autolysis is most successful in stage III or IV uninfected wounds and when exudate is light to moderate so that occlusive dressings can be maintained. Autolysis does not damage the periwound tissue, and it is an easy method of debridement, causing very little discomfort. However, it is slower than some methods, taking 72-96 hours before effects are demonstrated. Autolysis may be combined with other types of debridement, using autolysis first to soften and loosen eschar. Autolysis requires close monitoring of the wound, which may appear to enlarge as the eschar dissolves, showing the true dimensions of the wound.

PROCEDURES AND SELECTION OF AGENTS

Autolytic debridement requires a warm, moist, atmosphere, so occlusive or semi-occlusive dressings must be applied to the wound area. All moisture-retentive dressings promote autolysis to some degree, even when other methods of debridement are used, but as a sole means of debridement, it is recommended only for relatively small, uninfected wounds. The dressings most commonly used for autolytic debridement include:

- **Hydrocolloids** provide absorbency for wounds with small amounts of exudate, but may promote anaerobic infections if the dressing is occlusive.
- **Alginate dressings** provide added absorbency for wounds with large amounts of exudate, but require a secondary dressing to secure them.
- **Hydrogels** are particularly helpful when wounds are dry because they add necessary moisture and promote rapid autolysis.
- **Transparent films** promote autolysis for very small, shallow wounds or when used as a secondary dressing.

As the wound debrides, odor and drainage increase, so periwound tissue must be protected from exudate.

ENZYMATIC DEBRIDEMENT

Enzymatic debridement is a method of chemical debridement that can be used on any type of wound that has a large amount of necrosis and eschar, especially chronic wounds and burns. Enzymes either directly digest the fibrin, bacteria, leukocytes, and other cell debris that comprises slough or dissolves the collagen that secures it to the wound. Enzymes need a moist environment, so if enzymes are used to debride dry eschar, the eschar must be crosshatched through the upper layers with a scalpel to allow the enzymes to penetrate the eschar. Enzymes are selective and do not damage viable tissue although some people have local irritation from the enzymes, particularly if the enzyme contains papain. Enzymatic debridement is relatively fast-acting but can still take days to weeks to complete debridement, especially with large wounds, so it is slower than some other techniques.

PROCEDURES AND SELECTION OF AGENTS

Enzymatic debridement uses chemical enzymes. Enzymes can be used with any type of dressing, but the enzymes need to be applied to necrotic tissue 1-2 times daily, so long-term dressings are not cost-effective. Moisture-retentive dressings speed debridement. Two types of enzyme preparations are used:

- **Collagenase** (Santyl), derived from *Clostridium* bacteria, digests denatured collagen and is administered once daily by tongue blade into deep wounds or applied to gauze for shallow wounds. It is inactivated by low pH (optimum range is 6-8) hexachlorophene and heavy metal ions, including mercury, zinc, silver, and Burow's solution.
- **Papain/urea** combinations (Accuzyme, Panafil White, Panafil, Gladase), derived from papaya, with or without chlorophyllin copper complex sodium, which reduces inflammation and odor. This enzyme digests nonviable protein composing the necrotic tissue. It is applied 1-2 times daily and is inactivated by hydrogen peroxide and salts of heavy metals, including lead, silver, and mercury. It works at a pH of 3-12.

BIOLOGICAL DEBRIDEMENT WITH MAGGOTS

Maggot debridement is inexpensive, faster than other non-surgical therapies, and effective, but it is usually saved for cases not responding well to other therapy. Sterilized maggots (blowfly larvae) secrete proteolytic enzymes, including collagenase, which debrides the wound, as well as growth factors and cytokines, which increase healing. The teeth of the maggots penetrate the eschar, aiding the enzymes. While the FDA has approved Medical Maggots only for debridement, numerous reports indicate that they also are effective against wound infections, such as MRSA. Antibiotics are often given concurrently with infected wounds because maggots can pick up pathogens in the wound and spread them in the tissue and to the bloodstream. Maggots are effective for many wounds, including pressure and stasis ulcers and burns. Maggots cannot be used with hydrogels. Periwound tissue must be protected from exudate. Large numbers of maggots should not be used in areas where blood vessels are exposed or damaged to prevent bleeding. Those on anticoagulants must be observed for bleeding.

PROCEDURE

Medical Maggots are applied to the open wound. The periwound tissue must be protected. The procedure is as follows:

1. A wound pattern is transferred onto a hydrocolloid pad, the opening is cut, and then the pad applied to the skin with the wound exposed. The pattern is used to cut an opening in a semi-permeable film for an outer dressing.
2. Maggots are wiped from the container with a saline-dampened 2X2 gauze (about 5-10 maggots per cm^2 wound size). The gauze is loosely packed into the wound.
3. A porous mesh (Creature Comfort) is placed over the wound and secured to the hydrocolloid with tape or glue, creating a maggot cage.
4. Transparent film is placed over the hydrocolloid, making sure that the cutout area is over the cage so that the maggots have air and drainage can escape. Saline-dampened gauze is placed loosely over cage.
5. Dry gauze is used for the outer dressing and changed every 4-8 hours as needed.
6. Maggots are wiped from the wound after 48 hours, and the wound is irrigated with normal saline.

Wound Care: Intervention and Treatment

MECHANICAL DEBRIDEMENT
WET TO DRY

Wet-to-dry debridement is a common treatment in use for many years to debride wounds and absorb exudate, but it is non-selective in that it can pull healthy and granulating tissue from wounds as well. Treatment usually involves applying saline-moistened gauze to a wound and allowing it to dry for 4-6 hours and then pulling it off the wound. Using this approach to removing necrotic tissue can take days to weeks, depending upon the extent of the wound. It's important in wet-to-dry debridement that the dressings dry out completely, so the dressing should be moist but not saturated. One major drawback to wet-to-dry debridement is that it is quite painful, but wetting the gauze prior to removal to ease the pain decreases the effectiveness. This method requires frequent dressing changes and careful aseptic technique. Most experts in wound care no longer recommend wet-to-dry debridement or advise it only initially for heavily necrotic wounds.

SHARP DEBRIDEMENT

Sharp (instrumental) debridement involves the cutting away of necrotic tissue using forceps, scissors, and a scalpel. This is the most aggressive form of debridement that can be done by non-physician medical personnel, and regulations about doing this therapy vary from state to state. In some states, it is in the scope of practice for RNs while in other states it is within the scope of physical therapists' duties. Sharp debridement cleans the wound much faster than other non-surgical forms of debridement, promoting faster healing, and is selective as the person doing the debridement controls the type and amount of tissue that is removed. The procedure involves:

1. Using aseptic technique and sterile equipment.
2. Cleansing the site of debridement with an antiseptic.
3. Holding the tissue taut with forceps to establish a plane of dissection.
4. Dissecting carefully, avoiding vasculature.
5. Irrigating the wound with normal saline upon completion.

SURGICAL DEBRIDEMENT

Surgical debridement is instrumental dissection of necrotic tissue under general, spinal, or local anesthesia. It is most commonly used when very large amounts of tissue must be debrided, such as with extensive burns, or when there is a serious infection and immediate debridement is needed in order to effectively treat the wound infection. General anesthesia allows extensive debridement to be done without the patient suffering associated pain and trauma although postoperative pain is common. One advantage is that most debridement can be done in one procedure. Surgical debridement has been shown to stimulate healing in diabetic ulcers. However, there are risks associated with anesthesia and post-operative wound infections can occur. It is also much more costly than other methods. An alternative surgical method is **laser debridement**, which can cut away necrotic tissue. Pulsed laser beams are less damaging to adjacent tissue than continuous lasers.

CHEMICAL CAUTERIZATION

Chemical cauterization with silver nitrate is sometimes used to treat hypergranulation. Cauterization uses heat to burn or sear abnormal cells in order to destroy them. Silver nitrate sticks are wet with water to activate and are then gently rolled over the tissue to be treated for a short time. Chemical cauterization is used infrequently, for such things as treatment of nosebleeds and warts. The most common uses for chemical cauterization in wounds or skin lesions are to control hypergranulation tissue that grows in wounds, especially about stomas or to treat warts. Hypergranulation is excessive soft flaccid granulating tissue that is raised above the level of the periwound tissue, preventing proper epithelization, and it may reflect excess moisture in the wound. Hypergranulation tissue is often friable and bleeds easily. It may produce both exudates that interfere with healing and odor. Treatment may be repeated 2 times daily for 1-4 days until excess tissue sloughs.

Topical Agents

TOPICAL ANTIBIOTICS

Topical antibiotics may be used to treat localized wound infections based on results of culture and sensitivities so that the treatment is appropriate for the invading microorganism. Topical antibiotics include:

- **Cadexomer Iodine** (Iodosorb) is an iodine preparation formulated to be less toxic to granulating tissue. It can be applied as a powder, paste, or ointment. The ointment contains beads with iodine. The beads swell in contact with exudate, slowly releasing the iodine, which is affective against a broad range of bacteria, such as *Staphylococcus aureus, MRSA, Streptococcus, and Pseudomonas,* as well as viruses and fungi.
- **Gentamicin sulfate**, prepared as a cream or ointment, is a broad-spectrum antibiotic that is effective against both primary and secondary skin infections in stasis and other injuries or skin lesions. It is bactericidal against *Staphylococcus aureus, Streptococcus, and Pseudomonas,* but does not have antiviral or antifungal properties.
- **Metronidazole**, prepared as a gel or a wax-glycerin cream, is effective against MRSA infections.
- **Mupirocin 2%**, prepared in an ointment, is effective primarily against Gram-positive bacteria and is used primarily for *Staphylococcus, MRSA,* and *Streptococcus.* It is frequently used to treat nasal colonization of *Staphylococcus* because colonization is implicated in subsequent wound infections.
- **Polymyxin B sulfate-Bacitracin zinc-neomycin ointment** (Neosporin) is frequently used to prevent infections in small cuts and lacerations, but it can also be used in infected wounds and is active against *Staphylococcus aureus, Streptococcus and Pseudomonas.*
- **Polymyxin B sulfate-Gramicidin cream** is similar to that above except it is also effective against *MRSA.*
- **Silver sulfadiazine** (2-7%) is frequently used in burn treatment and has a strong antimicrobial action against *Staphylococcus aureus, MRSA, Streptococcus, and Pseudomonas.*
- **Silver (ionized)**, prepared in absorbent sheets and activated with sterile water, is effective against the same organisms as silver sulfadiazine. The moist environment increases re-epithelialization.

REGRANEX GEL TO STIMULATE WOUND HEALING

Regranex gel contains becaplermin, which is a recombinant human platelet-derived growth factor (Rh-PDGF). Regranex causes gathering and replication of cells to heal the wound and encourages granulation. Regranex gel is indicated for deep diabetic neuropathic ulcers, extending into or below subcutaneous tissue. It has not been studied for use with superficial diabetic ulcers or pressure injuries. The wound must have a good blood supply for the gel to be effective. The wound must also be debrided, infection must be controlled, pressure must be relieved, and the wound bed must stay moist for the best outcome. The wound should show improved healing within 10 weeks and be healed within 5 months. It should not be used if cancer is present at the site of the wound, sutures or staples are present, or if joints, ligaments, or tendons are exposed.

TOPICAL AGENTS FOR PERI-WOUND SKIN PROTECTION

MOISTURE BARRIER PASTE

Moisture barrier pastes are ointments with powder added to improve absorption and make them more durable and solid, providing a thick skin barrier. Many are zinc oxide based, making them somewhat difficult to remove. Mineral oil is often used to remove the paste. Some paste products now on the market are transparent so that the skin underneath can be monitored. Additionally, some pastes contain karaya or carboxymethyl cellulose to increase adherence to the tissue. Pastes are frequently used over denuded or excoriated tissue to absorb exudate and protect from drainage, urine, or feces, so they are used for both peri-anal and peri-wound tissues. While pastes are more resistant to drainage than ointments and adhere better to denuded skin, they do interfere with adhesion of dressings, and zinc oxide cannot be used with some wound care treatments. Pastes are usually reapplied with each dressing change without being completely removed first. Some **barrier pastes** include:

- Critic-Aid Skin Paste
- Ilex Skin Protectant Paste
- Remedy Calazime Protectant Paste

MOISTURE BARRIER OINTMENT

Moisture barrier ointments provide protection for the skin from moisture, exudate, urine, and feces with petrolatum or zinc oxide based-products packaged in tubes or small individual packets. These products, because of their greasy nature, can interfere with adhesion of the wound dressings, and some wound care products cannot be used with zinc oxide, so they have limited application. This type of barrier is frequently used with patients who are incontinent to prevent incontinence dermatitis, which can deteriorate into pressure injuries. Barrier ointments are usually reapplied with each dressing or adult brief change, so overall costs may be higher than with barrier films that can be applied less frequently. Some products contain karaya or carboxymethyl cellulose (hydrophilics) to improve adherence to the skin. Some **barrier ointment products** include:

- Calmoseptine Ointment
- Lantiseptic Skin Protectant
- Proshield Plus Skin Protectant
- Critic-Aid Clear Hydrophilic Ointment

SKIN SEALANTS

While a warm, moist environment is optimum for wound healing, the exudate poses a risk to adjacent tissue, which must be protected or it will macerate, potentially ulcerating and increasing the size of the wound. Various topical agents are used to protect peri-wound skin, including skin sealants, which are film-forming barriers composed of a polymer in a fast-drying solvent, applied every 1-4 days, depending on the product. When the sealant is applied to the skin, the solvent (often isopropyl alcohol) dissolves, leaving the transparent plasticized polymer barrier over the tissue. It may be applied to intact or irritated tissue although there may be some discomfort from the alcohol solvent with broken skin. Sealants can be used to protect skin from exudate, urine, stool, chemicals, and adhesive stripping. Sealants are applied with wipes, wands, or sprays. Some **sealant products** include:

- Skin Prep
- Shield Skin
- Bard Protective Barrier Film Wipe
- Allkare Convatec
- Cavilon No Sting Barrier Film (does not use alcohol)

SKIN BARRIER POWDERS

Skin barrier powders are used as an initial barrier on denuded skin to provide an adherent base for ointments, pastes, or solid skin adhesive barriers. The powder is sprinkled over the denuded area, and excess is removed before application of the second barrier. Powders should be applied thinly because excess will impair adhesion of other barrier products, and they should not be used on intact skin, as they will not properly adhere. Skin barrier powders contain powder pectin, karaya, gelatine, carboxymethyl cellulose or combinations. They are frequently used with ostomy products when the skin has become weepy. Warm moist areas are ideal for fungus growth, which causes burning and itching, so the addition of antifungal powder may be necessary as well to promote healing. Use of the skin barrier powders should be discontinued as soon as the skin heals. **Skin barrier powders** include:

- Stomahesive Protective Powder
- Karaya Powder
- Premium Powder

SOLID SKIN BARRIERS

Solid skin barriers are solid waterproof moldable adhesive skin barriers, usually in the form of rings, strips, or wafers that provide skin protection for moisture, exudate, urine, or feces. They may contain hydrocolloids, pectin, karaya, gelatine, carboxymethyl cellulose or combinations. They are frequently used with urostomies and ileostomies as a base to anchor appliances and protect the skin from discharge. They may be cut to fit snugly around wounds. While they are frequently left in place for days at a time, it is possible for drainage to leak under the barrier, so they must be checked. Some swell when in contact with discharge and have acidic pH to discourage growth of organisms. Solid skin barriers are more durable than ointments or pastes, but they must be removed carefully to prevent stripping of the skin, especially if they are applied in an area that receives pressure, such as the coccyx. **Solid skin barriers** include:

- Hollister Flextend
- Stomahesive
- Eakin
- Premium Skin Barrier

Wound Care: Intervention and Treatment

Skin Transfer and Surgical Closure

SKIN SUBSTITUTES

Tissue engineered skin and skin substitutes have been developed in spite of tremendous difficulties in the creation of non-contaminated cell cultures and the transport of these cells to operating rooms when they are needed. They are applied after the wound has been debrided:

- **Apligraf** is made of a bovine collagen mesh with living neonatal fibroblasts from neonatal foreskin. When applied, it looks like a mesh, and then it changes to a gel after about 7 days. It is a "living skin equivalent" that provides growth factors to the wound to stimulate healing. Apligraf is transported on media in a petri dish and must be kept warm until it is used. It is placed over a wound free from necrotic material and infection before a compression dressing is applied.
- **Dermagraft** is a cryopreserved skin substitute that also uses neonatal fibroblasts from neonatal foreskin but without the bovine material. It is used for diabetic foot ulcers.

SKIN FLAPS

A skin flap may be used to repair a wound that has a poor vascular supply. A section of skin is cut, leaving one end of the flap attached to its original site. The flap is then brought forward or twisted on its axis to reach the wound site. Some flaps are sutured to more distant sites, such as the arm to the face. The free end of the flap is sutured into the wound. When this end of the flap grows into the wound and new blood vessels are generated to support it, the other end of the flap is cut away from the donor site. The donor site is sutured or grafted. Sometimes the skin is stretched by the placement or injection of tissue expanders prior to raising the flap to increase the amount of skin available.

SKIN GRAFTS

Skin grafts speed healing and reduce fluid loss from burns and wounds. They enhance the wound cosmetically. Grafts may be taken from the patient's body (autograft), or from a cadaver (allograft). Skin substitutes (Apligraf or Dermagraft) or animal tissue, such as from a pig (xenograft), may also be used. Xenografts last 3-5 days before rejection and are used for partial wound healing and protection prior to permanent grafting with an autograft or allograft. Skin grafts may be partial or split thickness (epidermis and part of dermal layer) or full thickness (epidermis and entire dermis):

- **Partial thickness grafts** may not regain sebaceous or sweat glands, causing the area to be dry and to be warmer than the rest of the body. Hair follicles and nerves may regenerate in grafted areas.
- **Full thickness grafts** rely on neovascularization to stay vital and to grow into the defect. They provide the most natural appearance but can be used only in small areas, unlike a split thickness graft.

STAPLES

Staples may be used to close superficial wounds of the scalp, neck, axillae, extremities, trunk, or external genitalia. The procedure is as follows:

1. Position the patient so that the wound is easily accessed.
2. Irrigate the wound with NS, using a 10-mL syringe with an 18-gauge needle.
3. Wipe the skin in a 7-8 cm diameter area about the wound with an antiseptic.
4. Apply gloves and administer local anesthetic, typically 1% or 2% lidocaine.
5. Bring the skin edges together and place the stapling device over the edges, holding it perpendicular to the skin and depressing the lever.
6. Continue placing staples about every quarter inch.
7. Apply topical antibiotic ointment and dressing.

Staples should be removed within 7-10 days for staples in the limbs, hands, feet, and trunk, in 3-5 days for the face/neck, and 5-7 days for the ear or scalp as prolonged staple closure may result in scarring and increased risk of infection.

SUTURES

Sutures are used for superficial wounds of the scalp, face, nose, lips, mucous membranes, neck, axillae, trunk, extremities, and external genitalia, for superficial dehiscence, and for intermediate repairs with layer closures. The healthcare provider should determine the appropriate needle, suture material, and suturing technique. Procedure:

1. Position patient so that the wound is easily accessed.
2. Apply povidone-iodine with swab from wound edges outward to a circle of at least 4 cm beyond the wound on all sides.
3. Apply gloves and administer local anesthetic (usually lidocaine 1% or 2% with or without epinephrine).
4. Irrigate the wound with normal saline (60-100 mL NS), trim ragged edges with sterile scissors, undermine the edges if necessary to assure approximation.
5. Hold needle holder with suture in dominant hand and toothed forceps in the other to grasp the edges of the wound, and begin suturing with sutures about 0.5 cm from the wound edge.
6. Cleanse the suture line with NS and apply dry dressing.
7. Advise the patient of the length of time the sutures must remain in place.

Prior to suture removal, if the sutures are crusted, cleanse with a cotton-tipped applicator and hydrogen peroxide, remove hydrogen peroxide with applicator saturated with NS, and then dry with gauze.

Wound Care: Intervention and Treatment

117

SURGICAL/VASCULAR INTERVENTIONS FOR ARTERIAL INSUFFICIENCY/ULCERS

The goals of management for arterial insufficiency and ulcers are to improve perfusion and save the limb, but lifestyle changes and medications may be insufficient. There are a number of indications for surgical intervention:

- Poor healing prognosis includes those with ABI <0.5 because their perfusion is severely compromised.
- Failure to respond to conservative treatment (medications and lifestyle changes) even with an ABI >0.5.
- Intolerable pain, such as with severe intermittent claudication, which is incapacitating and limits the patient's ability to work or carry out activities. Rest pain is an indication that medical treatment is insufficient.
- Limb-threatening condition, such as severe ischemia with increasing pain at rest, infection, and/or gangrene. Infection can cause a wound to deteriorate rapidly.
- Surgical intervention is indicated only for those patients with patent distal vessels as demonstrated by radiologic imaging procedures.

SURGICAL/VASCULAR INTERVENTIONS FOR SEVERE ARTERIAL INSUFFICIENCY

Surgical/vascular interventions for treatment of severe arterial insufficiency include 3 different types of procedures:

- **Bypass grafts** in which a section of the saphenous vein or an upper extremity vein are harvested to use to bypass damaged arteries and supply blood to distal vessels. Because veins have valves, they must be reversed or stripped of valves prior to attachment. Synthetic grafts are also sometimes used, but they have a much higher failure rate.
- **Angioplasty** can be used if disease is not extensive (>10 in length), but arteries must be large enough to accommodate the procedure safely. Initial results are good but long-term rates have been less positive although the use of anticoagulants improves success rates.
- **Amputation** is the procedure that treatment tries to avoid, but it is sometimes required if ischemia is irreversible or if there is severe necrosis and infection that is life threatening.

Additional Wound Therapy Options

NEGATIVE PRESSURE WOUND THERAPY

Negative pressure wound therapy (NPWT) uses subatmospheric (negative) pressure with a suction unit and a semi-occlusive vapor-permeable dressing. The suction reduces periwound and interstitial edema, decompressing vessels and improving circulation. It also stimulates production of new cells and decreases colonization of bacteria. NPWT also increases the rate of granulation and re-epithelialization so that wounds heal more quickly. The wound must be debrided of necrotic tissue prior to treatment. NPWT is used for a variety of difficult to heal wounds, especially those that show less than 30% healing in 4 weeks of post-debridement treatment or those with excessive exudate, including the following:

- Chronic stage II and IV pressure injuries
- Skin flaps
- Diabetic ulcers
- Acute wounds
- Burns, both partial and full-thickness
- Unresponsive arterial and venous ulcers
- Surgical wounds and those with dehiscence

It is **contraindicated** in the below conditions:

- Wound malignancy
- Untreated osteomyelitis
- Exposed blood vessels or organs
- Nonenteric, unexplored fistulas

APPLICATION

Application of negative pressure wound therapy is done after the wound is determined to be appropriate for this treatment and debridement is completed, leaving the wound tissue exposed. There are a number of different electrical suction NPWT systems, such as the VAC (vacuum-assisted closure) system and the Versatile Implant (VI). Application steps include:

1. Apply nonadherent porous foam cut to fit, and completely cover the wound.
   a. **Polyurethane** (hydrophobic, repelling moisture) is used for all wounds EXCEPT those that are painful or have tunneling or sinus tracts, deep trauma wounds, and wounds needing controlled growth of granulation.
   b. **Polyvinyl** (hydrophilic), is used for all wounds EXCEPT deep wounds with moderate granulation or flaps and deep pressure injuries.
2. Secure foam occlusive transparent film.
3. Cut opening to accommodate the drainage tube in the dressing and attach drainage tube.
4. Attach tube to suction canister, creating closed system.
5. Set pressure to 75-125, as indicated.
6. Change dressings 2-3 times weekly.

Wound Care: Intervention and Treatment

Hyperbaric Oxygen Treatments

Hyperbaric oxygen therapy (HBOT) is treatment in a high-pressure chamber while breathing 100% oxygen, which increases available oxygen to tissues by 10-20 times. Blood that is saturated increases perfusion of the tissues. HBOT has shown considerable promise in reducing the need for amputation resulting from ulcerations of the lower extremities, but it is critical that treatment be instituted early enough while the potential for salvage remains. HBOT is used for a number of conditions, but is especially important for hypoxic wounds, such as those associated with peripheral arterial insufficiency, compromised skin from grafts, and diabetic ulcers. Treatment protocols vary according to the type of wound, but are limited to 90 minutes to avoid oxygen toxicity. HBOT has the following effects:

- Hyperoxygenation of blood and tissue
- Vasoconstriction, reducing capillary leakage
- Angiogenesis because of increased fibroblasts and collagen
- Increased antibiotic effectiveness for those needing active transport across cell walls (fluoroquinolone, amphotericin B, aminoglycosides)

Hyperbaric oxygen therapy (HBOT) supplies oxygen at pressures of 2-3 times that of the atmosphere. The patient is treated in a multi-person or single person chamber. This therapy is delivered by specially trained physicians since oxygen toxicity side effects are possible. Transcutaneous oximetry levels should reach >200 mmHg for HBOT to be effective. One or two hours of HBOT results in a higher amount of dissolved oxygen in the blood, and it remains for a prolonged period of time. HBOT is used for pressure injuries, burns, gas gangrene, radiation burns, skin grafts and flaps, vascular ulcers, osteomyelitis, and crush injuries.

Biophysical Technologies

Ultraviolet Light

Ultraviolet light B (UVB) can be used to induce inflammation, stimulate granulation, and decompose necrotic tissue. However, Ultraviolet light C (UVC) is the type most often used for wound healing, primarily for its bacteriocidal action, as it is effective against MRSA and other antibiotic-resistant bacteria (destroying 100%) and reduces overall bioburden in infected wounds. Most equipment comes with distance guides that help to ensure proper positioning in relation to the wound:

- Provide eye protection to the patient and the operator to prevent damage to the retina.
- Provide protection to periwound skin by applying petrolatum jelly.
- Position the light the proper distance (one inch) from the wound.
- Provide treatment according to manufacturer's guidelines.

UV light therapy is contraindicated if the patient has sensitive skin, or is taking medications that cause photosensitization such as tetracyclines, sulfonamides, quinolones, amiodarone, quinidine, phenothiazines, psoralens, and others.

Electrical Stimulation

Electrical stimulation (ES) is used to promote healing of a wound, as it stimulates proliferation of epidermal cells and activity of fibroblasts, which produce collagen. ES is most often provided by high voltage pulsed current (HVPC). It uses short pulses of current followed by longer pauses, which stimulates fibroblasts and growth factors. Tissue perfusion is improved with increased blood flow and development of new capillaries, and edema is decreased. ES promotes phagocytosis and has a bacteriocidal effect. It helps to relieve diabetic neuropathic pain. Treatments last 45-60 minutes and are given 5-7 times a week. Precautions include avoiding placement of the electrodes near the heart or larynx. Wounds treated with silver products must be rinsed thoroughly to remove all traces of silver before electrical stimulation is applied.

WATER-FILTERED INFRARED-A THERAPY

Water-filtered infrared-A (wIRA) uses heat radiation to help acute and chronic wounds heal. The infrared halogen light is filtered with water to increase humidity and prevent it from heating only the skin surface, causing skin irritation. Water-filtered infrared-A therapy acts by increasing the temperature in the wound, thereby increasing oxygen partial pressure and perfusion and thus the energy supply to the tissues. This treatment can be particularly useful in large wounds in which the center of the wound is hypoxic and has a positive effect on the amount of pain caused by the wound. The wIRA radiator does not contact the skin, the therapy is easily performed, and it is pain-free for the patient. It can be used on wound seromas and pressure injuries with good effect.

PHARMACOLOGIC MEASURES TO MAXIMIZE PERFUSION

The primary focus of pharmacologic measures to maximize perfusion is to reduce the risk of thromboses:

- **Antiplatelet agents** such as aspirin, Ticlid, and Plavix interfere with the function of the plasma membrane, interfering with clotting. These agents are ineffective to treat clots but prevent clot formation.
- **Vasodilators** may divert blood from ischemic areas, but some may be indicated, such as Pietal, which dilates arteries, decreases clotting, and is used for control of intermittent claudication.
- **Antilipemics** such as Zocor and Questran, slow progression of atherosclerosis.
- **Hemorheologics**, such as Trental, reduce fibrinogen, reducing blood viscosity and rigidity of erythrocytes; however, clinical studies show limited benefit. It may be used for intermittent claudication.
- **Analgesics** may be necessary to improve quality of life. Opioids may be needed in some cases.
- **Thrombolytics** may be injected into a blocked artery under angiography to dissolve clots.
- **Anticoagulants**, such as Coumadin and Lovenox, prevent blood clots from forming.

> **Review Video: <u>Antiplatelets and Thrombolytics</u>**
> Visit mometrix.com/academy and enter code: 711284

GROWTH FACTOR TREATMENTS

Growth factors are proteins that are necessary for growth and migration of cells, and are thus critical elements in healing of wounds. Growth factors may be isolated from tumor cells, platelets, macrophages, ovarian follicles, and the placenta. Recombinant DNA techniques have allowed production of synthetic growth factor from bacterial cultures or human cells with the growth factor genes. Growth factors are applied topically to the wound. There are a number of different **types of growth factors** in use or study, including:

- **Connective Tissue Growth Factor (CTGF)** is being studied for use to combat fibrosis.
- **Epidermal Growth Factor (EGF)** is used for burns and venous ulcers.
- **Fibroblast Growth Factor (FGF)** is used for burns and pressure injuries.
- **Insulin-Like Growth Factor (IGF)** is being studied as a means to reduce HbA1c in diabetes.
- **Platelet-Derived Growth Factor (PDGF)** is used for pressure and diabetic ulcers.
- **Transforming Growth Factor-Beta (TGF-β)** is used with chronic skin ulcers.

Wound Care: Intervention and Treatment

LEECH THERAPY

Leech therapy, known medically as hirudotherapy, is the practice of using leeches at the site of wounds to induce vasodilation, minimize coagulation (through the secretion of hirudin in their saliva), and decrease inflammation, thereby promoting wound healing. By maintaining a localized anticoagulated state, blood flow is sustained to the wound, helping to repair the tissue and prevent necrosis. The leeches also drain excess blood, which controls inflammation, another inhibitory mechanism for wound healing. Before considering leech therapy for wound healing or management of chronic wounds, active infection must be controlled, and circulation to the wound must be demonstrated. Laboratory work for hematocrit and hemoglobin should be drawn to ensure appropriate blood volume, as blood loss may occur with leech therapy, depending on the duration of the treatment, the surface area of the wound, and the number of leeches used.

MIST THERAPY

Mist therapy is an adjunctive therapy for wound healing that is meant to be used in addition to more traditional measures such as cleaning/debriding and dressing changes. This therapy involves the application of a saline-based mist to the wound surface and periwound area that is administered using a low-frequence ultrasound device. This therapy is both non-invasive and painless, which minimizes associated risks. The saline acts to reduce bacteria on and around the wound while stimulating blood flow to the wound, a necessary element of the healing process. Over time, the saline can also act as a mild debriding agent by removing necrotic tissue that is within the wound bed or margins.

Patient Comfort

Wound Care Environment During Wound Treatment

The wound care environment is important, especially when wound treatment is painful. The room should be clean, quiet, non-stressful, comfortably warm, and appropriately lighted. Privacy must be insured, and there should be no interruptions:

1. Explain the procedure to the patient.
2. Consider the need for another person to hold the patient's hand during the procedure.
3. Enlist help to minimize the time needed for the treatment.
4. Uncover only the area of the body with the wound.
5. Do not expose the wound until all preparations have been made and treatment is ready to begin.
6. Treat the wound as gently as possible and as little as possible to minimize pain.
7. Allow time-outs as needed to keep the patient comfortable.
8. Allow space in which to perform the procedure so that the wound is not accidentally bumped.
9. Check with the patient frequently during the treatment and allow breaks as needed for repositioning or relief from pain or stress.

Patient Comfort During Wound Treatment

Wound treatments may be very uncomfortable for the patient, so proper **premedication with analgesics** is important:

- Work with the patient to schedule the treatment for an appropriate time.
- Help the patient to use the restroom prior to treatment.
- Position the patient so that all parts of the body are supported, allowing the patient to relax as much as possible. Comfort will allow the patient to maintain the position that allows optimal access to the wound for as long as is necessary.
- Take time to check that the patient is comfortable and without pain before beginning the procedure.
- Check to see that breathing is unimpaired if the patient is lying prone. Small adjustments in position are important.

Removing a Dressing

The proper method to remove a dressing is described below:

1. Wash hands and don gloves.
2. Place open bag near the wound so the old dressing can be placed directly into the bag without leaking onto the bed linens or nearby surfaces.
3. Open plastic bag and fold top down so that only the interior of the bag is exposed.
4. Remove adhesive dressing slowly. Rapid removal can tear the top layer from periwound skin and from the wound bed. Dressings that are adherent should be soaked until easy removal is obtained. The use of chemical adhesive removers can cause the remover to leak into the wound, causing pain and destruction of newly formed tissues.
5. Place the dressing into the bag, remove the gloves, and put them into the bag also. Never reuse top layers of a dressing.
6. Grasp the bag by the outside and tie a knot in it.
7. Place it into a biohazard waste container.
8. Wash hands and don clean gloves to continue working with the wound.

Wound Care: Intervention and Treatment

Pain Management

CONSIDERATIONS REGARDING PAIN CONTROL MEASURES

Good wound care must include the assessment and management of pain. Dressing changes, especially, are often very painful. There are a number of considerations:

- Pain assessment should be done regularly, allowing the patient to describe the type and extent of pain as well as the patient's response to analgesia in order to manage pain optimally.
- Poor perfusion and infection increase pain, so measures should aim at increasing circulation/oxygenation of the wound, assessing for signs of infection, and instituting treatment.
- Increasing fluid intake and providing proper nutrition improve wound condition and reduce pain.
- Pain medications should be given as needed and prior to dressing changes. With severe pain, such as burns, patient-controlled analgesia (PCA) devices help the patient feel more independent and relieve fear of pain. Medications to relieve anxiety may potentiate pain medications.
- Fungating cancerous lesions may require modifications in dressing routines to decrease dressing changes and periwound care to prevent painful maceration.

INTERVENTIONS FOR NON-CYCLIC, CYCLIC, AND PERSISTENT WOUND PAIN

Non-cyclic pain occurs in specific non-routine situations, such as with periodic wound debridement. The patient should be provided pain medication prior to the treatment, and other pain relief methods, such as topical anesthetics may be considered. Surgical or sharp debridement may be avoided or decreased by using hydrogel, hydrocolloids, enzymatic agents, hypertonic saline, or transparent dressings.

Cyclic pain is predictable pain that occurs in a regular cycle, such as with daily changing of dressings. Pain should be managed with regular pain medications, and other methods of reducing pain may include using dressings that are less painful (avoiding wet to dry), scheduling wound care when the patient is not fatigued, soaking dressing before removal, keeping the wound bed moist, limiting packing, relieving pressure, taking time outs during procedures, and providing comfortable positioning.

Persistent wound pain requires regularly-scheduled pain control as well as other pain-reducing methods, such as relaxation and electrical nerve stimulation (EMS). The area may be splinted to decrease pressure. Antibiotics may be used to reduce infection.

PHARMACOLOGIC TREATMENT OF WOUND PAIN

TOPICAL ANESTHETICS

There are numerous different types of pain medications that may be used to control pain from wounds, including **topical anesthetics**:

- **Lidocaine 2-4%** is frequently used during debridement or dressing changes. Lidocaine is useful only superficially and may take 15-30 minutes before it is effective.
- **Eutectic Mixture of Local Anesthetics (EMLA Cream)** provides good pain control. The wound is first cleansed, and then the cream is applied thickly (1/4 inch), extending about 1/2 inch past the wound to the peri-wound tissue. The wound is then covered with plastic wrap, which is secured and left in place for about 20 minutes. The wrapped time may be extended to 45-60 minutes if necessary to completely numb the tissue. The tissue should remain numb for about 1 hour after the plastic wrap is removed, allowing time for the wound to be cleansed, debrided, and/or redressed.

REGIONAL ANESTHESIA

Regional anesthesia (injectable subcutaneous and perineural medications) is administered locally about the wound or as nerve blocks. Medications include lidocaine, bupivacaine and tetracaine in solution. Epinephrine is sometimes added to increase vasoconstriction and reduce bleeding although it is avoided in distal areas of the limbs (hands and feet) to prevent ischemia.

- **Field blockade** involves injecting the anesthetic into the periwound tissue or into the wound margins. The effect may be decreased by inflammation. The effects last for limited periods of time.
- **Regional nerve blocks** may involve single injections, the effects of which are limited in duration but can provide pain relief for treatments. Techniques that use continuous catheter infusions are longer lasting and can be controlled more precisely. Blocks may involve nerves proximal to affected areas, such as peripheral nerve blocks, or large nerve blocks near the spinal cord, such as percutaneous lumbar sympathetic blocks (LSB). Long-term blocks may use alcohol-based medications to permanently inactivate the nerves.

SYSTEMIC MEDICATIONS

Systemic medications may be given orally or by injection into muscles, subcutaneous tissue, or veins. The 3-step World Health Organization (WHO) "Analgesic Ladder" is frequently used as a point of reference. Combinations of drugs are often more effective than one alone:

- **Step 1**: Mild to moderate pain is treated with a non-opioid such as aspirin, acetaminophen, and NSAIDs.
- **Step 2**: Moderate to severe pain unrelieved by Step 1 medications may need opioids, such as codeine, tramadol, or Percocet.
- **Step 3**: Severe pain without relief from Step 1 or Step 2 medications may need stronger opioids, such as morphine, Dilaudid, or MS-Contin.

Note: Meperidine (Demerol) should not be used for long-term pain control because prolonged use may result in dependence, high doses may cause seizures, and a metabolite of meperidine (normeperidine) may accumulate. It is short acting and peaks quickly. It may be indicated for occasional use for the treatment of acute pain, such as that associated with dressing changes.

PAIN MEDICATION FOR DIFFERENT TYPES OF WOUND PAIN

Pain medication should be given on a regular schedule, not PRN, for pain that is cyclic or persistent. It should be given 30 minutes prior to painful treatments or dressing changes and again afterwards for non-cyclic pain. The patient should rate the pain before and after pain medication, and dosages should be increased until relief is obtained, or another analgesic should be tried or added to the pain medication regime. Pain medication should be given on schedule even if the patient can sleep, since this does preclude severe pain.

- **Nociceptive pain**, both somatic and visceral, responds to non-opioids, such as acetaminophen or the NSAIDs, and opioid medications, such as acetaminophen with codeine, hydrocodone with acetaminophen or ibuprofen, propoxyphene, morphine, fentanyl, or oxycodone.
- **Neuropathic pain** can be relieved with the adjuvants, such as the tricyclic antidepressants amitriptyline, nortriptyline, or desipramine. Anticonvulsants such as gabapentin or pregabalin are also helpful. Topical and local anesthetics may also be administered. Anesthesia may be indicated for treatments causing severe pain.

125

NON-ANALGESIC PAIN CONTROL MEASURES

Non-analgesic pain control measures begin with good communication between the patient and the healthcare provider and an assessment of the causes of pain, which can then be targeted for pain reduction.

- **Cleansing of wound**: Use normal saline and gentle flushing of wound rather than cytotoxic agents, such as antiseptics, which may cause burning and discomfort.
- **Peri-wound care**: Use skin sealants to protect intact skin from maceration and skin barriers over denuded skin.
- **Wound debridement**: Use autolysis when possible.
- **Dressings**: Select dressings with the goal of reducing pain as well as healing the wound. Moisture-retentive dressings often decrease pain. Avoid wet-to-dry dressings. Decrease frequency of dressing changes if possible.
- **Inflammation**: Elevate limb if indicated and provide medications to control inflammation.
- **Edema**: Elevate limbs and use compression dressings and sequential compression pumps as indicated.
- **Positioning**: Use body supports to stabilize wounds when possible, use turning sheets, and try splinting or immobilizing a wound area.

Infection Control

MINIMIZING RISK OF INFECTION

WOUND CARE MEASURES

Procedures for wound care should prevent infection of the wound and should prevent the spread of infection to others. A clean "no-touch" method for dressing changes and wound care is currently recommended. Clean gloves (rather than sterile) are used, but dressings, gauze, swabs, or solutions that directly contact the open area of the wound should be sterile. Any container, such as a syringe or squeeze bottle, used to irrigate the wound should be sterile as well. Wounds should be kept clean and debrided. Antimicrobials should be used as indicated and wound cultures done. Standard precautions should be used with handwashing both before and after treatment of a wound, even with glove use, and before contact with other parts of the body. If any wound irrigation is done that involves fluid under pressure, staff should wear personal protective equipment (gloves, gown, mask, and eye shield) to protect them and other patients from contamination with infective material.

CLEANSING PROCEDURES AND SOLUTIONS

Cleansing methods should remove surface bacteria, but cleansing must be done carefully to prevent damage to tissue. Wounds should be cleansed at each dressing change. Exudate may be removed carefully with soft gauze or swabs by wiping from the center outward, using a new piece of gauze or swab for each wipe. The wound should then be irrigated to mechanically remove exudate or debris. Irrigation under pressure has been found to cleanse wounds effectively while reducing trauma and infection.

- Optimum pressure is 8-12 psi
- <4 psi is inadequate
- >15 psi can cause trauma or force bacteria into tissue

Low-pressure irrigation with a 250 mL squeeze bottle delivers 4.5 psi while a 60 mL piston irrigation syringe delivers 4.2 psi. High-pressure irrigation (8-12 psi) utilizing a 35-cc syringe with an 18- to 19-gauge angiocath provides good cleansing. Irrigation solution should be sterile normal saline instead of antimicrobial/antibacterial solutions, which are cytotoxic and may delay healing.

STERILE AND CLEAN TECHNIQUES FOR WOUND CARE

Sterile technique is most commonly used in acute care facilities for procedures that are invasive and pose the risk of infection or that involve sharp debridement of tissue. It is important for those who are immunocompromised, chronically ill (e.g., diabetic), elderly, or children. A sterile field is prepared and sterile equipment and dressings are used, with care to maintain principles of sterility.

Clean technique can save money in supplies and time and will not increase the rate of infected wounds when done properly. It is most commonly used in the home environment, physician's offices, and long-term care facilities for dressing changes that do not involve debridement and with patients who are not considered high risk. A clean field is prepared and clean gloves used. If equipment, such as forceps, is used, it must be sterile, but the usual sterile-only-touches-sterile rules do not apply. Dressings may be clean or sterile.

Wound Care: Intervention and Treatment

PRINCIPLES OF STERILITY

Principles of sterility help to determine what things and areas are sterile and what types of activities constitute contamination:

1. Sterile only touches sterile.
2. Sterile objects should not be wet (poly-lined fields may be wet with sterile fluids only).
3. The outer wrapping of sterile packages is considered contaminated.
4. There should be a one-inch border between sterile and non-sterile area.
5. Sterile drapes hanging over the side of the table are considered unsterile.
6. One should always face the sterile field.
7. Sterile fields must be above the waist as anything below the waist is considered contaminated.
8. All sterile items, including gloved hands, must be held in front of the person and above the waist.
9. Avoid reaching or passing supplies over the sterile field.
10. When pouring sterile solutions onto a container on the sterile field, the bottle should not touch the container and should not splash.
11. Coughing or talking over a sterile field can contaminate the field.

STERILE FIELD

Two persons can prepare a sterile field. A sterile drape is first placed upon a surface that has been disinfected and dried. The drape is handled only by the edges and is placed upon the surface without touching the surface with the sterile gloves. Any overhang is considered not sterile. One person assists by using clean hands to open packages. The other person scrubs the hands and dons sterile gloves. The assistant opens packages so that the sterile provider may reach in to get the contents without contaminating them. The contents are then placed on the sterile field away from the edges. Items that are not sterile, such as medication vials, are held by the assistant so that the sterile provider may insert a needle without touching the vial to evacuate the contents. One person can prepare the field by placing a sterile drape on the surface and by opening packages and carefully dumping the contents on the drape, rearranging them later while wearing sterile gloves.

ADEQUATE DISINFECTION OF EQUIPMENT USED IN WOUND TREATMENTS

Most cases of nosocomial infections caused by equipment are a result of failure to follow **disinfection guidelines** established by the manufacturer or the facility. Studies have shown that up to 87% of healthcare equipment that was tested had contamination by bacteria. The nature of a device guides the disinfection and cleaning. Devices that are used during invasive procedures require the highest level of disinfection and sterilization. Equipment must first be cleansed of gross contaminants using chemical and mechanical means, then disinfected and sterilized as required by guidelines. Equipment that includes moisture is especially prone to harboring harmful microorganisms. Channels that contain moisture must be rinsed and dried with 70% alcohol solution and forced air. If a patient wound is infected, one must use equipment that can be dedicated to that patient or is disposable if possible.

STANDARDS AND PRECAUTIONS FOR PERSONAL PROTECTIVE EQUIPMENT

The CDC provides standards for the use of protective equipment, based on diagnosis and condition:

- **Standard precautions** (for all patients) include protection from all blood and body fluids and include the use of gloves, face barriers, and gowns as needed to avoid being splashed with fluids.
- **Airborne precautions** require respiratory precautions (a mask) to be worn if the patient has suspected or confirmed tuberculosis.
- **Droplet precautions** (measles, influenza, etc.) require staff and visitors who are within 3 feet of the patient to wear masks.
- **Contact precautions** (for those with infections, such as *Staphylococcus aureus*) include using gloves as for standard precautions, but they should immediately be removed and hands sanitized after contact with infective material. A clean protective gown should be worn inside the room for close contact with the patient and any type of patient care.

HAND HYGIENE STANDARD PRECAUTIONS

According to hand hygiene standard precautions, hands should be washed with soap and water for at least 15 seconds to remove visible soiling whenever exposed to patient-related surfaces, directly before patient contact, and before and after wearing gloves. When hands do not have visible soiling, they may be disinfected with the use of an alcohol-based hand rub. These rubs are more effective than soap and water when all surfaces of the hands are in contact with the rub. If there is a chance of spore contamination, the hands should be washed with antimicrobial soap and water. Healthcare workers in contact with patients who are at high risk for infection should not wear jewelry, artificial fingernails, or extenders. When dressing or treating a wound, hands should be washed before touching other portions of the patient or anything in the room. Surgical scrubbing should include using antimicrobial soap and the scrubbing of the hands and forearms for at least 2 to 6 minutes. This should be followed by an alcohol-based scrub and drying before donning sterile gloves.

CONTACT PRECAUTIONS

Contact precautions are used for patients with infected wounds that may contaminate the environment because of the virulent nature of the microorganism, uncontained drainage, or inability to cooperate on the part of the patient. The patient is placed in a private room or with patients with the same microorganism if possible. Gloves should be worn whenever entering the room and gloves removed and hands washed when exiting the room. A gown must be worn whenever there is a chance of touching the patient or surfaces in the room and always if there is uncontained wound drainage. The patient should only leave the room if it is unavoidable. If transporting, one must ensure wounds are well covered. Equipment should be dedicated to the patient and not shared. The room, furnishings and equipment must be cleaned and disinfected as needed and when the patient is discharged according to facility policy. Waste is double-bagged and handled as hazardous waste according to policy.

Wound Care: Intervention and Treatment

Exam Room Preparation and Cleaning

EQUIPMENT AND SUPPLY SET UP FOR BASIC WOUND CARE PROCEDURES

All necessary equipment and supplies should be gathered and ready for use before carrying out a wound care procedure, and the patient should be positioned so that the wound is clearly visible and easily accessible by the healthcare provider. The **equipment and supply set up** for basic wound care procedures may vary depending upon the type of wound, but generally includes:

- Adequate lighting (overhead, lamp)
- Hazardous waste container in which to place contaminated dressings and supplies
- Bedside stand or table on which to place supplies
- Irrigating set up with NS to cleanse the wound
- Antiseptic to apply about the wound perimeter
- Both sterile and non-sterile gloves as well as appropriate PPE
- Water-resistant under pads to place under the site of the wound, especially important if irrigating the wound
- Dressing supplies, including sterile dressings, cleansing swabs, and sterile field with sterile forceps (if needed)
- Any medications that may be utilized, such as lidocaine or enzymes

CLEANING OF THE PATIENT ENVIRONMENT

The facility policies for the cleaning of patient care areas must follow CDC guidelines for preventing the transmission of infectious agents in healthcare settings. This affects patients with uncontained wound drainage or wound infections. These patients should be in a separate room whenever possible, depending on the microorganism involved. Equipment and furnishings in the room should be cleaned of soil on a daily basis and as needed with an EPA-registered disinfectant. This includes all surfaces touched by the patient, including beds, bedrails, over-bed tables, bedside tables, phone, call bell, TV controls, and bathroom surfaces. Cleaning equipment should be dedicated to use in that room if possible. Terminal disinfection procedures should be followed when the patient is discharged.

CLEANING OF ROOMS BETWEEN PATIENTS

Patients with wounds are at high risk of developing infections with multidrug-resistant organisms and developing infections from environmental transmission (especially if patients have wounds that are draining) because they are often diabetic, paralyzed, and/or debilitated. **Treatment rooms** should be thoroughly cleaned and disinfected between patients, including not only horizontal surfaces but also high-touch surfaces, such as doorknobs, TV controls, call lights, handles, and faucets. If blood or body fluids are evident, these should be removed with wet soapy water prior to disinfection. Reusable equipment used with the patient during treatment, such as blood pressure cuffs, should be cleaned and disinfected. When possible, disposable equipment or individualized equipment should be used to decrease chances of cross contamination. Healthcare providers should utilize standard precautions, including face shields if splashing may occur and should wear appropriate gowns and gloves to avoid contamination of their clothing. Wound care supply carts should be left outside of the treatment room.

CLEANING A WHIRLPOOL TANK

The American Physical Therapy Association (APTA) guide for whirlpool cleansing should be followed:

1. Full personal protective gear should be worn by the person doing the cleaning.
2. Detergent is first used to scrub the inside of tanks, pipes, drains, thermometers, and turbines and all are rinsed.
3. The tank is then filled with hot water with a disinfectant and left for at least 10 minutes, after which it is drained and rinsed.
4. The agitator is immersed in a separate container with disinfectant and hot water and allowed to run for 10 minutes.
5. All equipment is dried with clean towels and then covered.

Hydrotherapy equipment, Hoyer lifts, and transfer equipment must also be cleansed after use. All other equipment and surfaces in the room should be wiped with a germicidal solution due to possible aerosol contamination during the whirlpool.

LEVELS OF CLEANING AND DISINFECTION

The levels of cleaning and disinfection include:

1. **Decontamination**: Makes equipment safe to handle while cleaning, uses 0.5% chlorine solution to decrease microorganisms.
2. **Cleaning**: The removal of gross contamination by using soap and water and scrubbing.
3. **Low-level disinfection**: The removal of SOME microorganisms by using disinfectant.
4. **Intermediate-level disinfection**: The removal of MOST microorganisms by using disinfectant.
5. **High-level disinfection**: The removal of ALL microorganisms (except spores) by using disinfectants, steam, or boiling.
6. **Sterilization**: The removal of ALL microorganisms by using high-pressure steam autoclave, dry heat, radiation, or chemical sterilants.
7. **Reprocessing**: The process that consists of cleaning, high-level disinfection, and drying.

Wound Care: Intervention and Treatment

Wound Care: Care Planning

Psychosocial Issues

EFFECTS OF WOUNDS ON PATIENT'S PSYCHOLOGICAL RESPONSE

The cause of a wound may affect the patient's and the family's psychological response:

- Traumatic wounds can serve to remind the person of the event involved with its occurrence. Each dressing change, pain, and disability from a wound reminds the person of this disruption in his or her life. Some patients may cope by refusing to see the wound or to be involved in its care until they have progressed to a more accepting phase in their adjustment. Some may react by demanding attention to the wound by others even if the wound is progressing.
- Cancer wounds may cause fear, anxiety, and depression, reminding the person of the disease.
- Wounds sustained through the fault of the patient or from carelessness may be embarrassing or shame producing. Family members may blame the patient.
- Patients coping with a disease or disability, such as quadriplegia, may not have the emotional energy to cope with the reality of a wound as well and may be overwhelmed.

PSYCHOLOGICAL SUPPORT NEEDED BY PATIENTS AND FAMILIES WHEN DIAGNOSED WITH A WOUND

Both the patients and families are in need of psychological support when a patient is diagnosed with a wound. The care provider must recognize that after diagnosis, patients and families may go through stages of anger, denial, fear, and frustration and may be psychologically unable to cope with caring for a wound. Patients need positive support and understanding during this period, helping them to reach acceptance and encouraging them to participate in wound care one step at a time. Patients and their families may have many concerns that they are afraid to address, so the care provider must openly address common concerns, especially fear of pain, disability, and disfigurement. Patients who have a plan for pain control and have realistic explanations about disability feel less threatened. Disfigurement must be discussed, and a plan for treatment that minimizes negative results must be developed. Reassurance that the wound will heal encourages hope and positive expectations that the entire ordeal will end at some point in the future.

SOCIAL ISOLATION DUE TO WOUNDS

Physical mobility may be affected by the wound and by pain, contributing to social isolation by keeping a patient close to home. The need to rest or elevate the wound cuts down on ambulation. Treatments or dressing changes can take much time out of the day. If patients must travel to a clinic or office to have these treatments, then this takes time from their normal schedule and responsibilities. Patients may experience fatigue from poor sleep and side effects from medications such as antibiotics or pain medication, making them less likely to seek social contact. The fear of further injury to the wound can restrict the person's activities and the places that they are willing to go. The appearance of the wound, dressings, or the type of clothes or shoes that are necessary may also limit the person's desire to go out in public.

PSYCHOSOCIAL ISSUES CAUSED BY WOUNDS WITH ODOR AND DRAINAGE

Wounds with odor and excessive exudate may have a profound psychological impact on the patient, who often feels embarrassed and ashamed. Some may try to mask the odor with cologne or perfumes, but this often compounds the problem. The patient may become depressed and avoid social interaction, becoming increasingly isolated. Family and friends may indicate that they find the odor or drainage offensive. The patient often feels a loss of self-esteem. Intimacy is often avoided by the patient or his or her partner, making the person feel unwanted. Cancerous wounds may serve as a constant reminder of impending death. With heavily draining wounds, the need for bulky dressings impacts the type of clothing the patient can wear, making the person feel unattractive. Patients need reassurance that the odor or drainage can be contained and need instruction in methods to manage the wound, such as cleansing the wound properly, using charcoal or special wound deodorants, and applying dressings that contain the drainage between changes.

PSYCHOLOGICAL EFFECTS OF ACUTE OR TRAUMATIC WOUNDS

An acute or sudden traumatic wound suddenly puts a person who is healthy into the role of a patient. The wound gets all of the patient and family's attention. The patient's role and responsibilities are impacted and changed by the presence of the wound. The traumatic wound may cause emotions that were previously hidden to emerge, stressing the patient's coping mechanisms and causing emotional crisis. It is not until the wound heals that the patient resumes being the "normal" individual that he or she was prior to the wound. The care provider can help the patient to learn coping mechanisms and ways to resume normalcy prior to complete healing to ease the feeling of being a different person due to the presence of the wound.

PSYCHOLOGICAL EFFECTS OF CHRONIC WOUNDS

A wound that is present for years can cause a loss of hope, depression, and lack of compliance by the patient who has no reward when the wound fails to heal. Activities are focused around the wound and planned around any pain or disability caused by the wound, such as difficulty walking. Sleep can be altered and lack of energy can hamper ADLs over time. Patients may go through the grieving process. Each dressing change is accompanied by relief if it is improved or depression if it is not.

- Patients may choose to live with the wound and continue with normal life activities, modified to accommodate the wound.
- Others may stay in and wait for wound healing to occur to resume life as before.
- Patients may find comfort from comparing themselves to others with wounds or chronic illnesses.
- Some may feel well except for the wound, and be able to continue life while coping with the healing process.
- Some may accept the wound as a part of life and growing old.

IMPACT OF WOUNDS ON FEMALES VS. MALES

Gender issues related to wounds are a matter of ongoing research. Studies have shown that males with wounds tend to report more of an impact from pain and limitations in mobility than females. They also lose more sleep when a wound is present and tend to be socially isolated by a wound. They may feel emotionally challenged more than females who have wounds. Females feel less energetic and less able to cope physically. They are also affected socially when a wound is present. However, studies of diabetic ulcers indicate that female gender along with small ulcer size and lack of infection was predictive of better healing. Additionally, females tend to have lower incidence of ulcers, possibly because of smaller size resulting in less pressure on the foot and less severe neuropathy.

EFFECTS OF AGE ON PSYCHOLOGICAL REACTION TO WOUNDS

Studies have indicated that younger patients tend to be more negatively impacted by wounds than older people, who may have more effective coping abilities and can more easily adapt to physical restrictions. Younger people are more active and social, and any activity restriction causes more of a change in their lifestyle. Young patients may not have had as many previous experiences in coping with illness or disability as older patients, and their expectations are often different. The support network for young patients may be narrower than for older, who may, for example, have children to assist them. Younger people often have less job and financial security, which increases stress. However, the group is not always an accurate representation of the individual. Some young people cope well while some older people react negatively to wounds.

HELPING PATIENTS WITH DISFIGURING WOUNDS

Disfiguring wounds take a daily emotional toll on the patient. Family reactions to the wound can adjust over time, but social encounters can result in stares and reactions of pity, disgust, repulsion, and disdain from others, causing a loss of self-esteem and negative feelings about the wound. Some disfiguring wounds, such as post-mastectomy, may impact a person's sexuality and self-identity. The care provider can provide acceptance,

133

treat the wound in a matter-of-fact way without negative reactions, and suggest practical ways to camouflage or minimize the appearance of the wound. The care provider can discuss reconstructive options and differences that will occur with healing such as less discoloration and swelling, provide encouragement and positivity about the healing process, and inquire about the patient's general well-being and any other problems the patient may have. This emphasizes that the patient is a person with a wound, not a wound alone.

IMPACT OF A WOUND ON FAMILY CAREGIVERS

The burden of caring for a loved one with a wound is stressful. Much time is spent on wound care and helping the patient with ADLs. Other family members may feel slighted or burdened with more chores and responsibility. **Caregivers** are conflicted by feelings of wanting to help the patient and yet resenting the need to spend so much time doing so. They may react with anger or even abuse. A lengthy healing period stresses coping and the caregiver may need to have help at times to allow time away from the patient or to take care of other matters. The patient may feel helpless and a burden or may be demanding and depend on the caregiver for emotional and physical support. Caregivers who are older or have their own health problems can be stretched to the limit. Providers can offer the caregiver an outlet for emotions and concerns and help them to find ways to meet their own needs as well as the patient's during this trying time.

FINANCIAL IMPACT OF WOUNDS AND ULCERS

The wound or ulcer may make it difficult for people to continue their jobs due to pain or the need to rest the limb. This can affect compliance with the healing regime. Patients without savings, another wage earner in the family, or other resources may have to tap into equity in their homes or take out loans to meet **financial obligations**. Patients may lose their jobs or be forced to quit or take early retirement. Even with health insurance, patients may have out-of-pocket expenses, such as for dressings, medications, the cost of transportation for treatments, and help for ADLs or housekeeping. Patients may be eligible for public assistance, but this may cause them shame and provide less income than they need. The care provider should assess financial status and make referrals as needed to local agencies that can help the patient. The choice of dressings and treatments needs to be made with the best option meeting the need for optimal healing combined with the need to contain costs for patients.

IMPACTS OF HEALTHCARE PROFESSIONALS ON PATIENTS' PERCEPTION

Healthcare professionals affect the patient's psychological reactions by their words, expressions, and actions concerning the wound. A reaction of disappointment, surprise, disgust, or disdain causes the patient to feel shame, embarrassment, imperfection, vulnerability, and other negative feelings. Caregivers also have these reactions. A healthcare professional may assume the patient has the level of knowledge needed to prevent such wounds, implying blame, when in fact the patient does not, but the patient may react with shame and guilt. Healthcare professionals who do not teach the patient about the wound or treatment, give results of tests or measurements, or include the patient in decisions or discussion about the wound can cause the patient to feel negatively towards the person and facility.

Patient-Centered Plan of Care

IDENTIFICATION OF PATIENT GOALS AND FACTORS AFFECTING CARE

It is easy to confuse healthcare provider goals with patient goals. Healthcare provider goals involve restoring a patient to the best health possible; however, patients' goals may be very different, or patients may lack defined goals. The only way to help patients to establish goals is to talk to them, helping them arrive at realistic short-term and long-term goals based on their condition and abilities. There are a number of **factors that can affect goals and care**:

- **Functional disability** may prevent a patient from taking the steps needed to reach a goal.
- **Mental status** may be such that a patient is not competent to set goals or to carry out needed actions.
- **Co-morbidity** may result in health problems that interfere with plan of care.
- **Low income** may prevent a patient from buying supplies or getting needed assistance.
- **Social circumstances** may be such that the patient lacks family support or is dependent on others.
- **Smoking** may impact healing.

PREVENTIVE, MAINTENANCE, AND CURATIVE GOALS

Goals should be set with the patient regarding prevention, maintenance, and cure:

- **Preventive goals**: Measures to prevent disease or disability or to prevent deterioration or complications of an existing disorder. May include screening (BP, Pap smear, mammograms, blood glucose), disease education, fall prevention, smoking cessation, substance abuse rehabilitation, vaccinations, nutritional counseling, and exercise.
- **Maintenance goals**: Measures to control an existing disorder in order to maintain status. May include therapy (OT, PT, ST), education, ongoing lifestyle changes, supervision, ongoing assessment, medications, blood glucose management, and treatment. Maintenance therapy may follow primary therapy for some diseases, such as cancer, in order to maintain status.
- **Curative goals**: Measures intended to cure disease rather than simply to alleviate symptoms or pain. May include medications, casting (as for broken limbs), radiotherapy, dialysis, transfusions, chemotherapy, physical therapy, rehabilitation therapy, and surgical interventions. *Note: Curative treatments without the intent to cure are also sometimes used for palliation.*

ACCESS TO CARE

A number of factors may influence a patient's access to care:

- **Proximity to medical services**: Some geographic areas have more medical services than others. For example, some rural areas lack both hospitals and physicians. Cutting-edge treatments may be unavailable in some areas.
- **Socioeconomic status**: Lack of insurance or money to pay for medical services prevents many people from seeking medical care or complying with treatments. Many cannot afford to pay for prescription drugs or supplies.
- **Language differences**: Non-English speakers may not be able to communicate needs or to understand information, such as the treatment plan.
- **Health literacy**: Some may have little knowledge and understanding of anatomy, physiology, disease, and medical treatments.
- **Disability status**: Disabilities may have a profound effect on access to care or very little, depending on the type of disability and the resources available, but some disabilities impair mobility and the ability to access care.
- **Transportation**: Private and public transportation may be unavailable or cost prohibitive.
- **Race and ethnicity**: Inequalities faced by minority populations often extend to medical services. Some individuals live in poor neighborhoods that provide little access to medical services.

Wound Care: Care Planning

135

ISSUES RELATED TO ASSESSMENT OF WOUNDS AT END-OF-LIFE

While the primary goals of skin care are to prevent and heal wounds, when patients are near the end-of-life there are a number of issues to assess:

- Hospice care
- Advance directives
- Best interests of the patient

Patients under hospice care are to receive palliative rather than curative treatment, but in the case of wound care, sometimes treatments that are essentially curative are appropriate if they reduce pain and discomfort. The Patient Self-Determination Act allows people to refuse treatment when they are competent to make that decision and to make advance directives about end-of-life care, and this must be respected in relation to wound care. As systems deteriorate near the end of life, patients are prone to pressure sores, so deciding what must be treated and what treatment is futile can be difficult. Frequently changing the patient's position to prevent pressure may increase pain and discomfort. These decisions must be individualized.

PALLIATIVE CARE

Palliative care is not curative (although it may be carried out in conjunction with curative treatments) but aims to provide emotional support and comfort measures, such as relief of pain, nausea, vomiting, dyspnea, and other symptoms. Palliative care is often carried out as part of hospice care but should be a consideration in the care of all patients. Palliative care may include oxygen, positioning, complementary therapies, analgesia, stool softeners, and antiemetics. Palliative wound care focuses on managing and preventing the symptoms associated with wounds, such as wound infections, discharge, and odor, rather than solely on healing the wounds. Skin breakdown is a common finding as patients near death and cutaneous perfusion decreases. Strategies should include measures to reduce risk of further skin and ulcer breakdown through proper positioning and application of appropriate dressings, to manage symptoms that are present, to attend to the emotional needs of the patient and the patient's family, and to provide care to existing wounds.

Therapeutic Relationships

RELIGIOUS OBJECTIONS TO TREATMENT
JEHOVAH'S WITNESSES

Jehovah's Witnesses have traditionally shunned transfusions and blood products as part of their religious beliefs. In 2004, the *Watchtower,* a Jehovah's Witness publication, presented a guide for members. When medical care indicates the need for blood transfusion or blood products and the patient and/or family members are practicing Jehovah's Witnesses, this may present a conflict. It's important to approach the patient/family with full information and reasons for the transfusion or blood components without being judgmental, allowing them to express their feelings. In fact, studies show that while adults often refuse transfusions for themselves, they frequently allow their children to receive blood products, so one should never assume that an individual would refuse blood products based on the religion alone. Jehovah's Witnesses can receive fractionated blood cells, thus allowing hemoglobin-based blood substitutes. The following guidelines are provided to church members:

Basic **blood standards for Jehovah's Witnesses**:

- **Not acceptable**: Whole blood: red cells, white cells, platelets, plasma.
- **Acceptable**: Fractions from red cells, white cells, platelets, and plasma.

CHRISTIAN SCIENTISTS

Christian Science, a religion developed by Mary Baker Eddy in 1879, promotes the belief that sickness is most effectively treated through prayer alone. While Christian Scientists do not avoid all medical interventions, their beliefs are conservative regarding medical treatment. Most notably, Christian Scientists, for the most part, do not believe in vaccinations and may only agree to such if required by law, as they do acknowledge the importance of community health. They have widely appreciated the use of exemptions from mandatory vaccines, but as these exemptions have become more limited, religious leaders have given their members the right to decide upon vaccinations.

IMPACT OF CULTURE AND RELIGION ON DIETARY PREFERENCES

When performing a dietary assessment, the nurse should remember that culture and religion might dictate which foods and spices are used. The manner in which food is prepared, cooked, and served may also be specified. The utensils used at the meal as well as the persons who may eat together may be important. Mealtimes and required fasts should be determined. Holidays may be accompanied by particular foods. Alcohol (including extracts made with alcohol) and caffeine may be prohibited. The culture may also consider obesity a sign of affluence and success. The nurse should evaluate the foods that are eaten in light of the patient's medical condition. The patient may not wish to eat the usual hospital fare and may need to have a special diet prepared or food brought from home. The nurse can guide the patient and family to foods that are acceptable and within the patient's requirements for health.

THERAPEUTIC COMMUNICATION
FACILITATING COMMUNICATION

Therapeutic communication begins with respect for the patient/family and the assumption that all communication, verbal and nonverbal, has meaning. Listening must be done empathetically. The following are some techniques that facilitate communication.

Wound Care: Care Planning

Introduction:

- Make a personal introduction and use the patient's name: "Mrs. Brown, I am Susan Williams, your nurse."

Encouragement:

- Use an open-ended opening statement: "Is there anything you'd like to discuss?"
- Acknowledge comments: "Yes," and "I understand."
- Allow silence and observe nonverbal behavior rather than trying to force conversation. Ask for clarification if statements are unclear.
- Reflect statements back (use sparingly): Patient: "I hate this hospital." Nurse: "You hate this hospital?"

Empathy:

- Make observations: "You are shaking," and "You seem worried."
- Recognize feelings:
    - Patient: "I want to go home."
    - Nurse: "It must be hard to be away from your home and family."
- Provide information as honestly and completely as possible about condition, treatment, and procedures and respond to the patient's questions and concerns.

Exploration:

- Verbally express implied messages:
    - Patient: "This treatment is too much trouble."
    - Nurse: "You think the treatment isn't helping you?"
- Explore a topic but allow the patient to terminate the discussion without further probing: "I'd like to hear how you feel about that."

Orientation:

- Indicate reality:
    - Patient: "Someone is screaming."
    - Nurse: "That sound was an ambulance siren."
- Comment on distortions without directly agreeing or disagreeing:
    - Patient: "That nurse promised I didn't have to walk again."
    - Nurse: "Really? That's surprising because the doctor ordered physical therapy twice a day."

Collaboration:

- Work together to achieve better results: "Maybe if we talk about this, we can figure out a way to make the treatment easier for you."

Validation:

- Seek validation: "Do you feel better now?" or "Did the medication help you breathe better?"

AVOIDING NON-THERAPEUTIC COMMUNICATION

While using therapeutic communication is important, it is equally important to avoid interjecting **non-therapeutic communication**, which can block effective communication. *Avoid the following:*

- Meaningless clichés: "Don't worry. Everything will be fine." "Isn't it a nice day?"
- Providing advice: "You should…" or "The best thing to do is…." It's better when patients ask for advice to provide facts and encourage the patient to reach a decision.
- Inappropriate approval that prevents the patient from expressing true feeling or concerns:
    o Patient: "I shouldn't cry about this."
    o Nurse: "That's right! You're an adult!"
- Asking for an explanation of behavior that is not directly related to patient care and requires analysis and explanation of feelings: "Why are you so upset?"
- Agreeing with rather than accepting and responding to patient's statements can make it difficult for the patient to change his or her statement or opinion later: "I agree with you," or "You are right."
- Making negative judgments: "You should stop arguing with the nurses."
- Devaluing the patient's feelings: "Everyone gets upset at times."
- Disagreeing directly: "That can't be true," or "I think you are wrong."
- Defending against criticism: "The doctor is not being rude; he's just very busy today."
- Changing the subject to avoid dealing with uncomfortable topics;
    o Patient: "I'm never going to get well."
    o Nurse: "Your family will be here in just a few minutes."
- Making inappropriate literal responses, even as a joke, especially if the patient is at all confused or having difficulty expressing ideas:
    o Patient: "There are bugs crawling under my skin."
    o Nurse: "I'll get some bug spray,"
- Challenging the patient to establish reality often just increases confusion and frustration:
    o "If you were dying, you wouldn't be able to yell and kick!"

COMMUNICATING WITH PATIENTS WITH DISABILITIES

Guidelines for communicating with individuals with disabilities:

- Do not assume that the person with disabilities also has impaired cognition.
- Always treat the person with respect and dignity.
- Use first names with the patient if asked to do so, but start out formally as with any patient.
- Offer to shake hands even when a prosthesis is present.
- Be patient if communication is impaired.
- Offer assistance, but allow the patient to tell you what is helpful; otherwise don't assist.
- When a wheelchair is used, sit down so the patient does not have to strain their neck to speak with you.
- If providing directions, consider the obstacles that may be in the way and assist the person to find an appropriate way around them.

Wound Care: Care Planning

COMMUNICATION WITH PATIENTS WITH COGNITIVE DISABILITIES

The person with cognitive disabilities may be easily distracted, so verbal communication should be attempted in a quiet area:

- Address people with dignity and respect.
- Do not try to discuss abstract ideas but stick with concrete topics.
- Keep words and sentences very simple and try rephrasing when necessary. People may have difficulty in distinguishing your spoken words and deriving the meaning from them.
- Be very patient with people's attempts to speak to you since they may have difficulty in processing thoughts and changing them into spoken words.
- Use objects around you and gestures to illustrate your words since the patient may also use pointing and gesturing when unable to find the words to communicate with you. The person may prefer written communication, although some may be unable to read.
- Use touch to convey your regard during communication, as this is recognized by the patient as reassurance of your care and concern for them.
- Give a few instructions at a time as to not overwhelm them.

COMMUNICATING WITH DEAF OR HEARING-IMPAIRED PATIENTS

Communicating with a person with deafness or hearing impairment:

- Try to communicate in a quiet environment if possible.
- Wave or touch the person to let him or her know you are trying to communicate.
- Determine the method the person uses to communicate: sign language, lip reading, hearing devices, or writing.
- Fingerspell or use some signs if able to do so.
- Address the person directly when you speak even though the person may be looking at an interpreter or your lips.
- Look at the person as the interpreter tells you what was said.
- Speak slowly so the interpreter can keep up with you.
- If the person reads lips, face the person and speak clearly and normally, using normal volume.
- If writing a communication, do not speak while writing.
- Do not be afraid to check that the person understands you, and ask questions if you do not understand the person.

COMMUNICATION WITH PEOPLE WITH LOW VISION OR BLINDNESS

Communicating with a person with low vision or blindness:

- Greet the person with low vision or blindness, identifying yourself and others present.
- Always say goodbye when you are leaving.
- Alert the person to written communications, such as warning signs or printed notices.
- Face the person and touch briefly on the arm to let the person know you are speaking to him or her if you are in a group.
- Speak at normal loudness.
- Make any directions given specific in terms of the length of walk and obstacles, such as stairs.
- Use the position of hands on a clock face to give directions (potatoes at 3 o'clock) as well as using *right* or *left*.
- Mention sounds that the person may hear in transit or on arrival at a destination.

COMMUNICATING WITH A PATIENT ON A VENTILATOR

When a patient on a ventilator is conscious, he or she may still be able to communicate by blinking, nodding, shaking the head, or pointing to a picture or word board:

- If the person is able to write, try to reposition the IV line to leave the dominant hand free to communicate.
- Discuss the need for communication with the physician and ask if a valve or an electric larynx can be used to permit speech.
- Help the patient practice lip reading of single words.
- Remember the patient's glasses or hearing aids when attempting to communicate.
- Enlist the aid of a speech therapist if there is frustration on the part of the patient and family due to communication difficulty.

COMMUNICATING WITH PERSONS WITH SPEECH PROBLEMS DUE TO A STROKE

Methods to communicate with stroke patients with speech problems:

- **Dysarthria**: Patients have problems forming the words to speak them aloud. Give them time to communicate, offer them a picture board or other means of communicating, and give encouragement to family members who are frustrated with the difficulty of trying to communicate.
- **Expressive aphasia**: The patients' efforts at speech come out garbled when they try to say sentences, but single words may be clear. Encourage the patients to try to write and to practice the sounds of the alphabet. Resist the urge to finish sentences for the patients.
- **Receptive aphasia**: The patients have a problem comprehending the speech they hear. Communicate in simple terms and speak slowly. Test comprehension of the written word as an alternative method of communication.
- **Global aphasia**: The patient has both receptive and expressive aphasia. Use simple, clear, slow speech augmented by pictures and gestures.

COMMUNICATION PROBLEMS OF PATIENTS WITH PARKINSON'S DISEASE

Parkinson's disease causes problems with speaking in the majority (75–90%) of patients. The reason for this is not clear but may relate to increasing rigidity and changes in movement. Speech is often very low-pitched or hoarse, given in a monotone and with a soft voice. Speech production may decrease because of the effort required to speak. **Speech therapy** can develop exercises for the patient that can assist them in remembering to speak slowly and carefully, as patients are not always aware that their **communication** is impaired:

- Allow time for the patient to communicate, asking for repetition if you do not understand the message.
- Help family by teaching ways to facilitate communication with the patient and encouraging them to assist the patient to do the exercises provided by the therapist.
- If speech volume is very low, suggest amplification devices that can be obtained through speech therapy.

Wound Care: Care Planning

COMMUNICATION WITH PATIENTS WITH PSYCHIATRIC PROBLEMS

Persons with psychiatric disorders appreciate being addressed with respect, dignity, and honesty:

- Speak simply and clearly, repeating as necessary.
- Encourage patients to discuss their concerns regarding treatment and medications to improve compliance.
- Use good eye contact and be attentive to your body language messages.
- Be alert, but unless the person is known to be violent, try to relax and listen to them.
- Don't try to avoid words or phrases pertaining to psychiatric problems, but if you do say something inappropriate, apologize honestly to the patient.
- Offer patients outlets for their thoughts and feelings.
- Learn more about their disorder and ways to use therapeutic communication to help them with their problem, such as re-orienting them as needed.

CULTURAL COMPETENCE

Different cultures view health and illness from very different perspectives, and patients often come from a mix of many cultures, so the nurse must be not only accepting of cultural differences but must be sensitive and aware. There are a number of characteristics that are important for a nurse to have **cultural competence**:

- **Appreciating diversity**: This must be grounded in information about other cultures and understanding of their value systems.
- **Assessing own cultural perspectives**: Self-awareness is essential to understanding potential biases.
- **Understanding intercultural dynamics**: This must include understanding ways in which cultures cooperate, differ, communicate, and reach understanding.
- **Recognizing institutional culture**: Each institutional unit (hospital, clinic, office) has an inherent set of values that may be unwritten but is accepted by the staff.
- **Adapting patient service to diversity**: This is the culmination of cultural competence as it is the point of contact between cultures.

CULTURAL CHARACTERISTICS

HISPANIC PATIENTS

Many areas of the country have large populations of Hispanics and Hispanic Americans. As always, it's important to recognize that cultural generalizations don't always apply to individuals. Recent immigrants, especially, have cultural needs that the nurse must understand:

- Many Hispanics are Catholic and may like the nurse to make arrangements for a priest to visit.
- Large extended families may come to visit to support the patient and family, so patients should receive clear explanations about how many visitors are allowed, but some flexibility may be required.
- Language barriers may exist as some may have limited or no English skills, so translation services should be available around the clock.
- Hispanic culture encourages outward expressions of emotions, so family may react strongly to news about a patient's condition, and people who are ill may expect some degree of pampering, so extra attention to the patient/family members may alleviate some of their anxiety.

Caring for Hispanic and Hispanic American patients requires understanding of cultural differences:

- Some immigrant Hispanics have very little formal education, so medical information may seem very complex and confusing, and they may not understand the implications or need for follow-up care.
- Hispanic culture perceives time with more flexibility than American culture, so if parents need to be present at a particular time, the nurse should specify the exact time (1:30 PM) and explain the reason rather than saying something more vague, such as "after lunch."
- People may appear to be unassertive or unable to make decisions when they are simply showing respect to the nurse by being deferent.
- In traditional families, the males make decisions, so a woman waits for the father or other males in the family to make decisions about treatment or care.
- Families may choose to use folk medicines instead of Western medical care or may combine the two.
- Children and young women are often sheltered and are taught to be respectful to adults, so they may not express their needs openly.

MIDDLE EASTERN PATIENTS

There are considerable cultural differences among Middle Easterners, but religious beliefs about the segregation of males and females are common. It's important to remember that segregating the female is meant to protect her virtue. Female nurses have low status in many countries because they violate this segregation by touching male bodies, so parents may not trust or show respect for the nurse who is caring for their family member. Additionally, male patients may not want to be cared for by female nurses or doctors, and families may be very upset at a female being cared for by a male nurse or physician. When possible, these cultural traditions should be accommodated:

- In Middle Eastern countries, males make decisions, so issues for discussion or decision should be directed to males, such as the father or spouse, and males may be direct in stating what they want, sometimes appearing demanding.
- If a male nurse must care for a female patient, then the family should be advised that *personal care* (such as bathing) will be done by a female while the medical treatments will be done by the male nurse.

Caring for Middle Eastern patients requires understanding of cultural differences:

- Families may practice strict dietary restrictions, such as avoiding pork and requiring that animals be killed in a ritual manner, so vegetarian or kosher meals may be required.
- People may have language difficulties requiring a translator, and same-sex translators should be used if at all possible.
- Families may be accompanied by large extended families that want to be kept informed and whom patients consult before decisions are made.
- Most medical care is provided by female relatives, so educating the family about patient care should be directed at females (with female translators if necessary).
- Outward expressions of grief are considered as showing respect for the dead.
- Middle Eastern families often offer gifts to caregivers. Small gifts (candy) that can be shared should be accepted graciously, but for other gifts, the families should be advised graciously that accepting gifts is against hospital policy.
- Middle Easterners often require less personal space and may stand very close.

Wound Care: Care Planning

143

ASIAN PATIENTS

There are considerable differences among different Asian populations, so cultural generalizations may not apply to all, but nurses caring for Asian patients should be aware of common cultural attitudes and behaviors:

- Nurses and doctors are viewed with respect, so traditional Asian families may expect the nurse to remain authoritative and to give directions and may not question, so the nurse should ensure that they understand by having them review material or give demonstrations and should provide explanations clearly, anticipating questions that the family might have but may not articulate.
- Disagreeing is considered impolite. "Yes" may only mean that the person is heard, not that they agree with the person. When asked if they understand, they may indicate that they do even when they clearly do not so as not to offend the nurse.
- Asians may avoid eye contact as an indication of respect. This is especially true of children in relation to adults and of younger adults in relation to elders.

Caring for Asian patients requires understanding of cultural differences:

- Patients/families may not show outward expressions of feelings/grief, sometimes appearing passive. They also avoid public displays of affection. This does not mean that they don't feel, just that they don't show their feelings.
- Families often hide illness and disabilities from others and may feel ashamed about illness.
- Terminal illness is often hidden from the patient, so families may not want patients to know they are dying or seriously ill.
- Families may use cupping, pinching, or applying pressure to injured areas, and this can leave bruises that may appear as abuse, so when bruises are found, the family should be questioned about alternative therapy before assumptions are made.
- Patients may be treated with traditional herbs.
- Families may need translators because of poor or no English skills.
- In traditional Asian families, males are authoritative and make the decisions.

Wound Care: Education and Referral

Patient Education

EDUCATION REGARDING RISK FACTORS AND PREVENTION STRATEGIES

Teaching patients and caregivers about risk factors and prevention strategies is an important part of wound management:

- **Limited mobility**: Referral for physical or occupational therapy may be indicated. If patients are unable to change position, caregivers must be taught proper skin care and positioning.
- **Diabetes**: Proper glucose monitoring and control is critical. Patients should avoid going barefoot and should inspect feet daily.
- **Impaired circulation**: Exercises may be indicated. Proper positioning to increase circulation should be stressed. Restrictive socks or clothing should be avoided.
- **Cognitive impairment**: Caregiver should be advised of all necessary treatments and may need to institute safety measures and assist patient with hygiene.
- **Malnutrition**: Diet should be planned and explained, and supplements should be provided. Meals-on-wheels or assistance for food preparation and eating may be necessary.
- **Fecal and urinary contamination**: Medical and dietary instructions should be given to control incontinence, including scheduled voiding. Skin barriers may be needed as well as assistance with hygiene and adult briefs.

RISK OF SKIN BREAKDOWN

Patient teaching points regarding the risk of skin breakdown include:

- Advise that skin over the tailbone, hips, shoulder blades, heels, inner and outer ankles, inner and outer knees, elbows, and the back of the head should be checked frequently for skin breakdown.
- Teach about the results of pressure on capillaries and the signs of early damage.
- Explain friction and shearing forces.
- Explain the action of urine and feces upon the skin and the need to keep the patient clean and dry.
- Teach techniques needed to move the patient in the bed using a lift sheet or trapeze.
- Stress the need to prevent skin breakdown to avoid lengthy and costly wound care.
- Recommend soaps and lotions, avoiding those that dry skin, based on the general skin condition and the patient's financial resources.
- Advise the patient and caregiver not to hesitate to call the nurse or physician to report any concerns about skin condition.

EDUCATION REGARDING LIFESTYLE CHANGES TO MAXIMIZE PERFUSION

The patient with arterial insufficiency must make lifestyle changes in order to avoid serious complications and/or amputation of the affected limb:

- Maintain adequate hydration to decrease blood viscosity, but avoid caffeine, which is vasoconstrictive.
- Keep pain under control in order to prevent further vasoconstriction.
- Stop smoking, as nicotine has vasoconstrictive properties.
- Begin a graduated walking program to improve tissue oxygenation, decrease pain, and increase activity tolerance.
- Avoid cold and constrictive clothing to avoid vasoconstriction.
- Do careful skin inspection and skin care: drying skin, using emollients and lamb's wool or foam between toes.
- Wear properly fitted, closed-toe shoes and avoid going barefoot.
- Have professional foot and nail care.
- Wear warm socks during cold weather, but avoid hot water bottles, heating pads, or hot bathing temperatures.
- Avoid the use of antiseptics or chemicals except as prescribed.
- Report even small injuries or changes in skin promptly.

ADDITIONAL MEASURES TO IMPROVE PERFUSION

There are a number of additional and more interventional measures which can improve the perfusion to wounds that the patient should be educated on:

- Management of diet and medication to control blood glucose levels, high blood pressure, and lipid levels.
- Aspirin therapy to reduce the danger of clot formation.
- Surgical revascularization to replace damaged vessels.
- Hyperbaric oxygen therapy, which increases available oxygen to tissues by 10-20 times. Blood that is saturated increases perfusion of the tissues. It is indicated for peripheral arterial insufficiency, compromised skin from grafts, and diabetic ulcers.
- Topical hyperbaric oxygen therapy has shown promise in increasing circulation and healing wounds. The topical oxygen increases perfusion to the wound bed itself rather than systemically.
- Circulator Boot therapy, an end-diastolic compression equipment system, is used to treat ulcers of the lower extremity. Compressions coordinate with the end of diastole to increase perfusion. It is FDA approved for the treatment of deficient arterial blood flow.

MANAGEMENT OF NUTRITIONAL FACTORS THAT AFFECT WOUND HEALING

Nutritional management must be designed according to individual needs based on many factors, such as age, weight, size, nutritional status, co-morbidity, and size and severity of wound. The average healthy person requires about 0.8 g of protein per kilogram every day (40-70 g). However, if a person has a wound, then not only must the person have adequate calories and general nutrition, but additional daily protein and vitamins as well:

- Protein amounts are increased to 1.25–2.0 g/kg
- Vitamin A 1600–2000 retinal equivalents
- Vitamin C 100–1000 mg
- Zinc 15–30 mg
- B vitamins 200% of RDA
- Iron 20–30 mg

Caloric and fluid intake should be monitored carefully to ensure that the person is eating the food that is served. Gastrointestinal tube feedings or parenteral feedings may be necessary if the person cannot take food and fluids orally. Prealbumin levels should be monitored regularly as well.

DIETARY CHANGES TO ADD PROTEIN, CALORIES AND NUTRIENTS

There are a number of dietary changes that can add adequate protein, calories, and needed nutrients to the diet. In some people, co-morbid conditions such as diabetes or high cholesterol should be considered because some foods, such as cheese, are high in sodium and fat, which may be restricted.

To **increase protein**:

- Add meat to vegetarian dishes, such as soups and pastas.
- Add milk powder to many foods during preparation.
- Substitute milk for water in soups, hot cereals, and cocoa.
- Add cheese to dishes, such as pastas and casseroles.
- Provide high protein drinks, such as High Protein Ensure.
- Use peanut butter on bread and apples.
- Add extra eggs to dishes, such as custards and meat loaf

To **increase calories**:

- Use whole milk or cream rather than low fat or non-fat milk.
- Add butter, sour cream, or whipping cream to foods.
- Provide frequent snacks.

NUTRITIONAL ADVICE FOR PATIENTS WITH ULCERS OR RISKS FOR SKIN PROBLEMS

Diabetic patients and those with ulcers or skin problems should have consultation with a dietitian for an individualized diet that meets healing needs without raising the blood sugar:

- Patients should be advised to drink at least 8 glasses of fluids per day unless there is a contraindication.
- Diets should have increased protein and iron for healing.
- Carbohydrates should be complex, and high-glycemic carbohydrates, which increase blood sugar, should be limited.
- Caloric intake should be determined by the dietitian.
- Eating small meals every few hours is preferable to 3 large meals.
- A dietary supplement may be prescribed up to three times a day to meet nutritional needs.
- Patients and caregivers should have lists of foods that help to provide the nutrients that the patient needs.

SKIN SELF-ASSESSMENT

The areas of the skin that are prone to breakdown should be assessed with the patient and caregiver present and unique findings discussed. This provides a baseline condition for them to reference when they do further assessments of the area:

- Teach how to blanch the skin and how to report signs of redness, abrasion, pallor, changes in skin texture or color, pain, bruising, or swelling.
- Provide pictures and color charts with demonstrations of skin abnormalities to watch for if possible.
- Show how to measure skin lesions or discolorations.
- Stress the importance of communicating areas of concern between caregivers so that changes are noted and monitored and action is taken to prevent breakdown and to bring the concern to the attention of the patient's nurse or physician.

Wound Care: Education and Referral

WOUND SELF-ASSESSMENT

The patient must learn to look at the wound and surrounding skin to assess for signs of infection or wound problems. The color of the tissues in the wound, and the amount, color, and odor of exudate should be explained. The patient must be taught to report pain in or around the wound or signs of redness, swelling, warmth, increased exudate or pus, or fever. The condition of the skin around the wound should be noted and reported if there are any signs of maceration or breakdown. The patient should also note whether the wound bed is dry or moist. The patient should be taught how to measure the wound consistently when dressings are changed. The signs of a beefy red healthy wound bed and of the various stages of a healing wound should be illustrated to the patient and caregiver to help them recognize and distinguish a healing wound from a non-healing or infected wound.

MEASUREMENT OF WOUNDS

The patient should be taught to measure the wound at the greatest length and width without touching the wound. The patient may also be taught to use two pieces of plastic wrap or a clean plastic bag to trace the wound with a permanent marker. The layers are laid on the wound and the edges are traced onto the top layer. After the ink dries the top layer of the bag is cut off or the top layer of plastic is removed. The patient should label each tracing with the date and time. The bottom layer touching the wound is then disposed of with the old dressing as hazardous waste. One can leave a form for the patient to record the date and measurements so that healing progress can be tracked.

CHANGING A DRESSING AT HOME

The patient should be alert and able to follow instructions regarding ulcer or wound dressings at home. A caregiver may be present to learn as reinforcement for the patient or to perform dressing changes and care for the patient. Teaching includes:

- Teach the importance of washing hands, using gloves, and disposing of hazardous waste properly.
- Demonstrate the dressing change using clean technique.
- Demonstrate the technique of removing the old dressing slowly to avoid trauma to the wound, then washing and regloving.
- Teach how to assess and measure the wound and the symptoms of infection to be reported. Demonstrate the technique to be used for wound cleansing or irrigation if needed.
- Show how to pad wounds if exudate is present.
- Finally teach the assessment of periwound tissues, how to apply skin protectant if needed, and how to secure the dressing to the site.

SELF-CARE OF COMPRESSION THERAPY

Teach patients to care for their compression stockings by maintaining two pairs, washing them according to manufacturer's instructions, and replacing them when they lose elasticity in 3 to 6 months. They should inspect skin of the legs and feet daily for breakdown or trauma. Stockings will dry the skin, so they should wash the feet and legs, dry them lightly, and apply a moisturizer without fragrance after removing the stockings for the night. Patients with lymphedema need to understand their disease and the need to control edema continuously. They should be taught skin care and how to apply special treatment when weeping dermatitis is present. Compression garments may be used after decongestive physiotherapy and massage brings edema under control. Exercises to gradually strengthen the calf muscles should be taught to the patient. Patients must comply with compression therapy and exercises to keep lymphedema under control.

POTENTIAL ADVERSE EFFECTS OF COMPRESSION THERAPY

There are a number of potential adverse effects of compression therapy that the patient should monitor for:

- Compression therapy could potentially restrict the blood flow to the distal portion of the extremity, ultimately causing tissue death, necrosis, and amputation. The skin color should be noted and reported if blue or pale. The patient should be aware of the need to report any numbness, tingling, excess warmth, or coldness in extremities during compression therapy.
- In those with cardiac disease, the fluid shift that occurs with controlling edema may cause cardiac failure and/or pulmonary edema, so patients must note increasing dyspnea, cough, or chest pain.
- Constriction caused by a bandage or compressive garment can restrict movement and cause contractions and skin trauma.
- Displacement of fluid may cause congestion proximal to the compressed legs, so the patient must report any swelling of the knee, thigh, or abdomen.
- Some people may develop sensitivity to materials in the compression material, resulting in itching and rash.

WOUND IRRIGATION AT HOME
PERSONAL PRECAUTIONS TO TAKE DURING WOUND CLEANSING IRRIGATIONS

Wound irrigation should be done in a small room with the doors closed, but not the bathroom. The patient should be seated comfortably or lying down, depending upon the site of the wound. The patient and/or caregiver should wash hands, apply clean gloves, and wear a mask during irrigation. Towels should be placed around the wound area with a basin below the wound to catch the returned solution. The patient should use a squeeze bottle to squirt normal saline on the wound to cleanse drainage and necrotic material, using care to avoid touching the wound with the irrigation tip or disturbing the wound. After irrigation, the hands should be washed and regloved and the wound dressed. The basin should be emptied in the toilet and towels washed. Surfaces in the room should be wiped with a disinfectant. The squeeze bottle and basin should be washed with hot soapy water, rinsed with bleach solution and hot water, then dried and covered with a clean towel until the next use.

MAKING SALINE IRRIGATING FLUID IN THE HOME SETTING

If the patient needs to use a quantity of normal saline to cleanse a wound by irrigation in the home setting, it may be advisable to make normal saline from boiled tap water and salt. A pot and quart glass jar or plastic container and lid should be washed with hot water, rinsed with diluted bleach water and then hot water, and dried (or a jar and lid can be boiled as for canning). Bring a quart of tap water to boil in the pot and keep it boiling for 5 minutes. Add two teaspoons of non-iodized salt and stir until dissolved. The solution should be allowed to cool completely before use. It can be stored in the clean covered glass or plastic container at room temperature and used for up to one week, after which it should be discarded.

AVOIDING WOUND INFECTIONS IN THE HOME

Patients should be aware of the need to avoid illness and infection when they have a healing wound and should take steps to prevent wound infections:

- Visitors should be screened for illness and advised to visit with the patient by phone until well.
- Family members who are ill should not be near the patient or prepare food for them.
- Those with coughs should wear a mask or should cover the mouth with a tissue and remain at least 3 feet from the patient.
- Patient and family should practice good hygiene and good handwashing techniques.
- Wound care procedures should be followed, and contaminated dressing supplies and outdated irrigation solutions discarded.
- Wound care, such as dressing changes, should be done in a clean environment.
- Pets should be groomed regularly and prevented from licking the wound area.

Wound Care: Education and Referral

REINFORCING SEATING AND TURNING SCHEDULES

The care provider should reinforce seating and turning schedules when educating the patient:

- Teach methods of turning and positioning the patient every 1-2 hours.
- Draw a clock face to post in the home to remind them to turn the patient, writing the position at the corresponding time on the clock. Time in a chair or in another upright position can be scheduled in the morning for AM care and at mealtimes, with side-lying and supine positioning in between. An alarm clock or timer can also help the patient and caregiver to remember to change position.
- Teach the 8 positions to use: supine with the knees elevated, supine tilted 30 degrees to the right or left, supine with a slight tilt off one sacral side, supine with the head elevated 30 degrees, and prone tilted 30 degrees to either side.
- Stress the prevention of skin breakdown and the fact that positioning is one of the most important components of prevention, along with nutrition, hydration, support surfaces, and cleaning and drying the skin after elimination.

SKIN TEMPERATURE MONITORING IN THE HOME

Temperature monitoring is a way to make early identification of areas of the foot that are experiencing tissue stress. This method uses special foot thermometers to identify compromised areas before subtle surface signs can be detected by the patient or caregiver. It is invaluable for patients who are at high risk for skin ulceration. The patient and caregiver are given a foot diagram with areas of the foot to be tested, including those that are problematic for this individual. They are instructed to let the bare foot come to room temperature for 5 or 10 minutes before testing. Temperature is then recorded on the diagram for each circled area. The time and date are also recorded. Temperature elevations of 3 degrees over the baseline obtained in the physician's office should be reported. The patient can also be taught measures to take when this occurs to provide immediate relief of pressure to the area. Serial temperature measurements can then be taken to see if these measures are working.

MANAGING INCONTINENCE TO PREVENT SKIN BREAKDOWN

Prompt cleaning after incontinence removes irritating urea and enzymes from the skin. The skin should be washed with soap and water or pre-moistened wipes. The area must then be dried thoroughly. A lubricating cream, such as zinc oxide, helps to protect the perineal areas. The patient may wear disposable briefs or use bed pads. Disposable adult briefs wick fluid away from the skin, but should be changed when wet. Scheduled toileting every 1 ½ or 2 hours, after meals, and before bedtime can decrease incontinence from occurring. Fluids should not be withheld to decrease incontinence because dehydration further compromises skin. Male external condom catheters may be used with a small leg collection bag. The condom must be removed for hygiene and to inspect skin on a regular basis. Stool softeners or fiber may help to regulate bowel movements.

TYPES OF MOISTURIZERS

Patients should be provided information about the different types of moisturizers in order to make the best for their skin. Moisturizing helps hydrate the skin, prevent dryness and cracking, and skin breakdown. It should be done after bathing and other times during the day. There are primarily 3 types although there are many varieties. Patients should use hypoallergenic moisturizers without added fragrance:

- **Lotions** contain a lot of water and must be applied often during the day.
- **Creams** contain water and oil and need to be rubbed into the skin 4 times daily.
- **Ointments** often consist of a petrolatum or lanolin combined with the least amount of water. They provide a protective layer over the skin that holds in moisture. They have the longest lasting moisturizing action of all three although they may be occlusive.

ENCOURAGING SMOKING CESSATION

Smoking directly affects vascular functioning, and patients must be encouraged to stop smoking in order to experience proper wound healing.

METHODS

Methods to encourage a patient to stop smoking:

- Discuss the social effects of smoking and the patient's feelings about smoking.
- List ways that smoking harms not only the patient but also family members and pets.
- Stress the use of smoking cessation aids and sources of support so that the patient doesn't feel that he or she must quit without help.
- Refer the patient to sources for free nicotine patches and tips on quitting.
- Enlist family members for support and encouragement.
- Teach the patient and family how smoking affects the patient's vascular problems, causing a high risk of wounds, ulcers, and poor healing.
- Help the patient to devise rewards at regular intervals for quitting.
- Enlist the aid of the physician as needed for pulmonary function testing, medications to use for cessation, and added encouragement and support with each clinic visit.

NICOTINE REPLACEMENT THERAPY

Nicotine replacement therapy (NRT) can increase the success of smoking cessation. Nicotine replacement is available in the form of an inhaler or nasal spray by prescription. It is also available over-the-counter in the form of gum, patches, and lozenges. The cost of replacement therapy is about the same as the daily cost of cigarettes, depending on the amount and type of nicotine replacement. Use of NRT will help the patient to avoid nicotine withdrawal symptoms such as tension and irritability, drowsiness, and problems with concentration. However, there can be side effects from NRT, including heartburn, hiccups, skin irritation from the patches, vertigo, tachycardia, sleeplessness, nausea, vomiting, aching muscles, and stiffness. Patients should be advised to consult with the physician before using nicotine replacement products. NRT should not be used when the patient is pregnant. Identify non-nicotine medications that can help the patient quit smoking.

NICOTINE PATCHES

Nicotine patches require three hours for the drug to be absorbed through the skin into the blood stream. Some patches are designed to be worn during waking hours and some for 24 hours. There are different strengths available for light and heavy smokers. Each patch contains an adhesive that causes it to adhere to the skin. The nicotine patch can cause skin irritation and may not adhere in humid weather or when the patient perspires heavily. The patch should be changed at the same time daily to keep the nicotine level in the blood at a constant state. The old patch should be discarded carefully by folding it and placing it in the trash so that children and pets are not able to access it. The patient should not use patches if they continue to smoke as this increases blood levels of nicotine.

NICOTINE SPRAY OR INHALER

The use of a nicotine spray or an inhaler as aids for smoking cessation:

- **Nicotine nasal spray** is absorbed rapidly through the nasal mucosa. The patient should deliver 2 sprays into each nostril up to 5 times per hour. Side effects include nose and throat irritation. Heavy smokers may succeed with this form of NRT since it reaches the bloodstream more quickly than other NRT.
- **The nicotine inhaler** uses cartridges of nicotine vapor that the patient puffs on for 20 minutes up to 16 times a day. Side effects are mouth and throat irritation and a cough, which decreases over time.

Both methods should be used consistently for effectiveness; however, they are more expensive to use than nicotine gum, patches, or lozenges.

Wound Care: Education and Referral

151

NICOTINE GUM AND LOZENGES

Patients should stop smoking when gum or lozenge therapy begins. Enough should be used to reduce craving and withdrawal symptoms, especially in the beginning. Patients should not eat or drink for 15 minutes prior to or while chewing the gum or using lozenges. Side effects are irritation of the mouth, throat, and gums. The gum is dense and may damage dental work. Both gum and lozenges should be disposed of safely out of the reach of children and pets. Both come in 2 mg and 4 mg strengths:

- **Nicotine gum** is chewed until tingling is felt, and then the gum should be parked between the gum and cheek. When the tingling sensation decreases, the gum is chewed a few times and parked again. This continues until the gum no longer produces the tingling sensation, and then it is discarded.
- **Nicotine lozenges** should dissolve slowly and must not be chewed or swallowed or heartburn and nausea may occur.

NON-NICOTINE MEDICATIONS THAT HELP PATIENTS QUIT SMOKING

Non-nicotine medications that help the patient quit smoking:

- **Zyban** (bupropion hydrochloride) has been used since 1977. It is also an antidepressant. The patient begins taking Zyban a week prior to quitting. During this time the drug begins to reach a stable level in the blood and the smoker will notice that cigarettes do not taste as good and are not as satisfying. Zyban helps to remove the urge to smoke but its exact action is unknown. Side effects include dry mouth, dizziness, and insomnia. It should be taken for 12 weeks to help the patient establish smoke-free behavior before stopping the drug.
- **Chantix** (varenicline) is a new drug that partially blocks nicotine receptors. It also reduces the pleasure of smoking while reducing side effects of nicotine withdrawal. It can be taken for 12 to 24 weeks. Side effects include nausea, vomiting, headache, flatus, insomnia, abnormal dreaming, and altered taste.

SELF-CARE FOR VENOUS INSUFFICIENCY

Venous insufficiency is a condition that occurs when the venous wall or valves in the leg veins are not working effectively, making it difficult for blood to return to the heart from the legs.

Points to teach the patient about self-care for venous insufficiency:

- Teach the patient about the disease, symptoms, and personal risk factors to modify, including smoking.
- Explain the reason for compression therapy and how to apply stockings properly.
- Teach skin assessment and care for the legs and feet. The patient should inspect the skin daily for any signs of trauma, redness, pain, or skin ulcer formation. Lubricants or emollients should be applied to the legs and feet at night to counteract the drying effect of compression stockings. The patient should learn to avoid crossing the legs and to elevate the legs when sitting several times a day.
- Stress the need to avoid injury to the skin of the legs and feet.
- Counsel the patient on improving nutritional intake.

SELF-CARE FOR ARTERIAL INSUFFICIENCY

Arterial insufficiency is any condition that slows or stops the flow of blood through the arteries, such as atherosclerosis.

Points to remember when teaching the patient about self-care for arterial insufficiency:

- Teach the patient the pathophysiology behind arterial insufficiency: hypertension, diabetes, and high cholesterol, signs and symptoms of these diseases, and personal risk factors that can be modified, including smoking and diet.
- Be sure the patient understands doctor's orders, including activity limitations and medications.
- Teach the daily inspection of the legs and feet to check for symptoms to report, such as redness, skin breakdown, and pain.
- Teach skin and toenail care, including washing and drying of the legs and feet, application of emollients, and filing of the nails straight across.
- Warn against going barefooted and review the proper fit for shoes and socks.
- Caution the patient to check bath temperature to avoid burning by bath water that is too hot.

MANAGEMENT OF IMMUNOSUPPRESSION

Immunosuppression may be the result of co-morbid conditions, such as AIDS, or medications, such as chemotherapy or steroids. Immunosuppression can decrease wound healing and increase the incidence of infection because the body can't destroy pathogenic agents through normal defense mechanisms. Careful management of immunosuppression is critical to healing:

- **Adjust dosages** or discontinue medications contributing to immunosuppression if possible, including steroid avoidance or steroid withdrawal regimens.
- **Monitor wound condition** carefully for changes or lack of healing response that may indicate infection because infection is the most common result of immunosuppression and may not be accompanied by increase of temperature or other usual indications.
- **Monitor immune status** with regular blood tests to determine changes.
- **Provide antimicrobials** as indicated prophylactically to prevent wound infections.
- **Maintain clean environment** and ensure staff use standard precautions.
- Observe for opportunistic infections, such as candidiasis.

EDUCATION FOR DIABETICS

GENERAL MANAGEMENT

Management of diabetes and maintaining glucose control for both Type I (insulin-dependent) and Type II diabetes may be the important determinant of the ability of the wound to heal. Plans should be individualized but usually include the following:

- **Establish goals**: HbA1c level of 6.5% or lower.
- **Maintain normal glycemic levels** during healing:
  - Monitor glucose 4 times daily up to every 4 hours.
  - Type I: Monitor food and insulin intake, adjusting as needed.
  - Type II: Focus on diet, medical control, weight loss, and maintenance of weight loss.
  - Avoid or limit use of alcohol because of unpredictable effects on glucose.
- **Institute exercise program**:
  - Type I: Increases general health and well-being.
  - Type II: Decreases insulin resistance.

Wound Care: Education and Referral

- **Treat co-morbid conditions**, such as atherosclerosis, hypertension, and early renal disease.
- **Cease smoking**, which interferes with circulation and damages vasculature.
- **Make lifestyle changes** that will promote long-term glucose control.

INFORMATION CONCERNING DIABETIC NEUROPATHY

The patient should be urged to contact the physician if signs of diabetic neuropathy, such as altered sensation, is detected in the lower extremities, including sensations of tingling, bugs crawling on the skin, burning, or numbness. The neuropathic foot can't adjust to painful areas with each step. The loss of sensation and pain makes injuries harder to detect, so the importance of daily checking the feet must be stressed. Motor neuropathy results in muscular, bone, and joint deformities. The loss of autonomic control causes the skin to become dry, scaly, and to crack from lack of nutrients and hydration. The presence of neuropathy greatly increases the risk of foot trauma so this patient must be extra vigilant. Neuropathy often leads to ulcerations that are deep and hard to heal. Rubbing from improperly fitted footwear, pressure on the bottom of the foot that isn't relieved, and injury from trauma are the main causes of foot ulcers and problems in this population.

PROPER SKIN-CARE TIPS

The diabetic should be taught to report skin problems as soon as possible, since there is a decreased ability to fight infections. Blood glucose should be regulated to help prevent dryness. The skin, especially skin folds and the feet, should be checked daily when bathing or undressing, and baths and showers should be less frequent, especially in the winter months. Baths should be warm, but not hot enough to burn skin. Only fragrance-free moisturizing soaps and mild shampoos should be used. Moisturizers that consist of a mixture of oil and water (such as Lubriderm or Alpha-Keri) should be used frequently to prevent dry, itchy skin, but not between toes to avoid fungal growth. Scratching damages skin and must be avoided. Powders may be helpful in areas where skin rubs together. Women should not use deodorant sprays in the vaginal area. Humidity in the home should be increased, especially in the winter months. Patients should not be hesitant to contact their physician, podiatrist, or dermatologist about any problem areas on the skin.

RISK OF FOOT ULCERS FOR PATIENTS WITH DIABETES

One should motivate diabetic patients to learn foot care by explaining their risks for foot problems. Patients should be taught that diabetes commonly causes foot and leg amputation in the diabetic patient but may be avoided with proper care. Foot ulcers and trauma are the cause for hospitalization in up to 25% of all diabetic admissions. Diabetics are up to 46% more likely to need an amputation, and if one is needed, another amputation on the same or opposite extremity is more likely. Survival up to five years after an amputation is 70% or below. Hispanics, African-Americans, and Native Americans have the highest amputation rates. The patient should be advised to see a podiatrist as needed. The importance of maintaining blood glucose control through diet, medication, and exercise to reduce risk factors for foot ulcers should be stressed.

FREQUENCY OF PODIATRY VISITS

Podiatrists inspect the feet and identify areas that need treatment or offloading to prevent ulcer formation. They treat calluses and trim thick or problem nails:

- The patient without altered sensation should be seen by a podiatrist yearly to ensure continued foot health.
- When nails are not ingrown, tented, or thick, the patient can use an emery board to keep them trim.
- The patient who has impaired sensation needs to have podiatry care at least twice a year. During this visit the patient can be advised on the type of shoes needed to ensure proper fitting and pressure relief as needed.
- A patient with neuropathy who also has another problem, such as decreased circulation or bony deformity, should be seen every 2 or 3 months and fitted with therapeutic shoes.
- A high-risk patient who has healed ulcers, a previous amputation, or nail problems needs to be seen by a podiatrist every 1 to 2 months to monitor conditions and for nail care.

SHOES FOR PATIENTS WITH DIABETES OR FOOT PROBLEMS

Any patient with diabetes or foot problems should be counseled to always wear shoes and not go barefoot to prevent trauma:

- Off the shelf shoes must be deep enough to accommodate deformed toes or other areas. They should be made of soft leather without stitching that will conform to foot shape and retain that shape. Shoes should allow space for an insole that can be modified to relieve pressure in troublesome areas on the bottom of the foot without redistributing pressure to the top of the foot.
- Patients should be taught how to trim insoles to provide off-loading to problem areas. If shoes or insoles are modified, the patient must monitor other areas for problems that can occur when windows are cut into shoes or insoles.
- Patients that must have custom-made shoes or orthotics should wear them at all times for walking. Patients should maintain shoes and insoles and replace them when worn.
- Patients who have Medicare Part B should be evaluated to determine eligibility for Medicare payment for shoes and inserts.

SOCKS FOR PATIENTS WITH DIABETES OR FOOT PROBLEMS

Patients with foot problems should be taught to buy socks without seams over the toes that can cause friction. Tube socks do not work because there are always folds formed that cause pressure and restriction. Socks should be replaced if they are worn out, not mended. They should be made of as much cotton as possible to absorb perspiration. They should fit well without extra material at the toes or heels and should fit smoothly across the top of the foot. Cushioned socks are best. Socks should not have a tight top that restricts circulation. Specialty socks with silicone padding or custom-made socks that fit a partial foot may be required. These socks may enclose each toe to decrease moisture. Two thin socks should be worn to break in new shoes to allow movement between the socks to avoid shearing pressure and blistering.

TEACHING DIABETIC FOOT CARE TO CAREGIVERS

Patients who are unable to inspect and care for their feet should have caregivers who can be taught to assume this duty:

- Patients who are obese or have mobility problems may not be able to get the feet into a position in which all areas can be inspected.
- Patients with visual problems need to have their feet inspected by others.
- Patients with cognitive problems, such as Alzheimer's disease, may lack adequate comprehension to manage skin care and need to have their skin care needs met by others as well.

Caregivers should be taught all aspects of foot and skin care and be willing to assume this responsibility. They should be encouraged to accompany the patients to physician and podiatrist visits so that ongoing education can be provided.

EXERCISE PRACTICES

The patient with neuropathy or other foot problems should be taught that walking causes 150% of the person's weight to rest on the foot with each step and jogging increases this to 300%. Therefore, the patient should not jog but should walk with slow, short steps only as needed and not for exercise. Appropriate exercise for these patients can include specialized low-impact aerobics and dance if appropriate. **Exercise** that is less stressful to the feet includes chair and mat exercises, swimming, or cycling. Isometric exercises can help to maintain muscle strength and can be done without weight bearing. The patient must be instructed to wear shoes while exercising and soft pool shoes when swimming to avoid injuries. The feet should be dried well after swimming.

Wound Care: Education and Referral

BARRIERS TO CARING FOR WOUNDS

Financial and psychosocial barriers to preventing and caring for wounds include:

- Low income, lack of insurance and resources, fear of being unable to provide for the self and/or family
- Inadequate diet and nutrition
- Lack of health literacy, illiteracy
- Lack of transportation options to healthcare providers (no auto, no public transportation, inability to afford options), distance from healthcare providers (such as in rural areas).
- Fear of doctors, phobias (needles, hospitals)
- Mental illness (bipolar, schizophrenia, depression), stress
- Religious beliefs (Christian Scientist, Jehovah Witness), cultural differences (including language)
- Lack of adequate housing, homelessness, unsanitary conditions
- Lack of family/friend emotional support
- Inadequate communication/coordination among healthcare providers
- Substance abuse, drug and/or alcohol use
- Threat to job security if absent from work
- Low expectation of recovery, perception of unfair treatment, uncaring healthcare provider
- Dysfunctional interpersonal relationships (friends, family, caregivers)
- Inadequate instructions for follow-up

Patient Adherence

PATIENT ADHERENCE TO WOUND CARE AND WOUND PREVENTION

If a wound is to heal and close, then patient adherence to wound care and preventive measures is a critical element. Patients who have had previous negative experiences, who lack support systems, who don't understand what they need to do, and who have lifestyle risks (homelessness, substance abuse, smoking) are especially at risk for nonadherence. Elements of the task may also affect adherence: complex tasks, inability to carry out the tasks, and aversion to the task because of pain or discomfort.

Methods to ensure adherence include:

- Provide step by step instructions and allow ample practice time.
- Provide emotional support and positive feedback when appropriate.
- Apprise the patient of progress, using pictures and/or diagrams.
- Encourage the patient to express feelings.
- Note early signs of nonadherence but avoid being judgmental: "I see that you weren't able to change the dressings every day."
- Provide continuity of care to allow the patient to establish a relationship with caregiver.

ENCOURAGING PATIENT COMPLIANCE WITH WOUND CARE REGIMEN

Methods to encourage patient compliance with wound care regimen:

- Take care to assess how the wound care regimen affects the patient.
- Refer to a social worker to help find resources to meet financial obligations and pay for medications, dressings, food, and bills.
- Assist to get help with ADLs, housekeeping, and other needs. This will help the patient feel that he or she can take the time from other obligations to heal.
- Teach about the healing process and how the wound care regimen encourages healing in the shortest time possible.
- Point out even minor improvements in the wound or ulcer to give them hope and encouragement to continue the regime. Keeping a wound progress chart can show tangible evidence of progress.
- Help establish realistic goals and enlist family members to help remind the patient of the goals and the ways to obtain them.
- Assess patient and family coping with each visit and teach as needed to help encourage compliance.

COMMON BEHAVIORS IN PATIENTS WITH WOUNDS

There is a wide range of behavior in patients with wounds:

- Some become deeply concerned about the wound and are motivated to learn about its cause, healing processes, and treatment. They maintain control by taking an active role in caring for the wound.
- Some react with denial and refuse to cooperate, sometimes worsening their condition by continuing, for example, to walk on an ulcerated foot.
- Some become belligerent and angry and lash out at family and caregivers.
- Some become depressed and withdrawn and may do nothing or react passively.
- Some say one thing and do another; for example, patients may state they have quit smoking while continuing to do so.
- Some set a goal for the healing to be completed, such as a social event that encourages them to learn and be compliant with treatment.
- Some patients may enjoy the attention and seek to continue getting this attention when the wound is healed.

Wound Care: Education and Referral

PSYCHOSOCIAL FACTORS AFFECTING CARE

Psychosocial factors affecting care include:

- **Ability to learn/perform care**: Cognitive impairment and hearing or vision deficits may interfere with the ability to learn, especially if appropriate educational materials are not available. Physical disabilities may make it difficult for patients to learn or perform some aspects of care. Language differences may result in impaired comprehension.
- **Economic implications**: Patients and families may be severely impacted if the wage earner is unable to continue to work or if they lack the resources (insurance, financial) to pay for needed care.
- **Education**: Patients may lack an adequate educational background to understand the implications of disease, to read materials, and to follow directions. Health literacy may be very low, so patients may have misconceptions about disease.
- **Mental status**: Patients often experience increased stress associated with illness, and this may interfere with functioning. Mental impairment may impact a patient's ability to participate in care. Additionally, depression is common, especially with chronic illness, and may cause patients to withdraw or fail to comply with treatment.

Patient Safety

PERFORMING PATIENT TRANSFER FROM CHAIR TO BED

Transferring a patient from chair to bed consists of the following steps:

1. Apply bed brakes and place the bed in the lowest position. A lift sheet should be on the bed.
2. Place the wheelchair next to the bed so the patient moves toward the stronger side if one side of the body is weak.
3. Lock brakes and remove the footrests.
4. Place a gait belt around the patient's waist.
5. Be sure the belt is not placed over a female patient's breasts.
6. Instruct the patient to push down on the arms of the chair if able to while standing up.
7. Perform a stand-pivot-transfer.
8. Seat the patient on the bed as far back as possible.
9. Help the patient turn onto the bed by lifting the legs as the patient turns.
10. Instruct the patient to press down on the bed during the turn to help prevent friction on the buttocks.
11. Two people should use the lift sheet to hoist the patient to the proper position in the middle of the bed.

PERFORMING PATIENT TRANSFER FROM CHAIR TO CHAIR

When transferring a patient from chair to chair, first instruct the patient in the transfer procedure. Position the chair that the patient is to be transferred to in a position that is slightly oblique to the first chair and lock the brakes if either chair is a wheelchair. The patient should be moving toward the strong side if one side of the body is weak:

1. Remove the footrests from the wheelchair.
2. Place a gait belt around the patient's waist.
3. Be sure that the belt is not placed over a female patient's breasts.
4. Instruct the patient to push down on the arms of the chair if able to while standing up.
5. Perform a stand-pivot-transfer.
6. Instruct the patient to reach down to grasp the arms of the chair as you help him or her sit.
7. Help the patient to readjust position until seated properly in the chair.
8. Reapply footrests to the wheelchair and position them so that the thighs are in a 90° angle to the body.
9. If the patient is paraplegic, use two people to accomplish the transfer.

PERFORMING PATIENT TRANSFER FROM BED TO STRETCHER

The following are steps for patient transfer from bed to stretcher:

1. Lower the side rails of the bed and lock the brakes.
2. Place the stretcher next to the bed and lock its brakes as well.
3. Raise the bed to the level of the stretcher.
4. While the patient is lying supine, instruct him/her to place the arms across the body.
5. One person should be next to the bed and two people should be on the outside of the stretcher.
6. On the count of three, all three people should lift the sheet slightly as the two next to the stretcher pull the patient across the gap and onto the middle of the stretcher.
7. Place a pillow under the patient's head and cover with a blanket.
8. Raise the head of the stretcher to a comfortable level.
9. Raise the side rails of the stretcher, unlock the wheels, and transport the patient.

Wound Care: Education and Referral

Evidence Based Practice

EVIDENCE-BASED RESEARCH AND WOUND CARE

For many years, common practice was accepted as evidence of effectiveness with little or no research to support or refute the perception; however, since the 1970s, when Archie Cochrane first advocated the need for research to support practice, evidence-based research has become one of the primary change agents in the practice of medicine. Evidence-based research provides information about the most successful approaches to wound care and also provides information about the areas of wound care that need further research. As part of evidence-based research, the researcher should review the current literature that is reliable and relevant, such as juried journals and collections, such as the Cochrane Collaboration, which provides metanalysis of similar studies to determine the most reliable information regarding outcomes. Relevant journals include *Advances in Wound Care; Journal of Wound Care; Advances in Skin & Wound Care; International Wound Journal; Journal of Wound, Ostomy, and Continence Nursing; Ostomy Wound Management;* and *The International Journal of Lower Extremity Wounds.* An online resource for peer-reviewed information is *World Wide Wounds.*

LEVELS OF EVIDENCE

Levels of evidence are categorized according to the scientific evidence available to support the recommendations, as well as existing state and federal laws. While recommendations are voluntary, they are often used as a basis for state and federal regulations:

- **Category IA** is well supported by evidence from experimental, clinical, or epidemiologic studies and is strongly recommended for implementation.
- **Category IB** has supporting evidence from some studies, has a good theoretical basis, and is strongly recommended for implementation.
- **Category IC** is required by state or federal regulations or is an industry standard.
- **Category II** is supported by suggestive clinical or epidemiologic studies, has a theoretical basis, and is suggested for implementation.
- **Category III** is supported by descriptive studies (such as comparisons, correlations, and case studies) and may be useful.
- **Category IV** is obtained from expert opinion or authorities only.
- **Unresolved** means there is no recommendation because of a lack of consensus or evidence.

RESEARCH METHODS FOR WOUND CARE PRACTICE

Various research methods can be applied to wound care practice. However, wound care practices should be based on evidence-based research already conducted as there must be justification for the interventions chosen. Clear definitions should be developed for inclusion, exclusion, and eligibility criteria, and guidelines for care should be outlined. **Methodologies**:

- Randomized controlled trial comparing different approaches to wound care.
- Blind randomized assessment of initial and final wound photographs: This type of research is done after-the-fact but assessment must have clear criteria because subjective evaluations may vary.
- Standardization of treatment so that all healthcare providers utilize the same steps and criteria for assessment, such as assessment by digital measurement, to determine if this makes a difference in outcomes.
- Comparing digital measurements with standard measurements to determine accuracy.
- Molecular level research utilizing tissue samples.
- Observational studies may include cohort studies, case-control studies, matched studies, and cross-sectional studies.

Multidisciplinary Team

MULTIDISCIPLINARY TEAMS

A multidisciplinary team is comprised of experts in a number of different fields, collaborating to address the complex problems associated with wound care and underlying pathology. Instead of the serial approach to problem-solving involved in the traditional model of care, where referrals are made in response to problems that arise with little communication among specialists, the multidisciplinary approach is to identify potential problems and institute preventive measures at their onset, with all members communicating and sharing information. Responsibilities of the wound care team include:

- **Prevention**: Establish standard risk assessment protocols and formulary. Incorporate national prevention guidelines.
- **Treatment**: Establish clinical protocols and product formularies in relation to national treatment practice guidelines.
- **Documentation**: Provide standardized methods.
- **Education**: Provide literature/training for patients and staff.
- **Quality Management**: Evaluate outcomes and disseminate findings.
- **Research**: Conduct clinical trials.
- **Care conferences**: Create individualized care plans.

ADVANTAGES

A team of individuals with expertise in wound care brings a combination of years of experience and skill to the patient's bedside. They use this skill to assess the wound and determine the range of treatments and dressings that would be effective. They consider the cost of the supplies and the patient's individual health, emotional status, and financial status when choosing treatments that will accomplish the goal of healing. The team may designate staff nurses to carry out treatments and assess the wound on a weekly and PRN (as needed) basis to evaluate the efficacy of treatment and to document wound progress. The team is able to evaluate progress consistently using the same people to assess wounds week after week. The team can also spot facility-wide needs in terms of skin trauma prevention, propose changes in techniques, procedures, and equipment, and evaluate the improvements. They can do research to determine new treatments available and do trials on wound care methods in the facility, contributing to evidence-based care.

INDICATIONS FOR REFERRALS TO SPECIALISTS

Various specialists may be indicated for referral in the care of specific patients:

- **Occupational therapist**: Patients with weakness, disability, or impairments may need OT to assist them in carrying out ADLs and IADLs and finding and using appropriate assistive devices.
- **Physical therapist**: Patients with physical weakness or disability may need PT to maintain or improve strength and mobility and to prevent further deterioration.
- **Nutritionist**: Patients may need nutritional guidance to ensure an adequate diet to meet specific needs, such as high protein diets for wound healing and low-calorie diets for obesity.
- **Diabetes educator**: Diabetic patients are at risk of multiple complications, so information about disease, diet, medications, lifestyle choices, foot/skin care, and preventive measures is critical.
- **Podiatrist**: Patients with poor mobility or vision, especially diabetics, should see podiatrists for routine nail trimming and foot care to prevent problems.
- **Dermatologist**: Patients with rashes or skin lesions need to be examined and treated and may need periodic skin checks.
- **Case manager**: The case manager serves as a resource for clients with multiple or chronic health problems and provides information to help them to make care decisions, to obtain healthcare services, and to achieve quality outcomes.

Wound Care: Education and Referral

REFERRALS FOR MEDICAL/SURGICAL INTERVENTIONS

Referrals for medical surgical interventions are an important part of wound care as healing requires that medical conditions be monitored carefully and treated, especially such disorders as diabetes and peripheral vascular disease, but this is also true of almost all acute or chronic disorders. Conditions that were stable prior to wound development may deteriorate or change in character in response to the body's needs during healing or infections that may occur. Patients may require referrals, such as to endocrinologists or infectious disease specialists. Wounds with extensive eschar may require surgical debridement in order to promote healing. It is important that the patient be an integral member of any planning and discussion. The patient must be apprised of the reasons for referrals and the types of testing, care, and procedures that will be done to ensure cooperation and to alleviate the patient's fears and anxiety.

HANDOFF/TRANSITION OF PATIENTS WITH WOUNDS

When a patient with a wound is to be transferred, such as to a different department, a different level of care, a different facility, or to the patient's home, **handoff/transition** should include complete documentation and verbal communication regarding:

- Demographic information, such as name, diagnoses, address, and telephone number
- List of medications and treatments
- Equipment/supplies needed for care
- Teaching strategies utilized with patient/caregiver and response
- Consultations/referrals, such as to social workers of specialists
- Follow-up needed, such as appointments and rehabilitation
- Documentation of all wounds, including discussion of location, size, depth, induration, drainage, granulation, infection, eschar, tunneling, and abscesses
- Notation of any high-risk pressure areas
- Explanation of all past and current approaches to wound therapies and patient/caregiver response
- Explanation of all past and current approaches to wound prevention (positioning, seat cushions, air mattresses and response)
- Psychosocial barriers to care or compliance, such as cognitive impairment, physical disabilities, poverty, and lack of support system
- Nutritional guidelines (high protein) to promote healing

Legal Concepts

PROTECTING PATIENT'S PRIVACY DURING WOUND CARE

Wound care should be done in a private area so others cannot observe the treatment. The room should have a door and a curtain around the bed area. One should always knock and wait for permission prior to entering the room or going behind a drawn curtain. When providing wound care, one should uncover only the part of body being treated, keeping the rest of the body covered and warm. Other people should not be in the room unless assistance is needed for the wound care, and the wound should not be discussed with others in the room without including the patient in the discussion. Schedules for turning or other wound care should not be posted in public areas. If the patient has visitors, one must not detail wound care or discuss other private healthcare matters with the patient in front of them.

STANDARD OF CARE REQUIREMENTS FOR DISCOVERY OF A PRESSURE INJURY

Upon discovery of a pressure injury, the actions of the facility and its providers are judged against a standard of care to determine liability. Swift action according to policy is the best defense:

- Measure and document the injury, including staging if possible.
- Conduct a pain assessment.
- Take action to dress the wound and take pressure off the area.
- Document physician notification, the response, and orders given.
- Clarify that the physician will notify the family.
- Implement treatment measures promptly and document them.
- Make referrals if needed to evaluate nutrition and hydration status or to do vascular studies.
- Add the new problems and interventions to the patient care plan.
- Consistently document the treatments, dressing changes, and wound status on a form and in narrative notes in one place on the chart.

LEGAL REQUIREMENTS FOR PRESSURE INJURY PREVENTION

A facility can be held liable for failure to prevent pressure injuries. There must be an effort to assess the patient for risk factors for skin breakdown at admission. When risk is found, the physician must be notified and treatment or preventive measures must be taken. Those measures must be evaluated for efficacy in prevention of breakdown and changed as needed. All interventions for risk factors must be incorporated in the patient's care plan and documentation must show that all interventions were employed as written. Pressure injuries can still develop on patients who are critically ill in spite of these measures, but when the facility can prove that preventive measures were routinely taken, they are not held liable. Medicare does not assign a higher-paying DRG for pressure injuries unless they were already evident on admission. Any organization that deviates from state or federal regulations related to prevention of pressure injuries may be legally liable.

TIME OUT PROCEDURE

A time out must occur just prior to a procedure, such as an incision or puncture of the skin of a patient or an insertion of a foreign body into the patient's body. During the time out, the participants in the procedure verify that it is the right patient and right procedure on the right portion of the body. Patient position is checked and the proper equipment and implants are verified for the procedure. Time out takes place in the room where the procedure is to be performed. This time out must be documented in the patient's record, including the names of the entire team who participate in the time out. The Joint Commission mandates the time out as part of the process developed to prevent medical errors. The other two steps in this process are pre-operative verification and marking of the correct portion of the body prior to the procedure. Time outs are NOT required before a venipuncture, urinary catheter insertion, or NG tube insertion.

Wound Care: Education and Referral

163

Certification and Government Regulations

Wound Care Certification

Wound Care Certification is available to licensed healthcare professionals, including those with an RN, LVN/LPN, PA, PT, PTA, OT, OTA, MD, DO, or DPM license, who meet both an education requirement and an experience requirement:

- **Education**: Either graduations from a skin/wound management educational program that meets certification criteria OR current active CWCN, CWON, CWOCN or CWS certification.
- **Experience**: Either 120 hours of hands-on clinical training with an approved preceptor (NAWCO) OR 2 years fulltime/4 years part-time experience in wound care, management, education, or research.

Applicants must pay a fee and pass the WCC certification exam. To renew the certification, the person must have a license in good standing, a current unexpired certification, and have completed 60 contact hours of approved continuing education in wound care in the previous 5 years. As with other licensed personnel, the scope of practice is determined by the state practice act appropriate to the discipline and duties may be further determined by the employing agency and job description.

Certified Wound Specialist

A Certified Wound Specialist is a licensed medical professional (OD, DPM, MD, NP, PA, PT, OT, PharmD, RD, or RN) with three or more years clinical experience working in wound care or one year of a fellowship in wound care. Candidates should have master level training in the management of wounds. While no specific wound care program is outlined, the candidate must submit documents detailing clinical experience as well as letters of recommendation. The candidate must also pass the certification examination if the clinical experience is accepted and the candidate is deemed eligible for certification. The CWS must renew certification annually by paying a fee and submitting proof of six hours of continuing education in wound care. The scope of practice may vary from state to state because it is determined by the state(s) in which the person is licensed to practice and the type of licensure. The CWS must retake the qualifying exam every 10 years.

Government Regulations Pertaining to Wound Care

Various government regulations pertaining to wound care management relate to licensure, who is allowed to provide wound care, price-setting (which may be based on outcomes), and quality measures. Regulatory bodies include OSHA (safety issues, infection control), the FDA (drugs and medical devices), and CMS (standards and reimbursement) as well as state boards of nursing, physical therapy, medicine, and osteopathy (scope of practice), but other organizations, such as the Joint Commission, WOCN society, and AAWC, provide rules and guidelines. CMS (Medicare, Medicaid) has a primary role in setting regulations that effect the entire medical and insurance industries. Reimbursement in most cases is now directly tied to the quality of care and to progress in wound healing. This has resulted in increased focus on accurate documentation and better methods of assessing and treating wounds in order to improve outcomes. Medicare regulations are consistent, although different types of facilities have different methods of reimbursement. Medicaid programs vary from one state to another, so the way in which wound care is reimbursed may also vary.

Medicare's Therapeutic Shoe Bill

Ill-fitting or stylish shoes may cause too much pressure on bony prominences or cause pressure that results in foot ulcers. Diabetic patients with Medicare Part B may be eligible for benefits under Medicare's Therapeutic Shoe Bill, passed by Congress in 1996. It is designed for diabetic patients who have inadequate circulation, foot deformities, calluses, peripheral neuropathy, a previous pre-ulcerative callus or foot ulcer, or an amputation of a portion of the foot or of the entire foot. Once a year, the patient is eligible for a combination of shoe inserts, custom made orthotics, modified depth shoes, or custom-made shoes to meet the individual's need to prevent foot ulceration. A physician, such as a podiatrist, must prescribe the shoes and specific insoles. Patients who are eligible should be informed of what is available to them under this bill to help them preserve their feet.

Ostomy Care: Assessment and Care Planning

Etiology, Risk Factors, and Screening

ANATOMY OF THE GASTROINTESTINAL SYSTEM

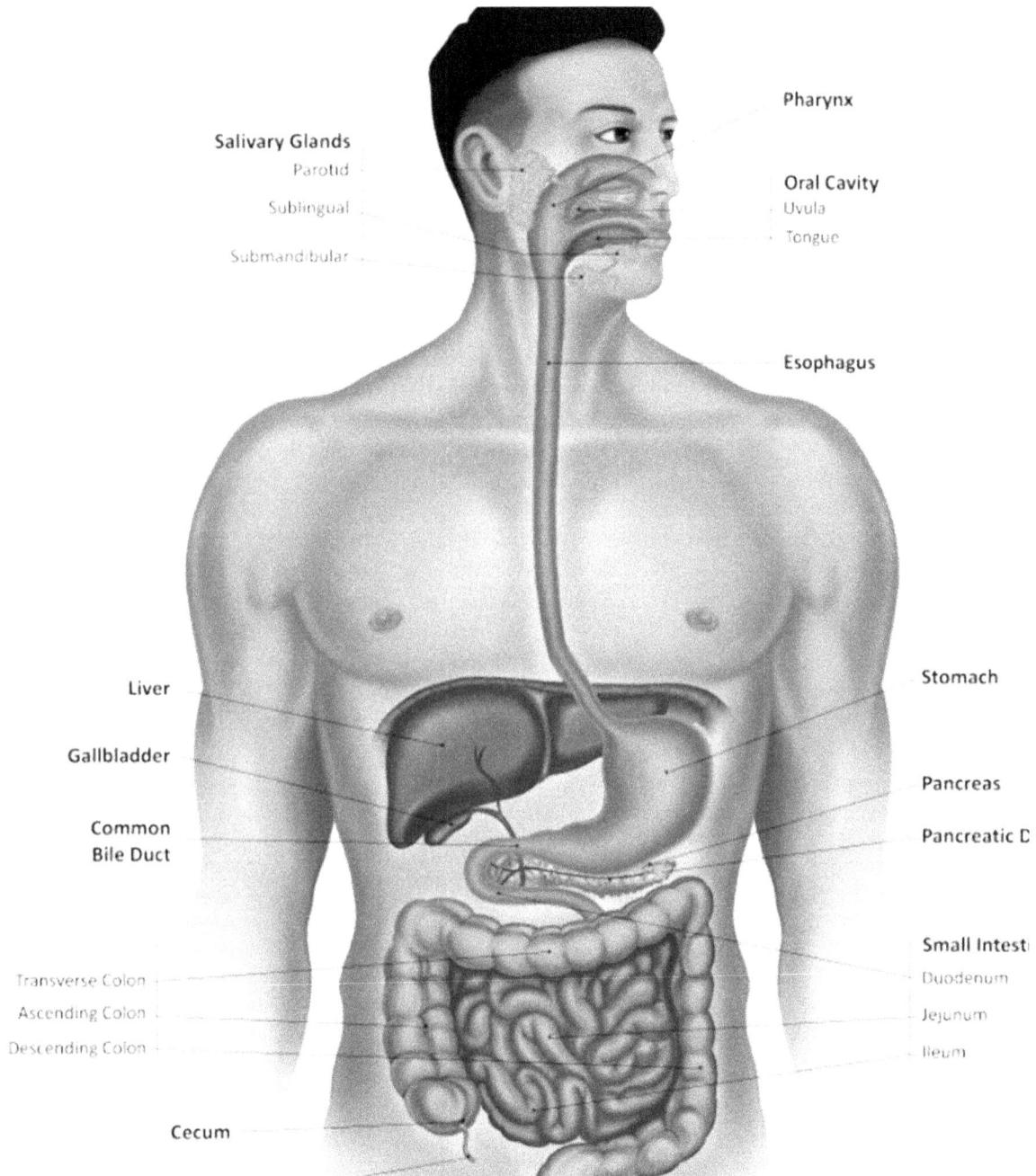

Anatomy of the Genitourinary System

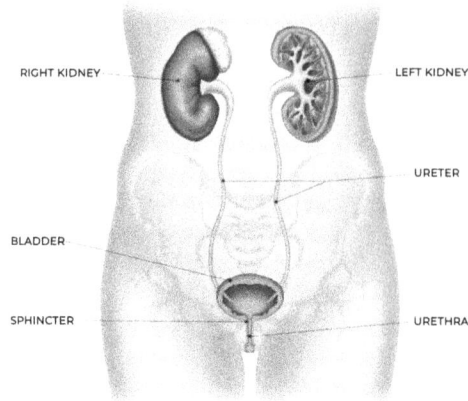

Urinary Incontinence

The different types of urinary incontinence are as follows:

- **Urge**: An urgency to urinate as soon as the bladder feels full, so person may urinate on the way to the toilet or in bed during the night. Diuretics may exacerbate urge incontinence.
- **Stress**: A sudden increase in bladder pressure from things such as coughing, laughing, or bending causes small amount of urinary leakage. It is common in people who are obese.
- **Overflow**: An overfull bladder causes dribbling of urine, usually in small amounts but the leakage can be almost constant.
- **Functional**: Incontinence caused by physical or mental impairment, such as dementia. May also be related to environmental barriers to urination, such as no accessible bathroom.
- **Reflex**: Loss of urine takes place without awareness of person because of fistula or bladder leak.
- **Mixed**: There may be more than one type of incontinence.
- **Induced**: Some surgical procedures (hysterectomy, prostatectomy, rectal surgery) can damage nerves or muscles that control urination.

Right-Sided (Ascending) Colon Cancer

Stool enters the cecum and ascending colon in liquid form, so cancers arising in these areas may grow to a large size before they cause obstruction and obvious symptoms. Lesions frequently grow into the lumen of the intestine and ulcerate, causing chronic bleeding that may not change the character or the appearance of stool. Liquid stool can pass through even a very narrow opening. 20% of colorectal tumors arise in the ascending colon.

Symptoms include:

- Fatigue: Generalized weakness.
- Pallor: Dull abdominal pain.
- Anorexia: Unexplained weight loss.
- Occult blood or melena (tarry stools).
- Hypochromic microcytic anemia.
- Chronic iron deficiency anemia.
- Palpitations or congestive heart failure related to anemia.
- Palpable abdominal mass may be evident with large tumors.

- Chronic diarrhea may rarely develop with some large right-sided lesions.
- Obstruction may occur in late stages.

TNM Staging for Adenocarcinoma of the Colon

Tumor, node, metastasis (TNM) staging is one method of staging cancer by examining the extent of the tumor, extent of lymph node involvement, and whether the cancer has metastasized. The scoring of each of those components combine to equate to the cancer's staging.

- **Stage 0**: Cancer cells are found in the lining of the intestine but have not spread to the outer layers or spread to the lymph nodes (carcinoma in situ).
- **Stage I**: Cancer has spread from the lining of the intestine into the submucosa layer and may extend into the muscle layer, but has not yet spread to the lymph nodes.
- **Stage II**: Cancer has spread to the muscle layer, the serosa, and invaded adjacent tissue, but has not yet spread to the lymph nodes.
- **Stage III**: Cancer has invaded all layers of the intestine, spread into adjacent tissue, and invaded some regional lymph nodes. The cancer has not spread to distant lymph nodes or organs.
- **Stage IV**: Cancer has spread, or metastasized, to other parts of the body, such as the liver, lungs, brain, or bones, with or without spread to the lymph nodes.

Diagnostic Testing for Bladder Cancer, Interstitial Cystitis, Refractory Radiation Cystitis, Neurogenic Bladder, and Prostate Cancer

Diagnostics for bladder cancer, interstitial cystitis, and refractory radiation cystitis include:

- **Urinalysis** identifies hematuria or other abnormalities of the urinary tract.
- **Urine culture** rules out or identifies infectious agents.
- Electrolytes, BUN, creatinine evaluates renal function.
- **CT scan/ultrasound** identifies cause of hematuria or other symptoms and identifies lesions.
- **Intravenous Pyelogram** identifies abnormalities within the entire urinary tract and rules out other causes of hematuria.
- **Cystoscopy** confirms a diagnosis, rules out other diseases, and views the type and extent of lesions.
- **Biopsy** determines the tumor grade and depth of lesion.

Diagnostics for neurogenic bladder include:

- **24-hour urine collection** determines volume and urine patterns.
- **Bladder stress test** determines reaction to full bladder while bending over, coughing, walking, or doing other activities.

Diagnostics for prostate cancer include:

- **Prostate-specific antigen test (PSA)** determines if cancer of the prostate has blocked the prostate ducts, causing an increase in blood levels of PSA.

AMERICAN CANCER SOCIETY'S RISK FACTORS FOR BLADDER CANCER

The American Cancer Society's risk factors for bladder cancer are as follows:

- **Smoking**: greatest risk factor; smokers have twice bladder cancer as nonsmokers. Carcinogens in lungs enter blood stream, are filtered by kidneys, and concentrated in urine, damaging bladder lining.
- **Occupational hazards**: exposure to aniline dye and aromatic amines and other organic chemicals.
- **Race**: Caucasians twice as likely to develop bladder cancer.
- **Age**: over 70% are over 65 years old.
- **Gender**: rate for men is 4 times that of women.
- **Chronic bladder inflammation**: especially with indwelling catheters or bladders left intact after urinary diversion.
- Previous bladder cancer: possible recurrence.
- **Congenital defects**: retention of urachus (connection between umbilicus and bladder) after birth. Exstrophy, defect in the bladder wall.
- **Genetics**: family clusters occur.
- **Chemotherapy/radiation**: high doses of cyclophosphamide and ifosfamide and radiation to pelvis.
- **Arsenic in drinking water**: risk depends upon water system meeting standards for arsenic consumption.
- **Low fluid consumption**: keeps chemicals in urine in contact with bladder.
- **Parasites**: schistosomiasis, worms lay eggs in muscle wall of bladder, causing chronic irritation.

BLADDER CANCER

Bladder cancer and most other urinary cancers begin in the inside lining of the urinary organs and then invade the deeper layers. The bladder wall and lining of urinary tract consist of several layers, from the inside wall to the outside lining:

- **Urothelium** (mucosa): Urothelial (transitional) cells line the inside layer of the urinary tract.
- **Lamina propria** (sub-mucosa): Thin layer of connective tissue.
- **Muscularis propria** (muscular): Thicker layer of muscle.
- **Serosa**: Fatty connective tissue covers superior surfaces.
- **Adventitia**: Covers areas with no serosa.

Symptoms include:

- **Gross hematuria**: Frank bright red blood may be evident. Sometimes urine brown or rust-colored. This is usually the first sign of bladder cancer. Blood in urine may appear, disappear, and reappear, usually without pain.
- **Microscopic hematuria**: Blood may be present but only visible under microscope examination.
- **Dysuria**: May have burning on urination or pain as well as feeling that bladder does not completely empty on urination, and frequency.

TYPES OF BLADDER CANCER AND CANCERS OF LINING OF OTHER URINARY ORGANS

Urothelial carcinoma: Cancer of urothelial (transitional) cells cause over 90% of these cancers, classified into subtypes:

- **Non-invasive**: Only in urothelium.
- **Invasive**: Spreads from urothelium to deeper layers.

- **Superficial**: Invasive and noninvasive cancers that have not spread or only invaded the lamina propria.
- **Flat**: Only grow in wall and may be noninvasive carcinoma affecting inner layer or invasive invading the deep layers, particularly the muscularis propria.
- **Papillary**: Tumors with finger-like projections usually growing into hollow center of bladder. Classified into subtypes:
  - Noninvasive: Only grow into center of bladder:
  - Papillomas: Benign.
  - Neoplasms: Low malignancy but may recur in more malignant form.
  - Carcinomas: Low grade rarely invade bladder wall but often recur; high grade may invade bladder wall and metastasize.
  - Invasive: Grow toward center and into wall.

Squamous cell carcinoma: Causes 4% of cancers, usually invasive.

Adenocarcinoma: Causes 1-2% of cancers; similar to intestinal cancers, invasive.

Small cell: Causes about 1% of cancers.

INTERSTITIAL CYSTITIS

Interstitial cystitis (painful bladder syndrome) causes chronic debilitating pain of bladder, urethra, and pelvic area as well as dysuria. May relate to congenital or traumatic injuries that cause inflammation and problems with urine storage and bladder emptying. The underlying cause is not known at this time. Does not respond to antibiotic therapy. Pain may persist after surgery. Affects women over men 9:1.

Symptoms include:

- Pain from mild to severe.
- Urgency.
- Frequency.
- The bladder wall may be irritated and scarred.
- Hunner's ulcers of bladder wall mucosa may occur.
- Glomerulations (pinpoint bleeding) on bladder wall.

Diagnosis is by:

- **Urinalysis**: To identify hematuria or other abnormalities of the urinary tract.
- **Urine culture**: To rule out or identify infectious agents.
- **Cystoscopy**: To confirm a diagnosis, rule out other diseases, and view the type and extent of lesions. Procedure done under anesthesia may include testing of maximum bladder capacity.
- **Biopsy**: To evaluate bladder wall.

Treatments for interstitial cystitis:

- Bladder distention sometimes relieves symptoms.
- Bladder instillation with dimethyl sulfoxide (DMSO) uses catheter to instill medication that is held for 15 minutes. Treatments every 1-2 weeks for 6-8 weeks and repeated as needed. May be self-administered.
- Medications may give relief: ASA, ibuprofen, pentosan polysulfate sodium (Elmiron).
- Transcutaneous electrical nerve stimulation (TENS) to lower back or above pubic area may relieve pelvic pain.
- Diet may affect pain. Elimination and reintroduction of foods can help to identify those exacerbating pain.

- Bladder training includes maintaining diary and scheduled voiding, gradually lengthening time between urinations.
- **Surgery** with different options available:
  - o **Fulguration**: Cystoscopic cauterizing of Hunner's ulcers to promote sloughing and healing.
  - o **Resection**: Cystoscopic resection of ulcers.
  - o **Bladder augmentation/reconstruction**: Ulcerated and inflamed tissue removed and piece of colon removed, shaped, and used to form part of bladder wall.
- Cystectomy with urinary diversion: If other treatments fail.

REFRACTORY RADIATION CYSTITIS

Refractory radiation cystitis: Damage from radiation of pelvic tumors resulting in intractable incontinence or urinary fistulas. Radiation may damage the bladder muscle or sphincter. This condition may relate to primary radiation for treatment of bladder cancer or incidental radiation from treatment of cancer in proximal areas. Treatment with both radiation and chemotherapy can increase the risk of developing this disorder. Radiation can cause damage to vessels, and deposits of collagen may result in scarring with further damage to blood vessel, which can result in tissue hypoxia and necrosis.

Symptoms may vary depending upon the degree of damage to the tissue. Early symptoms relate to submucosal inflammation, fibrosis, and ulcerations. Later symptoms related to occlusion of lumens, vascular ectasia (thinning), and vessel wall necrosis.

- **Acute/early**: Urgency, frequency, hematuria, dysuria.
- **Chronic/late**: Worsening of early symptoms and ischemia and fibrosis, leading to ulceration, fistulas, fecaluria, hydronephrosis, and incontinence.

DIAGNOSTIC PROCEDURES AND TREATMENTS

Tests are done to rule out other disorders:

- **Urinalysis**: To identify hematuria or other abnormalities.
- **Complete blood count**: To evaluate anemia/infection.
- **Urine culture**: To rule out/identify infectious agents.
- **Electrolytes, BUN, creatinine**: To evaluate renal function.
- **CT scan/ultrasound**: To identify cause of hematuria or other symptoms and identify lesions.
- **Intravenous pyelogram**: To identify abnormalities within the entire urinary tract and rule out other causes of hematuria.
- **Cystoscopy**: To confirm diagnosis, rule out other diseases, and view type and extent of lesions.

Medical management includes:

- **Anticholinergic agents**: Relieve frequency/urgency.
- **Conjugated estrogens**: Promote healing.
- **Hyperbaric oxygen therapy**: Repair vascular changes; will not reverse changes caused by significant fibrosis or ischemia. May preserve bladder function. Thirty treatments are usual.

Surgical management includes:

- **Cystoscopy with fulguration**: Treat lesions.
- **Percutaneous nephrostomy tube insertion**: Drain urine.
- **Bladder augmentation**: Correct small bladder.
- **Bladder irrigations and instillations**: Treat irritation.
- **Cystectomy with urinary diversion**: For severe cases non-responsive to medical treatment.

AMERICAN CANCER SOCIETY'S RISK FACTORS FOR PROSTATE CANCER

Risk factors for prostate cancer:

- **Age**: Risk increases after age 50 with two-thirds after 65.
- **Race**: African Americans are twice as likely to die of prostate cancer as Caucasians. Asians have the lowest rates for reasons unclear.
- **Nationality**: Most common in North America and northwestern Europe.
- **Family history**: Family clusters occur. A father or brother with prostate cancer doubles risk. Several affected relatives, especially with onset at early age, increases risk. Several inherited genes may increase risk, but genetic testing for these genes is not yet available.
- **Diet**: Diets high in red meat or high-fat dairy products with fewer fruits and vegetables may cause slight increased risk. Researchers are unsure which dietary factor raises risk.
- **Exercise**: Over age 65 may contribute to lower rate.
- **Vasectomy**: Research is inconclusive with some studies suggesting that men who have vasectomies before age 35 may have increased risk.

SMALL INTESTINE CANCER

The small bowel is part of the digestive tract, extending from the stomach to the colon. It is divided into three parts—duodenum, jejunum, and ileum—and is approximately 16 feet in length.

TYPES

The 4 main types of primary small intestine cancer are named for the type of cells from which they develop:

- **Adenocarcinomas**: Arise in lining of intestine and are the most common type, usually occurring in the duodenum.
- **Carcinoids**: Arise in hormone-producing cells in the small bowel, occurring most often in the ileum, but sometimes in the appendix.
- **Lymphomas**: Arise in the lymph tissue and are usually non-Hodgkin lymphomas, occurring most commonly in the jejunum or ileum.
- **Sarcomas**: Arise in the supportive tissues, such as fat and muscle. Leiomyosarcoma usually form in the muscle wall of the ileum. Gastrointestinal stromal tumors may develop in any part of the small intestine.

SYMPTOMS

The **symptoms of cancer of the small intestine** develop as the tumor grows, disturbing the natural functioning of the bowel. Cancer is often non-specific and vague and may resemble those of other disorders, but often worsens over time and lasts for many weeks. It is most common in people over age 50:

- Blood loss
  - Blood in stools or tarry stools from partially digested blood.
  - Anemia may develop from chronic bleeding.
- Discomfort
  - Abdominal discomfort, cramping.
  - Palpable mass may be evident.
- Inflammation
  - Chronic or recurrent diarrhea may occur.
  - Weight loss without dieting from malabsorption.
- Anorexia

- Obstruction: Complete/partial obstruction may result as cancer spreads; may be intermittent if no inflammatory disease.
  - Constipation. Nausea and vomiting. Abdominal distension.
  - Severe pain.
- Perforation (from obstruction)
  - Severe, acute pain. Hypotensive shock.
  - Abdominal distension. Peritonitis may occur.

COLORECTAL CANCER
RISK FACTORS
Risk factors for colorectal cancer include the following:

- **Adenomatous polyps**, especially large or multiple, can become cancerous.
- **Age**: Over 90% of people with colorectal cancer are over 50.
- **Alcohol intake**, especially heavy use, is linked to colorectal cancer, possibly due to alcohol's effect on folic acid.
- **Diet high in animal fats**, especially red meat, and low in fiber is a risk factor.
- **Family history** of colorectal cancer in first-degree relatives (parents, siblings, and children) is a risk factor for about 30% of those with colorectal cancer.
- **Genetic disorders** are related to cancer:
- **Familial adenomatous polyposis** (FAP) causes about 1% of colorectal cancers. Are related to this syndrome.
- **Hereditary non-polyposis colorectal cancer** (HNPCC) causes about 3-5% of colorectal cancers.
- **Inflammatory bowel disease** (ulcerative colitis and Crohn's disease) can lead to cancer.
- **Personal history** of colorectal cancer predisposes to recurrence.
- **Smoking** may account for 12% of colorectal cancers. Cancer-causing substances in cigarettes are swallowed and enter the digestive system.

SCREENING
Screening recommendations for colorectal cancer (according to the CDC):

- Screening should begin at age 45 for individuals without risk factors.
- Screening should begin earlier, generally at age 40, if risk factors are present, such as:
  - Family history of colorectal cancer in first or second-degree relatives.
  - Family history of genetic syndrome (FAP, HNLPCC).
  - Adenomatous polyps in first-degree relatives before age 60.
  - History of polyps or colorectal cancer.
  - History of inflammatory bowel disease.

Types of screening tests include:

- **Fecal occult blood**—yearly: Checks for blood in stool.
- **Flexible sigmoidoscopy**—every 5 years, or every 10 years with a fecal immunochemical test (FIT) annually: Scope to check for polyps or signs of cancer in rectum and lower third of colon. (Often done with fecal occult blood test.)

Ostomy Care: Assessment and Care Planning

- **Colonoscopy**—every 10 years or as follow-up for abnormalities in other screening: Longer flexible scope, usually with anesthesia, to check rectum and entire colon. It allows for removal of polyps, small cancerous lesions, and biopsies and provides surveillance of inflammatory bowel disease.
- **CT Colonography**—every 5 years: Digital scan using x-ray technology that captures images of the entire colon and displays them on the computer screen for analysis.

DIAGNOSTIC TESTING

Diagnostic testing for colorectal cancer includes the following:

- **Full colonoscopy** is more accurate than flexible sigmoidoscopy and better able to confirm the location of tumor and facilitate tissue biopsy and removal of polyps.
- **Double contrast barium enema** is useful with colonoscopy for right-sided lesions.
- **Complete blood testing** may indicate anemia from local blood loss. Liver chemistries may show hepatic metastasis, especially elevation of alkaline phosphatase, and tumor markers may indicate advanced disease. Carcinoembryonic antigen (CEA) may be elevated with colorectal cancer.
- **Chest x-ray** is used to rule out lung metastasis.
- **CT scan of chest** is needed if x-ray positive for added information about extent of lesions. CT of pelvic and abdominal area remains controversial for colon cancer because it does not always show liver metastasis and doesn't stage well.
- **CT scan/MRI of pelvic and abdominal area** is used for rectal cancer to verify absence of obvious metastasis.
- **Endoluminal ultrasound (ELUS)** is used to stage rectal tumors and to show extent of tumor invasion.

TYPES

Types of colorectal cancer include:

- **Adenocarcinomas** develop from epithelial tissue in adenomatous polyps and account for 90-95% of all colorectal cancers. There are two sub-types:
- **Signet ring** is a very aggressive form that is harder to treat but accounts for only 0.1% of adenocarcinomas.
- **Mucinous** is also an aggressive form that is composed of about 60% mucous, allowing the cells to spread faster and making it hard to treat. This form accounts for 10-15% of adenocarcinomas.
- **Sarcomas (Leiomyosarcoma)** develop from smooth muscle and account for less than 2% of colorectal cancers, but over 50% metastasize.
- **Carcinoids** are slow-growing tumors that rarely spread, most commonly found in the rectum and accounting for less than 1% of colorectal cancers.
- **Lymphomas** are rare and primary tumors occurring primarily in rectum while secondary metastatic tumors occur primarily in the colon.
- **Melanomas** are rare tumors usually metastasize from other parts of body; accounts for less than 2% of colorectal cancers.

DUKES' MODIFIED STAGING CLASSIFICATION

The **Dukes' staging system's original three classes have been modified to 6.** While this staging is still used, the TNM (tumor, node, and metastasis) staging is more common.

- **Class A**: Tumor invades only the mucosa of intestinal wall.
- **Class B1**: Tumor invades the muscle layer (muscularis propria) of intestinal wall, but doesn't go all the way through.

173

- **Class B2**: Tumor invades and goes all the way through the muscle layer (muscularis propria) of intestinal wall.
- **Class C1**: As in B1, tumor invades the muscle layer of the intestinal wall but doesn't go all the way through; however, there is evidence of cancerous cells in the lymph nodes.
- **Class C2**: As in B2, tumor invades and goes all the way through the muscle layer; additionally, there is evidence of cancerous cells in the lymph nodes.
- **Class D**: Tumor has metastasized beyond the lymph nodes to organs, such as liver, bones, or lungs.

TRANSVERSE, DESCENDING, SIGMOID, AND RECTAL CANCERS

Because some of the fluid in intestines is absorbed in the ascending colon, stool in the transverse and descending colon is more formed. Lesions arising in the transverse and descending colon tend to be annular constrictive lesions, encircling the intestine and leading to obstruction. Sigmoid and rectal tumors may cause pressure on adjacent structures, such as the vagina, prostate, and bladder.

Symptoms of transverse/descending cancers:

- Change in bowel habits may become evident.
- Abdominal cramping, especially left lower quadrant pain.
- "Pencil" stools from narrowing of lumen. Constipation.
- Abdominal distension. Intestinal obstruction.
- Perforation of bowel/peritonitis.

Symptoms of sigmoid/rectal cancers:

- Tenesmus (painful, ineffective straining to pass stool).
- Pain in rectal or perianal area. Feeling of fullness and incomplete evacuation of stool after bowel movement.
- Alternating constipation and diarrhea.
- Frank blood in stool, possibly blood clots.
- "Pencil" thin stools from narrowing of lumen.
- Abdominal pain and cramping.
- Urinary symptoms.
- Vaginal fistula.

NEOADJUVANT (PREOPERATIVE) RADIATION AND CHEMOTHERAPY
ADVANTAGES

A combination of radiation and chemotherapy given preoperatively has been shown to decrease the size of the tumor, allowing for more sphincter-saving procedures and a downstaging of the tumor grade. There is decreased seeding of the tumor in the operative site during surgery and less damage to the small intestine than is found with post-operative treatment. Reduction of the tumor results in better oxygenation to the surgical site. Studies have shown that neoadjuvant therapy is associated with a lower rate of metastasis and a higher rate of survival.

DISADVANTAGES

The primary disadvantage to neoadjuvant therapy is an increase in the risk of post-operative complications, such as wound infections, bowel obstructions, fistulas, ischemic ileostomy and peristomal hernia. Additionally, because it is difficult to accurately stage a tumor prior to surgery, some people may receive treatment intended for a higher stage than their actual tumor. Over-treatment with chemotherapy and radiation therapy can have long-term side effects.

Ostomy Care: Assessment and Care Planning

CROHN'S DISEASE

Crohn's disease manifests with inflammation in any part of the GI system. Inflammation is transmural, often leading to intestinal stenosis and fistulas. Inflammation is focal and discontinuous with aphthous ulcerations that progress to linear and irregular shaped ulcerations. Granulomas may also be present. The most common sites of inflammation are the terminal ileum and cecum. Condition is usually chronic, but an acute flare-up may mimic appendicitis. Children may have delayed development and stunted growth. There appears to be a genetic component to the disease.

Symptoms include:

- Perirectal abscess/fistula may be present in advanced disease.
- Diarrhea is usually present with colonic disease. May have nocturnal bowel movements, watery stools, and rectal hemorrhage.
- Anemia may develop with chronic bleeding.
- Abdominal pain is most common in lower right quadrant, usually indicates transmural inflammation; may include post-prandial pain and cramping

Other symptoms include nausea and vomiting (usually related to strictures of small intestine), weight loss (with small intestine involvement), fever, and night sweats.

ULCERATIVE COLITIS

Ulcerative colitis manifests with superficial inflammation of mucosa of colon and rectum, causing ulcerations in the areas where inflammation has destroyed cells. These ulcerations, ranging from pinpoint to extensive, may bleed and produce purulent material. The mucosa of the bowel becomes swollen, erythematous, and granular. Onset is usually between ages 15 and 30, and there is a genetic component. Ulcerative colitis may affect only the rectum (ulcerative proctitis), the entire colon (pancolitis), or only the left colon (limited or distal colitis).

Symptoms are as follows:

- Abdominal pain may be absent or mild unless disease is severe.
- Bloody diarrhea/rectal bleeding in absence of infection may result in anemia and loss of fluids and electrolytes. Diarrhea more frequent as colonic involvement increases.
- Fecal urgency and tenesmus (straining) may occur.
- Anorexia may result in weight loss, fatigue.
- Systemic disorders may manifest (eye inflammation, arthritis, liver disease, and osteoporosis) possibly because immune system triggers generalized inflammation.

DIAGNOSTIC TESTING FOR ULCERATIVE COLITIS AND CROHN'S DISEASE

Diagnostic testing for ulcerative colitis and Chron's disease includes:

- **Stool specimens** are examined for blood or pus or to rule out other disorders.
- **Flexible sigmoidoscopy** is useful for ulcerative colitis because the rectum is always affected. It can evaluate for mucosal inflammation, which is usually superficial.
- **Colonoscopy** shows extent of inflammation, especially for Crohn's disease.
- **Abdominal x-rays** can exclude complications.
- **Biopsy** shows tissue changes and lesions.
- **Technetium-labeled leukocyte scan** is used as less-invasive procedure for critically ill to determine extent of inflammation. It helps identify complications.
- **Complete blood testing** can show anemia, which may indicate chronic blood loss. Hypokalemia is related to chronic diarrhea. Hypoalbuminemia may reflect damage to mucosa of colon and/or malnutrition related to malabsorption.
- **Contrast radiography** with barium is useful for evaluating the upper GI tract for Crohn's disease.
- **CT scan, MRI, ultrasonography** may be used to identify complications
- **Serum anti-Saccharomyces cerevisiae antibody (ASCA) test** with positive finding is diagnostic of ulcerative colitis and indicative of Crohn's disease.

DIVERTICULAR DISEASE

DIAGNOSTIC TESTING

Diverticular disease is the abnormal presence of sac-like pouchings in the intestinal lining. Diverticular disease is diagnosed by a number of tests, some used to rule out other disorders:

- **CBC and liver function tests** show white count is usually elevated, but liver enzymes remain normal.
- **Urinalysis** is usually normal with diverticular disease despite dysuria.
- **CT scan with contrast of abdomen** will show inflammatory changes and rule out other abdominal disorders.
- **Barium enema** may be used to show diverticula.
- **Ultrasound** uses high-frequency sound waves and a computer to create images of the soft tissue of the intestines. It may be used to rule out gall bladder disease or obstruction.
- **Colonoscopy/flexible sigmoidoscopy** can be used only when diverticulitis is NOT present to establish extent of disease. It is the most commonly used test for diverticular disease as it allows direct visualization as well as biopsy and surgical excision.

RISK FACTORS AND SYMPTOMS

Risk factors for diverticular disease include:

- **Age**: Incidence increases with age, affecting over 50% of those over 60.
- **Nationality**: More common in developed countries, such as the United States, England, and Australia where diets lower in fiber and high in processed carbohydrates are common. Diverticular disease is rare in Asian countries. People in Western countries primarily have diverticular disease in the left colon while Asians tend to have diverticular disease in the right colon.
- **Socioeconomic**: More common among those with lower income.
- **Genetics**: Occurs in family clusters.

Symptoms of diverticulosis (diverticula present but not inflamed):

- **Absent**: May have no symptoms at all.
- **Abdominal**: Cramping and distention.
- **Intestinal**: Constipation or diarrhea. Muscles spasms in colon.

Symptoms of diverticulitis (diverticula inflamed):

- **Systemic**: Fever, chills
- **Gastrointestinal**: Nausea, vomiting, constipation, GI bleeding, blood in stool, rectal bleeding.
- **Abdominal**: Mild to severe cramping, pain (especially in left lower quadrant), abdominal tenderness.
- **Urinary**: Dysuria may be present.

NEUROGENIC BLADDER

Neurogenic bladder is bladder dysfunction from lesions of peripheral or central nervous system, related to traumatic or congenital etiologies or develop from cerebrovascular accident or diabetic neuropathy. Nerve damage can cause underactive bladder unable to contract to effectively empty the bladder or overactive bladder that contracts frequently and ineffectually. **Symptoms** vary:

- **Underactive**: Incontinence, dribbling, straining or inability to urinate, retention.
- **Overactive**: Frequency, urgency, dysuria, urinary tract infection, fever.

Diagnosis is by:

- **Neurological testing (x-rays, MRI, and EEGs)**: To determine etiology. 24-hour urine collection: To determine volume and urine patterns.
- **Bladder stress test**: To determine reaction to full bladder while bending over, coughing, walking, or doing other activities.

Treatment includes:

- **Antibiotics**: To control infections.
- **Clean intermittent catheterization** (CIC): To empty bladder.
- **Endoscopy**: Combined with cutting of external sphincter or injecting sphincter with paralytic agents to allow urination.
- **Surgical repair**: Placing of permanent stents at bladder neck, bladder augmentation to increase bladder size, repair of vesicoureteral reflux, or urinary diversion.

DIAGNOSTIC TESTING FOR RADIATION ENTERITIS, ISCHEMIC COLITIS, INTESTINAL OBSTRUCTION, AND GASTROINTESTINAL TRAUMA

Radiation enteritis:

- **Endoscopy** is used to examine intestinal mucosa for changes consistent with radiation enteritis.

Infectious enteritis:

- **Stool specimens** are examined for occult blood, ova and parasites, other organisms, and white blood cells to determine infecting agent.
- **Endoscopy** provides direct examination of the lumen of the intestines.
- **Biopsy** is done for tissue analysis and culture to identify the infecting agent.

Intestinal obstruction:

- **CT scan of abdomen** helps identify causes and location of obstruction.
- **Complete blood testing** helps to eliminate infections and other diagnoses.
- **Laparoscopy** allows direct visualization of obstruction to determine best procedure for correction.

Intestinal trauma: Tests relate to severity and location of trauma and may include a wide range, including.

- **CT scan** is done to determine the extent of the injury and complications.
- **Complete blood testing** is done to determine blood loss, clotting times, and oxygen saturation.

HIRSCHSPRUNG'S DISEASE

Hirschsprung's disease is a congenital disorder in which infants are born without intestinal ganglion nerve cells in part or the entire colon, causing mechanical obstruction. It may be an acute life-threatening or chronic condition.

Normally, nerves signal the colon to contract, pushing the stool through the colon, but the absence of propulsion in the segments without ganglions causes the fecal material to accumulate. Affected areas almost always include the rectum and distal colon, but in rare instances can skip segments and involve the entire colon, including the small intestine. As fecal material collects, the segment of the bowel proximal to the defect distends, creating megacolon. The internal rectal sphincter may fail to relax as well, preventing evacuation and contributing to obstruction. Hirschsprung's disease accounts for about 25% of all neonatal obstructions, is 4 times more common in males than females, may have a genetic link, and is more common in children with Down syndrome.

The **symptoms** of Hirschsprung's disease in the neonatal period, infancy, and childhood are as follows:

- Neonatal period:
  - No meconium within 24-48 hours after birth, although rectal stimulation during the physical exam after birth may cause a small amount of meconium to be expelled.
  - Reluctance to nurse/bottle feed. Vomitus stained with bile. Abdominal distension from gas and accumulated fecal material.
- Infancy:
  - Underweight/failure to thrive. Chronic constipation.
  - Abdominal distension. Episodes of diarrhea and vomiting.
  - Loud bowel sounds with gurgling. Enterocolitis—fever, explosive watery diarrhea (stool frothy, green with foul odor), severe prostration with symptoms of sepsis.
- Childhood:
  - Thin, poorly nourished appearance. Anemia. Chronic cycles of constipation. Foul stools with ribbon-like appearance.
  - Abdominal distension with visible peristaltic waves. Fecal masses palpable in abdomen.

Diagnosis is based on symptoms, which may vary, so diagnosis may be delayed until infancy or childhood when acute enterocolitis occurs. Procedures include:

- Abdominal x-rays. Barium enema done without preparation.
- Anorectal manometry. Full-thickness rectal biopsy showing absence of ganglion cells.

IMPERFORATE ANUS

Imperforate anus (anorectal malfunction) is a congenital abnormality where the rectum is absent, malformed, or displaced from normal position. It may include disorders of the urinary tract. Imperforate anus occurs in 1 in 5000 births, more commonly in males than females. Imperforate anus may include stenosis or atresia of anus. There are 3 main categories, classified according to relationship of rectum to puborectalis musculature:

- **Low anomalies**: No external opening, but rectum is otherwise in normal position through the puborectalis muscle, with normal function, and no connection to the genitourinary tract.
- **Intermediate anomalies**: Rectum is at or below the level of puborectalis muscle and an anal dimple is evident. The external sphincter is in normal position.
- **High anomalies**: Rectum ends above the puborectalis muscles, and internal sphincter is absent. Frequently, there is a rectourethral fistula in males or a rectovaginal fistula in females. There may be fistulas to the bladder or perineum.

Symptoms include:

- **Absence of anal opening**: No meconium in 24-48 hours, Abdominal distension, and vomiting.
- **Rectovaginal fistula or rectourethral fistula**: Symptoms may not be evident at first because stool passes through fistula.
- **Fistula between the rectum and the bladder**: Gas or fecal material may be expelled per the urethra.
- **Displacement of the anus**: Chronic constipation develops over time.

Diagnosis includes:

- Physical examination.
- Digital or endoscopic examination.
- Contrast radiography with the infant inverted and an opaque marker at the anal dimple will outline the location of a pouch in relation to the normal position of the anus.

Most forms of **treatment** require surgery, type depending upon extent of abnormality:

- Simple excision for anal opening may suffice.
- 2-3 step procedures for higher anomalies in which a colostomy is first performed with later reconstruction of the anus in the proper position, involving anoplasty and pull through procedures.
- Manual dilation may treat stenosis.

NECROTIZING ENTEROCOLITIS

Necrotizing enterocolitis is acute inflammatory disease of bowel, especially in preterm and high-risk infants, resulting in necrosis and frequent perforation, affecting large or small intestines or both and often the ileocecal area. "Skip" areas of necrosis may be present, making surgical treatment difficult. The causes of necrotizing enterocolitis are not completely clear, but vascular compromise occurs, often related to an episode of hypoxia or sepsis or post blood transfusion. The hypoxic condition in the intestines causes damage and necrosis to mucosal cells so bowels can't secrete protective mucus, making the intestine susceptible to bacterial infection. Three factors are implicated: feeding, injury to intestinal mucosa, and bacterial infection.

Symptoms usually appear 3-10 days after childbirth and range from mild Abdominal distension to severe sepsis:

- Hypotension.
- Apnea.
- Decrease in urinary output.
- Vomiting/gastric retention.
- Temperature fluctuations.
- Irritability.
- Lethargy.
- Blood in stools or gastric aspirate (occult or gross).
- Poor feeding.

Diagnosis includes:

- **Careful physical examination**: Observing for signs of peritonitis
- **Monitoring of abdominal girth** to determine degree of distention.
- **Laboratory findings**: Neutropenia, thrombocytopenia, and metabolic acidosis. Abdominal x-rays: One every 6-8 hours to observe for perforation. Contrast studies: Carry risk of perforation, but are occasionally done with water-soluble contrast medium.

Treatment:

Both **medical** management and **surgical** repair may be needed although severely compromised infants are not good surgical candidates:

- **Medical treatment**: Discontinuation of oral fluids and administration of intravenous fluids. Nasogastric decompression. Correction of fluid and electrolyte imbalances. Oxygen to correct hypoxia. Systemic antibiotics for infection. Transfusions.
- **Surgical treatment**: Varies, depending upon extent and location of necrosis, and may involve creation of ileostomy, jejunostomy, or colostomy as permanent or temporary diversion. Some surgeons remove clearly necrotic tissue while others avoid resection. One or more stomas may be established. Closure of stoma is usually done 1-4 months after initial surgery.

MALROTATION AND OMPHALOCELE

Malrotation is an abnormality during fetal development in the rotation and fixation of the midgut area. With ischemia or bowel necrosis, pre- or post-operatively, fecal diversions may be needed.

Omphalocele is a congenital herniation of intestines or other organs through the base of the umbilicus with a protecting amniotic membrane but no skin. The sac may contain only a loop or most of the bowel and the internal abdominal organs. This sac differentiates gastroschisis from omphalocele. Diagnosis is usually with fetal ultrasound.

Symptoms vary widely. Maintaining integrity of tissues by keeping exposed sac or viscera moist and providing intravenous fluids is important. Small omphaloceles are repaired immediately, but more extensive repair is usually delayed until the infant is stable if the sac is intact. Silvadene® cream toughens the sac, which is usually covered with a Silastic® (plastic) pouch to protect the tissue. The abdomen may be unusually small, making correction difficult, so surgeons may wait 6-12 months while the abdominal cavity grows. Surgical repair may be done in stages over 8-10 days.

GASTROSCHISIS

Gastroschisis is extrusion of the non-rotated midgut through the abdominal wall to the right of the umbilicus with no protective membrane covering matted, thickened loops of intestine. The abnormality is usually small, but the stomach and almost all of the small and large intestines can protrude. Because the intestines float without protection in amniotic fluid, there may be severe damage to the intestines with bowel atresia and ischemia. Gastroschisis is usually diagnosed with fetal ultrasound and is obvious at birth. These infants lose body temperature, fluids, and electrolytes and receive intravenous fluids. The exposed organs are covered with sterile plastic film for protection and to prevent fluid loss and a nasogastric feeding tube is inserted. Primary closure is done when the infant stabilizes for small abnormalities. Larger abnormalities may require stages with only part of organs returned to the cavity and the remaining covered with a Silastic pouch until the abdominal cavity grows and surgical repair can be completed.

UMBILICAL HERNIA

An umbilical hernia is a skin-covered herniation of intestine and omentum through an abdominal wall defect near the umbilicus caused by an incomplete closure of the umbilical ring. The herniation may range from 1-5 cm in size and may be obvious on physical examination or felt on palpation. It may appear flat when the child is supine but protrude when the child is upright or crying. Approximately 1 in 6 infants are born with umbilical hernias. Symptoms are usually absent unless strangulation of the hernia occurs, and then the infant may cry with pain, feed poorly, vomit, and have an increase in temperature. The abdomen may become distended. In this case, emergency surgical repair must be done. Treatment usually involves just observing the hernia for complications as, in most cases it will reduce on its own. If the hernia is still present at 3-4 years, a simple surgical repair of the hernia may be done.

MESOCOLIC PARADUODENAL HERNIA

Mesocolic paraduodenal hernia is an internal herniation of the small intestinal loops in the paraduodenal area due to incomplete rotation of the small intestine, resulting in intestinal loops becoming trapped in the mesentery of the descending colon. Right and left hernias are separate entities. Right (Waldeyer's hernia) results in the small bowel being trapped behind the mesentery of the right and transverse colon. With left, the herniated sac is to the left of the duodenum and the inferior mesenteric vessels are on the anterior margin. Some infants are asymptomatic and the condition may go undiagnosed. Infants may have frequent indigestion, and some go on to develop chronic digestive problems, but acute bowel obstruction with strangulation and perforation may occur. Radiographic studies with contrast are done for diagnosis. Surgical reduction with repositioning of the bowel is done to repair the hernia if there are no complications, such as strangulation, which may require more extensive repair.

CONGENITAL DIAPHRAGMATIC HERNIA

Congenital diaphragmatic hernia is herniation of abdominal contents into chest cavity. During fetal development, a hole in the diaphragm that should close at about 3 months stays open, allowing loops of the intestine or the stomach to herniate into the chest and preventing adequate development of the lungs (pulmonary hypoplasia) and/or heart. The infants are usually very dyspneic at birth and may need to be ventilated. They may need temporary heart/bypass as well. The kidneys are often enlarged. Radiographic studies are done to show the extent of the abnormality, usually showing a high gastrointestinal obstruction, often at the duodenum. A nasogastric feeding tube is inserted and an intravenous line. Supportive treatment is given for dyspnea as well as correction of acidosis. Surgical repair may be done after birth or delayed for weeks until child stabilizes. Surgical repair may be done in one stage or more, depending upon the degree of abnormality.

INTUSSUSCEPTION

Intussusception is telescoping of one portion of intestine into the next, usually distal small intestine near ileocecal junction moving into the ascending colon and causing obstruction, inflammation, edema, and ischemia of the involved intestine. It usually occurs between 5-10 months, but can occur from 3 months to 6 years. It occurs 3-4 times more frequently in males.

Symptoms include:

- Acute onset of severe intermittent abdominal pain.
- Loud frantic crying with knees drawn to chest.
- Vomiting.
- Bloody mucoid stool resembling currant jelly.
- Sausage-like abdominal mass, usually in right upper lateral region and along transverse colon.

Diagnosis is by physical examination, abdominal x-rays or ultrasound, and contrast enemas.

Treatment includes:

- **Non-surgical**: Hydrostatic reduction using barium or air if no evidence of peritonitis or gangrene.
- **Surgical**:
  - Laparotomy with manual reduction.
  - Resection and anastomosis: Irreducible areas dissected.
  - Fecal diversion (rare): If bowel ends too inflamed and swollen for anastomosis.

Meconium Ileus

Meconium ileus is the obstruction of the ileum with inspissated (thick) mucilaginous meconium that clings to the side of the narrowed lumen of the intestine and forms hard pellets in infants with cystic fibrosis. This is usually the first clinical sign of cystic fibrosis. A complicated meconium ileus may involve volvulus, gangrene, perforations, peritonitis, or bowel atresia. Meconium ileus must be differentiated from Hirschsprung's disease, which presents with similar symptoms.

Symptoms include:

- **Uncomplicated**: Abdominal distension, vomiting, no meconium in first 24-48 hours.
- **Complicated**: Pain, fever, erythema, and edema of abdominal wall consistent with peritonitis.

Diagnosis is by abdominal x-rays to show air-fluid levels and contrast enemas to show obstruction.

Treatment:

Contrast enema with water-soluble contrast: May relieve obstruction by emulsifying fecal material. 10-15 cc small volume enemas: To flush stool, especially after contrast enema. Enterotomy: With proximal instillation of wetting agent. Resection of colon/fecal diversion: For perforated or gangrenous bowel.

Persistent Cloaca

Persistent cloaca is a condition in females with an **imperforate anus** and the rectum, vagina, and urethra forming a **single channel**, with a rectal fistula attached to the posterior wall of the channel. Diagnosis is made with a physical exam showing a single perineal opening. An abdominal mass (hydrocolpos— distended bladder) may occur. A voiding cystourethrogram (VCUG) will show bladder abnormalities if catheterization is possible.

Treatments include:

- **Colostomy**: Fecal diversion in neonate prevents fecal material from entering urinary system and causing infection.
- **Decompression of vagina**: Decompression prevents infection and scarring and relieves obstruction of urinary tract.
- **Posterior sagittal anorectovagino-urethroplasty (PSARVUP)**: This is usually done 2 months after colostomy. The rectum is separated from the vagina, the vagina is separated from the urethra, the urethra is reconstructed, the vagina is reconstructed, and the rectum is reconstructed with anoplasty.
- **Postoperative anal dilation**: Dilation begins 2 weeks after surgery until final size is reached.
- **Cystoscopy/ vaginoscopy**: Check for urethrovaginal fistula.
- **Colostomy removal**: Anastomosis of colon and rectum and colostomy removed.

CLOACAL EXSTROPHY

Cloacal exstrophy is a rare and complicated disorder of pelvic area, usually including multiple abnormalities, such as omphalocele with abdominal viscera covered by thin membrane outside of abdomen; exstrophy of bladder, which is bivalve and surrounds the intestinal mucosa at midline and communicates with the rectum; imperforate anus; spinal defects; and genital abnormalities, such as vaginal duplication, agenesis, or atresia. May also include multiple urinary, spinal, and skeletal abnormalities. **Symptoms** vary widely depending on abnormalities. **Diagnosis** is made by physical examination and renal ultrasound to assess kidneys.

Treatment:

Surgical repair is done in stages, beginning with separation of urinary and intestinal systems and creation of intestinal stoma. If possible, primary closure of bladder and repair of omphalocele are done with initial surgery. Reconstruction of urinary and reproductive system is usually done when the child stabilizes and weight is ≥9 kilograms. The intestinal stoma is permanent, but urinary continence may be through urinary diversion or reconstruction.

BLADDER EXSTROPHY

Bladder exstrophy is eversion of posterior wall of the bladder through anterior wall of the bladder and through the lower abdominal wall with bladder and urethra exposed, a wide pubic arch, anterior displacement of the anus, renal disorders, and abnormalities of reproductive organs in both males and females. **Symptoms** include urinary and bowel problems related to specific anomalies. **Diagnosis** is by physical examination to assess abnormalities. Renal ultrasound is done to determine the number of kidneys and presence of hydroureteronephrosis.

First stage treatment includes:

- **Primary closure of bladder**: No ostomy necessary if done within 72 hours of birth. Procedures include ureteral stents and suprapubic urinary drainage.
- **Bilateral iliac ostomies**: Necessary after 72 hours because pelvic ring is not malleable.
- **Epispadias repair**: May be done in first or second stage.

Second stage treatment includes:

- **Epispadias repair**: Usually done between 6-12 months.

Final stage of treatment includes:

- Bladder neck reconstruction and reimplantation of ureters.
- Permanent urinary diversion: Required by 10-15%.

MEGAURETER

Megaureter is dilation of ureters from the normal 3-5 mm to more than 10 mm in diameter with or without obstruction and/or reflux from abnormality of ureters or secondary causes:

- **Primary obstruction**: At point where ureter joins bladder; can cause kidney damage.
- **Refluxing**: Backward flow of urine from bladder to ureters.
- **Non-obstructing/non-refluxing**: Dilated ureters without blockage may resolve over time.
- **Obstructed/refluxing**: Ureters continue to dilate with blockage.
- **Secondary**: Ureters enlarge because of other conditions, such as neurogenic bladder.

Symptoms include urinary tract infection, dysuria, back pain, and fever.

Diagnosis is by:

- **Fetal ultrasound**: in utero diagnosis
- **Ultrasound**: To evaluate appearance of urinary tract
- **Voiding cystourethrogram (VCUG)**: To check for reflux
- **Diuretic renal scan**: To check for obstruction
- **Intravenous pyelogram**: To view urinary system

Treatment includes:

- **Antibiotic prophylaxis**: Until surgery.
- **Ureteral implantation**: Trimming widened portion of ureter; removing obstruction and reattaching.

PRUNE BELLY (EAGLE-BARRETT) SYNDROME

Prune belly (Eagle-Barrett) syndrome is a group of abnormalities involving lack of developed abdominal muscles, undescended testicles, and urinary tract problems. Urinary abnormalities may include large, hypotonic bladder, dilated ureters, and prostatic urethra. Males comprise 96-99% of cases. It may include anomalies of the pulmonary, cardiac, skeletal, and GI tracts.

Symptoms vary widely, frequently including cardio-pulmonary complications:

- **Prune-like appearance of abdomen**: From fetal Abdominal distension. After birth, abdominal fluid is lost and abdomen develops wrinkled "prune" appearance, noticeable because of undeveloped abdominal muscles. Undescended testicles: Bilaterally.
- **Urinary tract abnormalities**: Urinary infections, obstruction, and chronic renal failure. Diagnosis is by physical examination, chest x-rays to evaluate pulmonary problems, renal ultrasound to evaluate kidneys, and voiding cystourethrogram (VCUG) to evaluate urinary defects.

Management includes the following:

- Monitor condition. Antibiotics, therapeutic and prophylactic.
- Intermittent catheterization. Surgical repair to correct genitourinary defects varies according to abnormality. Procedures may include: Vesicostomy, ureterostomy, or pyelostomy.

Ostomy Care: Assessment and Care Planning

- Reduction cystoplasty, urethroplasty.
- Abdominoplasty.

URETEROPELVIC JUNCTION OBSTRUCTION

Ureteropelvic junction obstruction (UPJ) is congenital obstruction at the point where the ureter connects to the renal pelvis, unilaterally or bilaterally, causing inadequate urinary flow and hydronephrosis. Some children improve markedly within the first 18 months, but others require surgery.

Symptoms include:

- Urinary tract infections.
- Abdominal or flank pain
- Palpable mass from hydronephrosis.
- Vomiting.

Diagnosis is based on:

- **Fetal ultrasound**: in utero diagnosis.
- **Renal ultrasound**: To show dilation of renal pelvis.
- **Intravenous pyelogram (IVP)**: To identify obstruction.
- **Renal isotope scan**: To evaluate and measure kidney function.

Treatment includes:

- **Fetal urinary diversion**: Remains controversial.
- **Pyeloplasty**: Open surgical procedure where ureteropelvic junction is excised and ureter reattached to renal pelvis with wide junction, allowing adequate drainage.
- **Laparoscopic pyeloplasty**: Through abdominal wall and abdominal cavity with internal excision of ureteropelvic junction.
- **Insertion of wire through ureter**: To cut ureteropelvic junction from inside with a ureteral drain left in place for a few weeks.

VESICOURETERAL REFLUX

Vesicoureteral reflux is an abnormality where urine flows from the bladder back up the ureter. Reflux is graded on a scale of 1-5, depending upon the degree of dilation of the ureter and renal pelvis.

- **Primary**: Congenital defect with impaired valve where ureter opens to bladder. The ureter may be too short so the valve doesn't close properly.
- **Secondary**: Caused by infection or other cause of obstruction.

Symptoms of urinary tract infection are most common:

- **Neonates**: Fever, irritability, lethargy, emesis.
- **Older infants, children**: Abdominal pain, emesis, diarrhea, fever, dysuria with enuresis, frequency, urgency, cloudy/foul urine.
- **Late symptoms**: Hypertension, dysuria with difficulty urinating, proteinuria, chronic renal insufficiency.

Diagnosis is by:

- **Ultrasound**: Evaluate appearance of urinary system.
- **Voiding cystourethrogram (VCUG)**: Identify reflux (after infection has cleared).
- **Intravenous pyelogram**: Reveal obstructions.
- **Nuclear scans**: Show urinary functioning
- **Cystoscopy**: View bladder interior.

Treatment includes:

- **Antibiotics**: For infection.
- **Surgical repair/reconstruction**: Usually involves severing ureter from bladder and reattaching at a different angle to prevent reflux.

EPISPADIAS AND HYPOSPADIAS

Epispadias is a condition in which the urethral orifice is in an abnormal position with a widened pubic bone. In boys, the urethra may open on the top (dorsum), the sides, or the complete length of the penis. In girls, the urethra, with a urethral cleft along its length, usually bifurcates the clitoris and labia but may be in the abdomen. Boys may have a short, wide penis with abnormal chordee (curvature). Epispadias is 3-5 times more common in males than females. Hypospadias, which occurs only in males, is a condition in which the urethral orifice opens onto the ventral surface of the penis.

Diagnosis is by physical exam and endoscopy to evaluate bladder neck and external sphincter. Intravenous pyelogram evaluates the urinary tract.

Symptoms for both conditions include urinary incontinence, infections, and reflux nephropathy (backward flow of urine to kidneys). **Treatment** is surgical repair to lengthen the urethra (and penis, in males) and reconstruct the bladder neck. Multiple surgical procedures may be required for both males and females. Urinary diversion may be necessary if incontinence cannot be corrected.

MYELOMENINGOCELE WITH LIPOMA AND TETHERED CORD

Myelomeningocele is meninges and spinal cord herniating (neural tube defect) through bony defect in the vertebra (spina bifida) anterior or posterior, with protrusion usually in the lower back, with or without lipomas (fatty lesions that grow around the spinal cord) and/or tethered cord (fatty tissue at base of spinal cord that "tethers" the vertebra, stretching it as the child grows). May also have scoliosis, kyphosis, or lordosis.

Symptoms include:

- **Hydrocephalus**: Affects about 30%.
- **Urinary incontinence**: Most have constant leakage of urine but may not empty bladder completely. Others have detrusor-sphincter dyssynergia (sphincter fails to relax).
- **Neurogenic bowels**: Chronic constipation with altered sensation and sphincter control, fecal incontinence.

Diagnosis is by physical exam with posterior lesions evident and MRI for diagnosis of anterior lesions, lipomas, and tethered cord.

Treatment includes:

- **Surgical repair** of neural tube defect/Ventricular-peritoneal shunt.
- **Urinary care**: Clean intermittent catheterization (CIC).
- **Vesicostomy/continent urinary diversion**: To manage incontinence.

- **Bowel management**: Diet and habit training.
- **Appendicostomy**: To allow easy irrigation of bowel.

POSTERIOR URETHRAL VALVES

Posterior urethral valves (PUV) are a urethral abnormality in males where urethral valves have narrow slit-like openings that impede urinary flow and allow reverse flow, damaging urinary organs, which swell and become engorged with urine. Thirty percent with PUV will develop long-term kidney failure. **Symptoms** vary depending upon severity:

- **Dysuria**: Pain, weak stream, frequency.
- Hematuria. Urinary retention. Incontinence. Enlarged bladder palpable as abdominal mass. Urinary infection (most common symptom after 1 year of age). Sepsis, metabolic acidosis, and azotemia (increased blood levels of urea and other nitrogenous compounds) may develop.

Diagnosis consists of the following:

- Fetal ultrasound.
- Voiding cystourethrogram (VCUG): Evaluate extent of valvular abnormality and other urinary defects.
- Endoscopy: Examine inside of urinary tract/take tissue samples. Blood tests: Assess kidney function and electrolytes.

Treatment includes:

- Supportive care, antibiotics, electrolytes, Foley catheter.
- Urinary diversion: Usually closed after valve repair.
- Endoscopic ablation/resection: Examine obstruction and remove valve leaflets.

HEREDITARY NON-POLYPOSIS COLORECTAL CANCER (HNPCC)

HNPCC is an inherited autosomal-dominant syndrome where people develop a few polyps and cancer at about age 40. Two clinical variants exist:

- **Lynch I** is early onset of cancer, usually in proximal bowel.
- **Lynch II** is nonpolyposis colon cancer with cancer of endometrium, ovary, small bowel, and urinary tract.

There are **two criteria for genetic testing**:

- **Amsterdam** determines if family members need testing. At least 3 relatives (2 first degree) in 2 successive generations have colorectal cancer, one before 50.
- **Bethesda**—one of following criteria means the person with colorectal cancer should have cancer cells checked for microsatellite instability (MSI)—changes in DNA of cells, giving rise to mutations:
  - Colorectal cancer before 50.
  - History of another cancer associated with HNPCC.
  - History before 60 of cancer with characteristics of MSI.
  - First-degree relative before 50 has non-colorectal cancer often found in HNPCC carriers.
  - Two or more second-degree relatives have HNPCC-related tumor at any age.

Familial Adenomatous Polyposis (FAP)

FAP is an inherited autosomal-dominant syndrome where people develop hundreds to thousands of colorectal polyps between ages 5-40 with cancer usually in one or multiple polyps by about age 20. Between 20-40, virtually everyone develops cancer. A genetic factor predisposes people with this genetic mutation to other malignancies, especially in duodenum and stomach. They may develop Gardner syndrome with congenital hypertrophy of retinal pigment (CHRP), sebaceous cysts, desmoid tumors (fibrous tumors arising in tissue covering intestines), and benign bone tumors. Identifying FAP before colorectal cancer develops is critical as prophylactic colectomy may be indicated with high risk. People with familial history of FAP should have genetic testing.

Variant forms of FAP:

- **Attenuated familial adenomatous polyposis** has delayed polyp growth, with onset of colorectal cancer at about 55 years of age.
- **Autosomal recessive familial adenomatous polyposis** typically causes fewer than 100 polyps and is caused by mutation on different gene than other forms.

Anorectal Fistulas (Fistula-In-Ano)

Anorectal fistulas are those extending from the anal canal to the perineal skin. Most anorectal fistulas originate in the anal glands, which are located between the layers of the anal sphincters and drain into the anal canal. If the glands become blocked and an abscess forms, it can begin to tunnel toward the surface of the skin. There may be only one tunnel or tract, but there may also be multiple. Abscesses can become recurrent if they heal over at the surface. As purulent material collects beneath the healed surface, pressure builds, and it breaks through again. Anorectal fistulas are common in those with Crohn's disease and can occur with rectal cancer or after radiation.

Symptoms include:

- Swelling, pain, and discharge (purulent or sanguinous).
- Diarrhea.
- Anal bleeding.
- External opening of fistula.

Treatment includes:

- **Antibiotics**: To treat infection/abscesses.
- **Seton**: Suture holding fistula opening (draining seton).
- **Fistulotomy/fistulectomy**: Excision (most effective but contraindicated with Crohn's disease.)

Enterocutaneous Fistulas

Enterocutaneous fistulas are those extending from the intestine to the skin. The most frequent causes are Crohn's disease, cancer, anastomotic leak, bowel obstruction, and sepsis. They may develop post-operatively or spontaneously. If excess pressure develops on an anastomosis, a fistula can develop. Malignancy, infection, steroids, and poor nutrition are all contributing factors. Fistulas seek weakness in tissues and thus may exit through wounds, incisions, drain sites or compromised tissue.

Symptoms include:

- **Local**: Erythema, evident opening, purulent/sanguinous discharge.
- **Systemic**: Sepsis, fever, electrolyte imbalance, anemia, malnutrition, dehydration.

Treatment includes:

- **Decrease secretions**: Restrict fluids, Somatostatin to decrease small bowel secretions.
- **Nutritional support**: Enteral (if only colon affected) or total parenteral support.
- **Surgery**: Surgical closure may be done if spontaneous closure unlikely. Usually delayed for 6 to 8 weeks after sepsis controlled to allow for spontaneous closure if possible and reduce the risk of peritonitis. May be done in stages for complex fistulas.

COMMON CAUSES OF FISTULAS

Common causes of fistulas include:

- **Intestinal diseases**: Inflammatory bowel disorders such as ulcerative colitis and Crohn's disease as well as diverticulitis are associated with inflammation, infection, and ulceration, leading to formation of fistulas.
- **Cancer**: Rectum, colon, bladder, or any cancer in the abdomen or pelvic area can cause trauma that result in fistulas.
- **Abscess**: About 50% of abscesses develop fistulas, regardless of the cause of the abscess, so they are always a cause for concern.
- **Surgery**: Any surgery involving the pelvic organs or the intestines can result in fistulas, especially with infections and abscess formation. Cholecystectomy is a common cause of fistula formation.
- **Radiation**: Pelvic radiation, especially, is a common cause of vesicovaginal fistulas.
- **Trauma**: Fistulas are a possibility with many types of traumatic injuries. Trauma from obstructed labor during childbirth is a frequent cause of vesicovaginal and rectovaginal fistulas. Rape, especially gang rape, has been implicated as a frequent cause of fistulas.

Obtaining the Health History

INTERVIEW PROCESS

The nurse should review previous medical records and have a clear idea of the purpose of the **interview** and should outline questions. If possible, the patient should be interviewed alone or should be asked if he/she wants family members present. Both verbal and nonverbal responses should be observed during an interview. Important factors include

- **Initial introductions**: Make introductions by name and explain roles and the purpose of the interview, asking how the patient wishes to be addressed and avoiding using familiar terms, such as "dear," which may be considered condescending. Stress the confidential nature of the interview and explain who will receive the information.
- **Interview structure**: The interview may be somewhat unstructured, guided by patient responses, or may be very structured with the nurse asking a list of questions, but the nurse must remain flexible while still guiding the discussion in order to accommodate different communication styles.
- **Appearance**: The nurse should be professionally dressed and wearing a clear nametag. The patient's appearance should be observed non-judgmentally for clothes (loose/tight clothes may indicate weight change), cleanliness (dirty clothes/skin/hair may indicate cognitive or physical impairment or poverty), and demeanor (calm, fidgeting, nervous).

INITIAL ASSESSMENT OF PATIENT REQUIRING FECAL AND/OR URINARY DIVERSION

History and presentation: The initial assessment will focus on everything that has led the patient to needing a fecal and/or urinary diversion. This can include other treatments that have been utilized if there is a chronic disease involved, or the details of an acute event or trauma that has occurred.

Comorbidities: Any other disease states that may affect the patient's ability to recuperate from the surgery should be considered. This can include cardiovascular disease or diabetes. Chronic conditions that may impair a patient's ability for self-care are also important considerations.

Age: The impact of having a permanent fecal or urinary diversion can vary at different points in a person's life. Young patients that are otherwise healthy may have a different prognosis than elderly patients with comorbidities. Age may also obstruct the ability to self-care or retain education received regarding the fecal/urinary diversion.

Medications: Reviewing all medications that a patient is taking before surgery is important. For example, a patient who is taking medication for Crohn's disease may not require this after a fecal diversion is placed. Depending on the location of the diversion and the type of medication, absorption rates may be affected. It is important for the patient to review all medications with their provider or pharmacist prior to surgery.

Psychological issues: The stress of undergoing surgery, along with the impact the diversion will have on the patient's life, should be considered. Any issues of depression or anxiety should be addressed with appropriate referral to a mental health professional if necessary.

INTERPRETING LAB VALUES FOR OSTOMY PATIENT

Hemoglobin – Carries oxygen and is decreased in anemia and increased in polycythemia. Used to assess bleeding. Normal values:

- Males >18 years: 14.0-17.46 g/dL.
- Females >18 years: 12.0-16.0 g/dL.

Hematocrit – Indicates the proportion of RBCs in a liter of blood (usually about 3 times the hemoglobin number). Used to assess bleeding. Normal values:

- Males >18 years: 45-52%.
- Females >18 years: 36-48%

Glucose – High levels are indicative of diabetes, which predisposes to skin injuries, slow healing, and infection:

- Normal values: 70-99 mg/dL.
- Impaired: 100-125 mg/dL.
- Diabetes: ≥126 mg/dL.

Serum creatinine – Increases with impaired renal function, urinary tract obstruction, and nephritis. Level should remain stable with normal functioning.

- Normal values: 0.6-1.2 mg/dL.

Blood urea nitrogen (BUN) – Increase indicates impaired renal function, as urea is end product of protein metabolism.

- Normal values: 7-8 mg/dL (8-20 mg/dL >age 60).

White blood cell (leukocyte) count is used as an indicator of bacterial and viral infection. WBC is reported as the total number of all white blood cells.

- Normal WBC for adults: 4,800-10,000.
- Acute infection: 10,000+; 30,000 indicates a severe infection.
- Viral infection: 4,000 and below.

The differential provides the percentage of each different type of leukocyte. An increase in the white blood cell count is usually related to an increase in one type, and often an increase in immature neutrophils (bands), referred to as a "shift to the left," is an indication of an infectious process:

- Normal immature neutrophils (bands): 1-3%. Increase with infection.
- Normal segmented neutrophils (segs) for adults: 50-62%. Increase with acute, localized, or systemic bacterial infections.
- Normal eosinophils: 0-3%. Decrease with stress and acute infection.
- Normal basophils: 0-1%. Decrease during acute stage of infection.
- Normal lymphocytes; 25-40%. Increase in some viral and bacterial infections.
- Normal monocytes: 3-7%. Increase during recovery stage of acute infection.

MEDICAL TREATMENTS FOR URINARY INCONTINENCE

Medications for urinary incontinence:

- **Antispasmodics (tolterodine, oxybutynin, hyoscyamine)**: for overactive bladders. These drugs may cause thirst, so longer-acting preparations of these drugs, which have fewer side effects, may be better for some people.
- **Antidepressant (imipramine)**: to relax the bladder and contract the muscles at the bladder neck:
- **Hormone replacement therapy**: Administered as a vaginal cream, ring, or patch to protect bladder and urethral mucosa. Oral estrogen may not be as effective as topical for incontinence.

191

- **Antibiotics**: To treat infections that may be causing or worsening incontinence.
- Some medications, such as sedatives, may increase or cause incontinence, so all medications should be assessed.

Medical devices:

- **Catheters**: Clean intermittent catheterization to empty bladder.
- **Penile clamps**: Apply pressure around the penis to clamp the urethra.
- **Pessaries**: A stiff ring inserted vaginally to treat bladder prolapse.
- **Urethral inserts**: Urethral inserts may be inserted temporarily during times of activity that may prompt incontinence.

FOODS THAT CAN CAUSE OR RELIEVE PROBLEMS WITH OSTOMIES AFTER BOWEL SURGERY
Foods that may cause obstruction include:

- **Fruits**: Dried fruits, fruits with seeds (such as pomegranates and figs) and skin (such as cherries), large servings of raw fruit.
- **Nuts**: Tree nuts (such as walnuts and almonds), peanuts, and popcorn.
- **Vegetables**: Whole corn, bean sprouts, bamboo shoots, large servings of raw vegetables, celery, mushrooms.

Foods that may cause diarrhea/loosening of stool include:

- **Fruits**: Juices (especially apple and prune juice), prunes, fresh fruit.
- **Vegetables**: Broccoli, cabbage, raw vegetables.
- **Other**: Spicy foods, fried foods, baked beans, sugar-free gum.

Foods that may cause constipation/thickening of stool include:

- **Fruits**: Applesauce, bananas.
- **Proteins**: Cheese, creamy peanut butter.
- **Starches**: Potatoes (without skins), rice, pasta, whole wheat bread, tapioca pudding, marshmallows.

Foods that may cause gas/odor include:

- **Vegetables**: Cabbage, broccoli, kale, cauliflower, kohlrabi, Brussels sprouts, asparagus, onions, dried peas, rutabagas, and turnips.
- **Proteins**: Dried beans fish, strong cheeses, and eggs.
- **Other**: Spicy foods, chewing gum.
- **Drinks**: Beer, carbonated beverages (such as sodas or juices).

DIET AND FLUID MODIFICATIONS
AFTER CONTINENT CUTANEOUS FECAL DIVERSIONS AND ILEAL POUCH ANAL ANASTOMOSIS
After continent cutaneous fecal diversions (continent ileostomy) and ileal pouch anal anastomosis, the pouch will stretch and consistency of stool will thicken in the months following. Monitoring diet and fluids can control bowel movements and prevent dehydration. Meal times may need to be adjusted for better control, especially at night.

- **Eat**: Regular meals are important. After surgery, eating helps to stretch the pouch and food will slow down the frequency of bowel movements. Gas forms when bowels are empty, so eat small frequent meals.

- **Add foods**: Try one new food at a time to determine tolerance. Many people are lactose intolerance, so be careful with dairy products. Cheese can help to slow stools.
- **Starch**: Rice, potatoes, and pasta once a day can help to slow stools.
- **Potassium**: Foods high in potassium, such as bananas and potatoes, can help to prevent hypokalemia from diarrhea.
- **Simple sugars**: Can cause diarrhea, so limit.
- **Fluids**: Drink 6 to 8 glasses of fluid a day, but not with meals.

PEOPLE WITH CONTINENT CUTANEOUS URINARY DIVERSIONS

For individuals with **continent cutaneous urinary diversions**, it is important to maintain adequate kidney function by drinking 8-10 glasses of fluid daily. The pH of the urine ranges normally from 4.6-8, in the acidic range and an effort should be made to maintain acidity. Alkaline urine is more likely to become infected and develop crystals. Most meats and cereals produce acidic urine, but most fruits and vegetables produce alkaline urine.

- **Odor-producing foods**: Fish, asparagus.
- **Acid foods**: Grains and cereals, meats, cheese, corn, crackers, cranberries, eggs, pasta, nuts, rice, prunes, plums, fish, and poultry.
- **Alkaline foods**: Bananas, beans, beets, milk, greens, most fruits (including citrus fruits such as oranges and lemons), most vegetables.

Including acid foods as part of daily diet and making some substitutions, such as drinking cranberry juice instead of orange juice, can help to keep the urine acidic. Taking daily vitamin C, with permission of physician, can also help to keep the urine acidic.

ENVIRONMENTAL, SOCIAL, AND OTHER FACTORS THAT IMPACT PATIENT'S ADAPTATION

Environmental factors such as living alone or being homeless can add to the burden. Lacking a support system or having non-supportive family and friends may increase fear and depression.

Social factors such as low income or lack of insurance make the cost of colostomy supplies prohibitive.

Cultural factors also have an impact. Mexican families are often patriarchal with the eldest male in the family consulted first. Asians often believe people should not receive bad news about their health and may want to keep diagnostic information secret. Religion is also a consideration. Muslims may be concerned about the gender of healthcare providers. Jews, Hindus, and Muslims may want the body to remain intact. Hindus and Buddhists may believe their condition is related to karma. Folk beliefs must be respected and an attempt made to integrate into plan for care.

Other factors include **language barriers**. A translator and the use of teaching materials in other languages may be required.

PSYCHOSOCIAL FACTORS AFFECTING CARE

Psychosocial factors affecting care include:

- **Ability to learn/perform care**: Cognitive impairment and hearing or vision deficits may interfere with the ability to learn, especially if appropriate educational materials are not available. Physical disabilities may make it difficult to patients to learn or perform some aspects of care. Language differences may result in impaired comprehension.
- **Economic implications**: Patients and families may be severely impacted if the wage earner is unable to continue to work or if they lack the resources (insurance, financial) to pay for needed care.

- **Education**: Patients may lack an adequate educational background to understand the implications of disease, to read materials, and to follow directions. Health literacy may be very low, so patients may have misconceptions about disease.
- **Mental status**: Patients often experience increased stress associated with illness, and this may interfere with functioning. Mental impairment may impact ability to participate in care. Additionally, depression is common, especially with chronic illness, and may cause patients to withdraw or fail to comply with treatment.

COPING STRATEGIES FOR FECAL OR URINARY INCONTINENCE WHILE IN SOCIAL SITUATIONS

The following are coping strategies that people with fecal or urinary incontinence can use to manage when they are outside of the home in social situations:

- Plan:
  - Schedule activities, if possible, at times with less chance of fecal/urinary incontinence. Use the toilet before leaving home.
  - Wear an incontinence pad or disposable underwear as needed.
  - Wear clothing that is comfortable and not constricting.
  - Carry pre-moistened wipes, extra pads, ostomy supplies as needed. Keep extra clothes, supplies/disposable underwear somewhere that is easily accessible.
- Survey environment:
  - Locate the bathrooms before an urgent need arises so they can be accessed easily.
  - If more than one bathroom is available, determine which provides the most privacy.
- Practice prevention:
  - Sit so exit to the bathroom is convenient, at end of a row or table rather than in the middle.
  - Use toilet periodically at whatever schedule gives best control, probably at least every 2 hours.
  - Avoid foods or drinks, such as carbonated beverages, that may cause gas or stimulate bowels/bladder. Foods to avoid are often individual based on experience.

Ostomy Care: Assessment and Care Planning

Surgical Indications and Procedures

SURGERY FOR COLORECTAL CANCER

Indications for colorectal surgery include:

- **Prophylactic**: To prevent cancer, often for precancerous polyps.
- **Diagnostic**: Biopsy to confirm diagnosis and determine type of cancer. Various surgical techniques may be used.
- **Staging**: To determine extent of malignant invasion. Surgical staging is more accurate than imaging or laboratory findings.
- **Curative**: Removal of tumor to affect a cure. It is considered the primary treatment but may be done in conjunction with chemotherapy or radiotherapy.
- **Cytoreductive**: Debulking removes all possible tumors without damaging organs or surrounding areas and may be done when it's impossible or too dangerous to remove entire tumor. It may be followed by chemotherapy or radiotherapy.
- **Palliative**: To alleviate symptoms or discomfort; not curative.
- **Supportive**: To assist with other treatments. May include installation of catheter port into large vein for delivery of chemotherapy or blood testing.
- **Restorative**: To restore function, as when colostomy is removed and bowel reattached.

SURGICAL OPTIONS FOR HIRSCHSPRUNG'S DISEASE

Surgical treatment for Hirschsprung's disease used to always be done in two stages, with a temporary colostomy performed proximal to the aganglionic segment to allow the bowel to heal and regain tone prior to the final surgical procedure. However, earlier diagnosis has resulted in most children having one-step procedures. All procedures are pull-through in that the aganglionic portion is removed and the functioning portion of bowel is "pulled through" and attached to the anus:

- **Swenson procedure**: This procedure retains a small 1-2 cm section of aganglionic sleeve through which the functioning bowel is pulled through and sutured to the anus.
- **Duhamel procedure**: This procedure uses a stapler to connect aganglionic segment to functioning bowel so that the aganglionic segment constitutes the anterior wall but the posterior wall has enervation.
- **Soave procedure**: This procedure brings the functioning bowel down through the sleeve of the rectum where it is attached to the anus.

SURGICAL TREATMENTS FOR URINARY INCONTINENCE

There are over 200 different surgical procedures to treat disorders that cause incontinence. Common options include:

- **Artificial urinary sphincter**: Fluid-filled ring placed around bladder neck to keep the sphincter closed. A valve under the skin is pushed to deflate the ring to allow urination. Procedure is rarely done on women.
- **Augmentation cystoplasty**: A section of the colon is removed, shaped, and sutured into the bladder wall to expand the bladder capacity.
- **Injections of bulking agents**: Collagen is injected to the tissue around the urethra or urinary sphincter to tighten the sphincter for women. Must be repeated every 6-18 months.
- **Sacral nerve stimulation**: Small device is implanted in the abdomen with a wire to the sacral nerve to stimulate the bladder.

- **Sling procedure**: Abdominal, donor, or synthetic tissue placed under the urethra, acting like a hammock and compressing urethra to prevent leakage for women.
- **Urinary diversion**: Cystectomy with urinary diversion as last resort for intractable incontinence.

INDICATIONS FOR FECAL DIVERSION SURGERY

Indications for fecal diversion surgery are as follows:

- Inflammatory bowel disease:
  - **Crohn's disease** may affect any part of the GI system, especially the ileum. It may cause swelling and lesions that involve all layers of the intestinal wall.
  - **Ulcerative Colitis** causes inflammation and ulceration of the large intestine, but only in the top layer of the intestinal wall.
- Gastrointestinal cancers:
  - Rectal or colon cancer may metastasize or obstruct.
  - Rectal obstruction may result from metastasis of advanced pelvic cancer
- Gastrointestinal and non-gastrointestinal etiologies:
  - **Diverticular disease** with complications may result in abscess, obstruction, fistula or perforation of intestine. Radiation enteritis may cause malfunction from intestinal damage. Ischemic colitis most often of the left colon may cause irreversible damage.
  - **Infectious enteritis** may be caused by bacteria, viruses, parasites, or fungi. Hospital stay and/or antibiotic use may lead to Clostridioides difficile infection, which may lead to severe complications. Intestinal obstruction, mechanical or non-mechanical, can lead to necrosis. Gastrointestinal trauma related to blunt or penetrating injuries may damage part of intestine.

INDICATIONS FOR URINARY DIVERSION SURGERY

Bladder cancer with cystectomy results from either primary bladder cancer or cancer originating in pelvic organs. Bladder cancer may result from chronic irritation caused by indwelling catheters or when bladders are left intact after urinary diversion surgery.

Prostate cancer may advance to cause ureteral obstruction from lymph node involvement or from invasion of the base of the bladder.

Neurogenic bladder, bladder dysfunction from lesions of the peripheral or central nervous system, may be related to traumatic or congenital etiologies. It may also develop after cerebrovascular accident or from diabetic neuropathy.

Interstitial cystitis causes chronic debilitating pain of the bladder, urethra, and pelvic area as well as dysuria. It may relate to congenital or traumatic injuries that cause inflammation and problems with urine storage and bladder emptying. Pain may persist after surgery.

Refractory radiation cystitis is damage caused from radiation treatments, resulting in intractable incontinence or urinary fistulas.

PROCEDURES FOR HARTMAN'S POUCH AND COLONIC J POUCH

Hartman's pouch: To create a Hartman's pouch, the intestine is severed, usually with removal of a part of the distal segment because of a cancerous lesion. The proximal end is brought through the abdominal wall to form a stoma for fecal drainage. The non-functioning distal end of the colon with the rectum intact is stapled or stitched to close and then left in place, forming a non-functioning pouch.

Colonic J pouch: To create a colonic J pouch requires a two-step procedure. In the first step, a temporary loop ileostomy is performed for fecal diversion above the surgical site, and a newly constructed pouch from a 6-10 cm segment of colon is attached to the rectal stump after removal of a cancerous lesion, creating the J pouch. In the second step, after about 2-3 months, the ileostomy is reversed and anastomosis is done to re-establish intestinal continuity.

OPERATIVE PROCEDURES FOR RECTAL CANCERS/COLOSTOMIES

Abdominal peritoneal resection: The rectum, anus, and sphincter are removed and the distal end of the sigmoid colon is used to form a stoma in the left lower quadrant. Used commonly for low rectal cancers.

Coloanal anastomosis: This sphincter-preserving procedure entails removal of cancerous bowel proximal to the rectum and then anastomosis of the distal end of the remaining colon to the rectum, above the levator ani muscles, leaving a 1-2 cm distal margin. Best for women with gynecoid pelvis and people who are not obese and lack complications or pre-surgical fecal incontinence.

Low anterior resection: The lower rectum is left intact and an anastomosis is done below the peritoneal reflection. Used for cancers in the upper and middle thirds of the rectum.

Combined low anterior resection with coloanal anastomosis: This combination procedure is usually done with anastomosis completed after temporary fecal diversion gives tissue time to heal.

COLOSTOMY IRRIGATION

The following considerations should be made as it relates to colostomy irrigation:

- **Type of colostomy**: People who had regular bowel habits before surgery and have permanent colostomies in the descending or sigmoid colon are good candidates for irrigation because the stool is usually formed rather than liquid at this part of the colon.
- **Contraindications**: People with prolapse or hernia should not irrigate as the irrigation may worsen the conditions.
- **Motivation**: Irrigation requires people to be committed to and be physically able to perform the procedure by themselves or with the assistance of caregivers on a regularly scheduled basis.
- **Constipation**: Since constipation and impaction can still occur, this must be managed as well by medications, such as stool softeners, or diet, fluid, and exercise. Irrigation can help relieve chronic constipation.
- **Regulation**: Irrigation is usually done every 1-2 days. Once the ostomy is regulated, without fecal leakage between irrigations, a stoma cap can be used between irrigations rather than a pouch.

LOW ANTERIOR RESECTION (LAR)

Low anterior resection is a sphincter-sparing procedure for rectal cancer (stage I, II, or III) occurring in the anterior portion of the rectum. LAR may be done as an open surgical procedure or through a minimally invasive laparoscopic procedure with site election guided by ultrasound and MRI. LAR involves removing the rectum (completely or partially) about the lesion and lymph nodes and then attaching the remaining rectal tissue to the colon. The procedure avoids creation of a permanent colostomy although some patients may require a temporary ileostomy to allow the tissue to adequately heal, especially those who have undergone radiotherapy and/or chemotherapy. However, complications may occur and may impair the quality of life. LAR syndrome, which occurs when the anal sphincter is injured or innervation impaired, may result in chronic leakage of fecal material, urgency, frequent bowel movements, constipation, or impaction. These symptoms may persist for years or become permanent. Treatment includes Kegel exercises, medications (loperamide, psyllium), biofeedback, stool training, and emotional support.

TOTAL PROCTOCOLECTOMY

A total proctocolectomy is removal of the entire rectum, colon, and anus through an open surgical procedure or minimally-invasive laparoscopic procedure. Total proctocolectomy may be done for cancer, severe inflammatory bowel disease (Crohn's disease, ulcerative colitis), toxic megacolon, uncontrolled GI bleeding, or intestinal perforation. Total proctocolectomy requires an alternate method of fecal evacuation, so this may involve creation of an ileostomy or, in some cases, a J pouch. If the total proctocolectomy is combined with an ileostomy, the ileostomy is created during the initial surgical procedure. However, if a J-pouch is constructed (most common for ulcerative colitis), two or three stages are utilized. In the first stage, the rectum is retained but is later removed and the J-pouch created along with a temporary loop ileostomy to allow the J-pouch to heal. Complications of total proctocolectomy may include postoperative ileus, infection, hemorrhage, necrosis, intestinal obstruction, and sepsis. With a pouch, pouchitis, and pouch-anal/vaginal fistulae may also occur.

CONTINENT CUTANEOUS FECAL DIVERSION (CONTINENT ILEOSTOMY)

Continent ileostomy: May be done after proctocolectomy; the lower part of the small bowel is used to create an internal reservoir for collection of fecal material. This pouch is created from the small intestine and has a leak-free nipple valve inside the abdominal stoma, also created from the intestine to prevent leakage of stool, with an intestinal conduit leading to the pouch.

This type of pouch is a **Kock pouch**, named after the physician who developed the procedure. The valve-modified T-pouch or Barnett pouch is also sometimes used. It is usually done for either ulcerative colitis or familial adenomatous polyposis (FAP). Pouch is emptied 4 times daily through a plastic catheter. The continent ileostomy has been superseded by newer techniques, such as the restorative proctocolectomy with the J pouch, but it is still useful for those over 50, those who are incontinent, or those whose J pouches have failed.

INTUBATION AND DRESSING SUPPLIES FOR CONTINENT CUTANEOUS FECAL DIVERSIONS

Choice of supplies depends on personal preference as well as factors such as mucus production or leakage of stool:

- **Intubation supplies**: Most people use a 30-34 Fr. catheter to drain continent ileostomies. There are a number of brand names, such as Marlen, Medina, Weber and Judd and Mentor. Some have a bullet tip with holes on the side. Others have a rounded tip with a hole at the tip and on the side. Some catheters are straight, and others are curved, but all are flexible. If straight catheters are stored coiled for a length of time, they tend to stay curved. They range from 12-18 inches in length and can be trimmed to preferred length.
- **Dressing supplies**:
  - Absorbent pads with hypoallergenic adhesives, often 4x4.
  - Stoma caps in various shapes and sizes, look like flesh-colored adhesive bandages.
  - Nursing pads/eye pads are inexpensive, easily available substitutions for stoma dressings.

ILEAL POUCH ANAL ANASTOMOSIS (IPAA)

Ileal Pouch Anal Anastomosis: Involves leaving rectal sphincter intact with excision of colon and creation of temporary ileostomy. A reservoir (pouch) is constructed of small intestine pulled down and sewn or stapled to the anal muscles.

- Ileo-anal pull-through: Distal end of small intestine is pulled through rectal stump and sutured to the anus.
- The J, S, and W (named because of the appearance of the looped intestines) pouches are made by looping the intestine side-by-side, detubularizing, and then suturing together to make a larger pouch.

Ostomy Care: Assessment and Care Planning

- ○ J Pouch—2 limbs of small intestine are used to create a pouch.
- ○ S Pouch—3 limbs are used.
- ○ W Pouch—4 limbs are used.

The ileostomy is taken down after about 2 months, giving the pouch the time to heal. The reservoir capacity will be small at first with 10-12 stools per day, but the pouch will stretch and frequency will decrease to 4-5 stools per day.

DETUBULARIZATION

Detubularization refers to the preparation that takes place to prepare an intestinal segment for use in the construction of a urinary reservoir. The intestinal segment is divided and then sewn back together to create a spherical rather than tubular reservoir. Intestinal segments have a muscular layer which contracts to carry out peristalsis and propel the fecal material through the intestines. When a segment of the intestine is removed and attached elsewhere in the body, the intact tubular intestine retains the ability to contract, and this would apply too much pressure within the reservoir and prevent adequate stretching. To accommodate this intestinal characteristic, the tubular intestinal segment is opened lengthwise along the anti-mesenteric border to reduce or eliminate muscle tone. It is sutured together again in such a way as to interfere with peristaltic activity. This effectively decreases the pressure generated by the newly-formed reservoir and increases its capacity.

ORTHOTOPIC NEOBLADDER

Orthotopic neobladder is the creation of a reservoir to serve as a urinary bladder in the normal bladder position. The bladder is usually removed, and a urinary reservoir is made out of segments of the ileum or colon, including the ileocecal valve. The long intestinal segment, usually from the ileum, is detubularized before being shaped into a pouch. The ureters are attached superiorly in a refluxing manner. Sometimes, the ureters may be anastomosed to a short limb of the small bowel, a configuration known as the Studer pouch, and allowing easy conversion of neobladder to an ileal conduit if necessary. The urethra is anastomosed to the reservoir. During surgery, a urethral catheter is placed to drain urine and perform as a stent. There are ureteral catheters and often a suprapubic catheter and drains in place as well; all drains except for Foley catheter are usually removed before discharge. Foley remains about 3 weeks.

SURGICAL PLACEMENT METHODS FOR GASTROSTOMY TUBES

Gastrostomy is a permanent or temporary opening into the stomach. While percutaneous endoscopic gastrostomy is standard for feeding tubes, with hypopharyngeal or esophageal carcinomas, stenosis may prevent oral feeding and endoscopy, so surgical methods are used.

- **Janeway** is a laparoscopic procedure where the gastric mucosa is sutured/stapled to the abdomen, creating a permanent continent gastrostoma in the left upper quadrant through which intermittent catheterization provides long-term feeding.
- **Stamm** is an open procedure where a midline incision opens to the anterior aspect of the stomach with a stab incision into which a balloon catheter is inserted with purse-string sutures to tighten the opening around the catheter. The stomach wall is sutured to the anterior abdominal wall at the exit site, providing a secure opening for catheters.
- **Witzel** is an open procedure where a serosal tunnel of tissue in the gastric wall covers 4-6 cms on the implanted tube, making a permanent tract and securing the tube.

PLACEMENT FOR GASTROINTESTINAL FEEDING TUBES

The three types of placement for gastrointestinal feeding tubes are summarized below:

- **Surgical placement**: There are both open and laparoscopic surgical techniques for tubes to the stomach or jejunum. The three most common methods are the Janeway, the Stamm, and the Witzel techniques.
- **Endoscopic placement**: Percutaneous endoscopic gastrostomy (PEG) involves intubation of the esophagus with the endoscope and insertion of a sheathed needle with a guidewire through the abdomen and stomach wall so that a catheter can be fed down the esophagus, snared, and pulled out through the opening where the needle was inserted and secured. Similar endoscopic procedures can be done in the jejunum.
- **Radiologic placement**: Through fluoroscopy, ultrasound and/or CT, gastrostomy tube is inserted through the epigastrium and secured with a balloon and external bumper or disk. Insertion into the jejunum is done in a similar manner through the duodenum into the jejunum. A gastrojejunostomy tube, which both drains the stomach and feeds the jejunum, is another procedure.

SURGICAL JEJUNOSTOMY FOR FEEDING TUBES

Jejunostomy: Creation of an opening into the jejunum beyond the ligament of Treitz for insertion of feeding tube.

- **Indications**: This procedure is indicated for those with high risk of aspiration (such as those with neurologic disease or decreased awareness), esophageal or gastric cancer, oropharyngeal dysmotility, or previous surgery of stomach, duodenum, or pancreas. Those suffering from dysphagia should be evaluated as potential candidates for jejunostomy rather than gastrostomy. Jejunostomy decreases the risk of aspiration pneumonia.
- **Procedures**: Open surgical or laparoscopic techniques may be used to create the jejunostomy. Both the Stamm and the Witzel procedures that are used for gastrostomy may be modified to use with jejunostomy. With the Stamm procedure, the jejunum is secured to the abdominal wall to make a secure opening for the balloon feeding tube. With the Witzel procedure, a seromyotomy creates a tunnel by involuting the jejunal wall over the tube.

BOLUS/SYRINGE, GRAVITY DRIP, AND PUMP FEEDINGS PER ENTERAL TUBES

Feeding tubes should be checked and flushed before infusion. The type and amount of feeding solution is prescribed by physician.

- **Bolus/syringe feedings** use a 60-cc catheter tip syringe attached to the end of the feeding tube. The tube is clamped until the formula is poured into the syringe, unclamped, and the formula allowed to flow in by gravity. Raising or lowering the syringe will speed or slow flow.
- **Gravity drip feedings** use a feeding bag filled with formula from the top. The measures are marked on the outside to help monitor inflow. Roller clamps control the rate of flow. Feedings may be continuous or for a prescribed number of hours. The bag should be changed at least every 24 hours to prevent bacteria from growing.
- **Pump feedings** use an electrical or battery-powered device to control rate of infusion when the tubing is fed through the device, allowing precise control of the infusion rate.

INSERTION OF BALLOON REPLACEMENT GASTROSTOMY TUBE

Insertion of a balloon replacement gastrostomy tube:

1. Gather supplies, position patient to 30 degrees, wash hands.
2. Inject 20 mL sterile water into balloon port to check balloon leaks. Withdraw water and retain filled syringe.

3. Apply gloves and move external disk to near distal end.
4. Lubricate catheter tip with water-based lubricant.
5. Cleanse peristomal area with normal saline in spiral movement. Dry skin.
6. Insert tube gently to pre-measured distance. Do not force. Turn tube if resistance met or withdraw and try different angle until in place. (If unable to insert, call physician.)
7. Inflate balloon through balloon port, using correct amount of water.
8. Gently pull tube until resistance met. Slide external bumper to 1.5 cm from skin surface.
9. Rotate tube in circular motion to ensure free rotation.
10. Use 30-60 mL syringe to aspirate gastric content. Flush tube with water.
11. Clean skin, apply barriers as needed, and mark exit measurement with tape flag or indelible ink.

REMOVAL OF BALLOON REPLACEMENT GASTROSTOMY TUBE

Removal procedure:

1. Gather the supplies for a clean procedure. Sterile gloves are not necessary.
2. Reassure patient that the procedure is not painful and explain the steps. If reinsertion is to be done, explain that procedure as well.
3. Position patient's head no higher than 30 degrees.
4. Wash hands.
5. Schedule removal for 2 hours after continuous feeding or prior to bolus feeding so residual feeding solution doesn't drain onto the skin as this could cause irritation.
6. Using a 20 mL Luer-Lok syringe inserted into the balloon port, slowly deflate the internal balloon.
7. Measure extracted fluid to make sure the balloon is completely deflated, and then gently pull the tube out. If resistance is met, rotate tube and try again.
8. Cover stoma with gauze pad until reinsertion of new tube. Reinsertion should immediately follow removal of tube to prevent tract closure.

MANAGING FECAL/URINARY DIVERSIONS IN SPECIAL POPULATIONS

NEONATAL

Education will be geared toward the parents/caregivers of the infant. With fecal diversions, a pouch that will accommodate increased gas should be used. Any changes in the stoma size should be regularly assessed, also, as this will change the barrier and pouch sizes as the infant grows.

PEDIATRIC

Once a child reaches 5 or 6 years of age, they can usually start learning how to care for a diversion. Size and fit should be considered, especially as the child begins to be more active. Issues with body image will begin as the child matures.

ADOLESCENT

Body image issues are a major concern at this age as the adolescent patient matures and lives with a fecal or urinary diversion. The patient can learn how to care for the diversion on their own. Support groups consisting of other adolescents with fecal/urinary diversions can be very helpful at this age, when social acceptance is a priority.

BARIATRIC

Body habitus can affect the stoma size and location. Larger patients with multiple skin folds can increase the risk of skin breakdown or skin infection. If morbidly obese, there may also be issues of the patient performing self-care of the diversion.

ASSESSING ABILITY TO PROVIDE SELF-CARE

A number of issues are important when assessing the patient's ability to provide self-care:

- **Manual dexterity**: Both fine and gross manual dexterity should be assessed to determine the patient's ability to carry out any necessary treatment and to perform procedures. Additionally, the patient's manual dexterity may impact the person's ability to perform ADLs. Testing may include asking patients to pick up small items with tweezers, place pins in a pegboard, grasp, lift, and throw.
- **Vision**: The patient should wear glasses when vision is assessed. Impaired vision can impact the patient's ability to safely take medications, carry out ADLs, and do treatments. Testing may include asking the patient to read and to describe something at a distance.
- **Cognition**: Impaired cognition may interfere with all aspects of self-care. If a patient has mild cognitive impairment, instructions may need to be broken down into very simple steps, but with more severe impairment, the patient may need assistance. Testing may include questions (name, birthdate, residence, date), simple memory tasks (remember 3 items after a few minutes), drawing (face of a clock), and talk back (asking patient to demonstrate or explain to show understanding).

Focused Assessment of Urinary and Fecal Diversions

Ostomy Care: Assessment and Care Planning

CONTINENT CUTANEOUS URINARY DIVERSION

Continent urinary diversion: Involves construction of a urinary reservoir to which ureters are attached. The reservoir has some type of valve inside the stoma to prevent leakage. There are a number of different types of pouches, which are modifications of the original Kock pouch, which has 3 segments: a nipple made by intussuscepting 17 cm of small bowel to form a 5 cm segment. A second small intestinal segment is used to create a stoma in the abdominal wall. The third segment is a 78 cm segment that is looped into a u-shape, opened, and sutured together to create a U-shaped pouch to which the ureters are implanted. The ureters also have valves to prevent backflow.

Other pouch techniques: Several pouches involve the use of part of the right colon as well as the small intestine: Indiana, Florida, Miami, and Mainz pouches. The Florida pouch has consistently the highest degree of continence.

UROSTOMY

A urostomy is a procedure by which urine is redirected to a stoma in the abdominal wall. This type of urinary diversion drains urine constantly and requires the use of a pouch.

There are **two main types of urostomies**:

- **Ileal conduit**: This is the oldest urinary diversion procedure and has few complications. In this procedure, about a 12 cm loop of ileum (or in some cases colon) is cut from the intestine and the intestine is then reconnected. One end of this intestinal "tube" is sutured to the abdominal wall to create a stoma and the ureters are attached to the other end, thus creating an ileal conduit for urinary flow. Stents are usually placed in the ureters to maintain patency.
- **Ureterostomy**: This procedure is rarely done now except as a temporary measure in pediatric patients. In this procedure, the ureters are directly connected to the abdomen, creating one or two small bud stomas.

COLOSTOMY

A colostomy is the general term that involves removal of part of the colon with the end of the remaining colon sutured to the abdominal wall to create a stoma, or opening, through which stool can pass.

The following are terms related to colostomies:

- **Permanent**: A permanent colostomy is usually done after part of the colon, usually the rectum and lower colon, is excised without plans for reanastomosis.
- **Temporary**: A temporary colostomy allows the part of the colon distal to the stoma to rest or heal until the two parts of the colon can be reattached or reconstruction completed.
- **End**: An end colostomy is a temporary (as above) procedure or a permanent procedure where a stoma is created proximal to an inoperable carcinoma to allow for fecal diversion and to prolong life.
- **Ascending**: An ascending colostomy creates a stoma from the ascending portion of the colon on the right side of the abdomen.
- **Descending/sigmoid colostomy**: The descending or sigmoid colostomy is the most common type and creates a stoma from the end of the sigmoid (descending) colon, usually in the lower left abdomen.
- **Loop**: A loop colostomy creates one stoma with two openings, one for stool and the other for mucus, usually in the transverse colon. May have a supporting rod in place. This is a common procedure for short-term fecal diversion.

- **Transverse**: The transverse colostomy creates one or two stomas from the transverse colon, usually in the upper abdomen in the middle or on the right side.
- **End-loop**: Loop of intestine is brought to abdominal wall with both proximal and distal end stomas side by side. Often used as a temporary procedure for obstructed colon.
- **Hidden colostomy**: A loop of intestine is retained in subcutaneous fat and left for easy access in case a colostomy becomes necessary at a later date.

Ileostomy

The following are the two main types of ileostomy:

- **End (standard, Brooke's)**: The end of the ileum is brought up through the abdominal wall to create a stoma, usually after the colon and rectum are surgically removed. If some colon and the rectum remain but are sutured closed and left below the surface, this type of ileostomy is a temporary procedure. The stoma is usually small and round and fairly easy to pouch.
- **Loop**: A loop of the ileum is brought through the abdominal wall. A rod may be placed beneath the loop to keep it elevated above the skin. The loop is opened to allow for fecal drainage from the proximal portion of the loop and mucus from the distal portion. The loop is usually temporary, allowing the colon to heal, and this construction allows for easy closure of the ileostomy. Loop ileostomies tend to have larger misshapen stomas that are more difficult to pouch.

Absorption Concerns for Medications for Those with Continent Cutaneous Fecal Diversions

Because of the loss of the colon and less time in the intestine, enteric-coated medications or time-release capsules may not be absorbed completely or at all. Uncoated tablets or liquid medications usually are absorbed; however, if the food is passing through the ileostomy undigested, there may be decreased absorption of even these medication forms.

- **Antacids**: Magnesium can cause diarrhea.
- **Antibiotics**: May cause diarrhea and dehydration.
- **Antidiabetics**: Glucophage may not be absorbed properly.
- **Birth control pills**: May not be completely absorbed, making them unreliable.
- **Corticosteroids**: Can cause sodium retention and fungal infection under faceplate of pouch because of suppression of immune system.
- **Diuretics**: May cause electrolyte imbalance.
- **Laxatives**: Should NOT be taken. Can cause electrolyte imbalance.
- **NSAIDs**: May cause gastric bleeding or duodenal-gastric irritation. Take with food.
- **Sulfa drugs**: Usually cause no problem.
- **Vitamins**: Liquid form is absorbed best. Vit B-12 should be given by injection or nasal spray.

Fecal Diversion Pouchitis

Pouchitis is a non-specific inflammation of the mucosal lining of the internal (ileo-anal, Kock, J, W, S) pouch created from part of the small intestine after colectomy. It usually occurs during the first two years after surgery. It is most common among those with ulcerative colitis, affecting 20-30%. About 5-7% of those with pouchitis will have chronic recurring episodes. Pouchitis rarely requires removal of the pouch. Acute episodes last fewer than 4 weeks; chronic, more than 4 weeks.

Symptoms include:

- **Stools**: A steady increase in the frequency of stools is the most common problem. The person affected may also develop incontinence of stools, watery, or bloody stools. A feeling of urgency is also common.

- **Pain**: May have crampy abdominal pain.
- **Systemic**: Fever, dehydration from excessive loss of fluids.

Treatment includes:

- **Antibiotics**: 1-2 weeks course of metronidazole or ciprofloxacin.
- **Probiotics**: Replacement of normal intestinal flora.
- **Steroids**: Oral and topical, including budesonide.
- **Immunosuppressives**: Infliximab.

DEHYDRATION, HYPONATREMIA, AND HYPOKALEMIA

Electrolyte imbalance, especially loss of potassium and sodium, poses a problem for people with the large intestine removed. Any increase in fluid loss, such as diarrhea, perspiration, or vomiting, can exacerbate the imbalance. Generally, avoidance of a low salt diet and salting to taste helps to maintain sodium levels.

Dehydration:

- **Symptoms**: Thirst, dry mouth, loss of skin turgor, decreased urinary output, headache, lethargy, abdominal cramping.
- **Treatment**: Increase fluid intake to 8-10 glasses daily and include fluids high in electrolytes, like Gatorade.

Hyponatremia:

- **Symptoms**: Anorexia, headaches, drowsiness, cramping of legs and abdomen, dizziness, postural hypotension, arms, and legs feel cold.
- **Treatment**: Increase intake of high sodium foods and fluids, like canned soup, bouillon, ham, Gatorade, soy sauce, buttermilk.

Hypokalemia:

- **Symptoms**: weakness in muscles, fatigue, gas, Abdominal distension, shortness of breath, decrease in sensation of arms and legs.
- **Treatment**: Increase intake of orange juice, bananas, chicken, fish, pinto beans, potatoes, raisins, tomatoes, watermelon, yogurt, and Gatorade.

Stoma Complications

Assessment for Stomal and Peristomal Complications

Stoma assessment includes the following:

- **Type** of stoma may be fecal or urinary and constructed from small intestine, colon, bladder, or ureters. Diversion may be continent or incontinent.
- **Characteristics** of stoma include moist mucosa. Color depends on tissue used in construction. Stoma from intestines is red and beefy looking; from ureter or bladder, pale pink.
- **Edema** is usually present, so stoma should be measured routinely to determine changes.
- **Shape and size** may vary depending upon surgical technique and effects of peristalsis. Some are round; others, oval.
- **Protrusion** of stoma should be slightly above skin to provide for proper pouching, but stomas may retract below the skin or prolapse.
- **Function** depends upon type of ostomy and position. Urostomies produce urine immediately, but colostomies may not excrete stool for 4-5 days and ileostomies, 24-48 hours.
- **Peristomal skin** should be clear of irritation and intact with intact suture line.

Ostomy Signs and Symptoms That Require Follow-Up Care

Ostomy signs/symptoms requiring follow up care include:

- **Changes in functioning**: Any change in the normal function of an ostomy (constipation or diarrhea, change in character of stool/urine) or indications of blockage are a concern.
- **Changes in appearance**: The stoma, peristomal area, and any surgical incisions should be monitored carefully for changes. If the stoma becomes dusky, edematous, depressed, or prolapsed, this needs attention. The peristomal area should remain clear of any irritation.
- **Increase in pain**: Pain should decrease in the post-operative period, but if there is an increase in pain, especially with sudden onset, this could indicate an infection, obstruction, or other complications that need immediate attention.
- **Bloody or purulent discharge**: Stomas, peristomal areas, and discharge should be examined for signs of bleeding or infection. Any indication of blood or pus in feces or urine should be cause for concern.
- **Abdominal distension**: An increase in Abdominal distension, especially if accompanied by other symptoms such as pain or bleeding, may indicate complications.

Stomal Complications

Ischemia/Necrosis

Ischemia/necrosis is a lack of circulation resulting in cyanosis and discoloration of the stoma, from dark red to blue to black. Ischemia may occur within a few hours of surgery or up to 5 days postoperatively. It may be the result of too much mesenteric tension compromising circulation, which can result from edema, obesity, distention of the abdomen. It can also result from an embolism that impairs circulation. As condition worsens, it may be complicated by **mucocutaneous separation.** Sutures that are too constrictive have also been implicated. If necrosis is superficial, it may heal as necrotic tissue sloughs. However, with deeper necrosis or profound circulatory impairment, surgical repair is usually necessary to prevent infection or perforation. It's important to use clear pouches that are properly fitted after surgery so that ongoing assessment of the mucosa can be done in order to prevent deep necrosis and resulting complications.

Ileus

Ileus is the lack of intestinal contractions and bowel sounds because of paralysis of the bowel caused by excessive manipulation during surgery, prolonged period of anesthesia, or narcotic pain medications.

This can result in a non-functioning stoma, as the fecal material remains trapped. Individuals should be encouraged to exercise and roll from side to side frequently to stimulate contractions. Ileus may require nasogastric tube to decompress the stomach and prevent vomiting until normal bowel activity returns.

PERISTOMAL ABSCESS

Peristomal abscesses are characterized by open lesions that are painful with surrounding erythema. They are common when there is active Crohn's disease in the section of the bowel distant to the stoma. The abscess may need to be opened by the surgeon to promote drainage. Treatment will vary depending upon size and degree. Hydrophilic or hydrocolloid materials may be used as a barrier. A non-adhesive pouching system may be used during the healing process.

PROLAPSE

Prolapse is telescoping of the bowel 5 or more inches with mucosal edema, related to large fascial opening in abdominal wall, colostomy through abdominal incision, or obstruction at surgery. A pouching system should be used to accommodate the prolapse at its largest size, and pouches with rigid rings should be avoided. The person should be taught techniques to reduce the prolapse, such as lying flat, applying pressure/ice pack. The person should be taught signs of ischemia.

HEMORRHAGE

Hemorrhage is active bleeding with considerable blood loss and is usually caused by an open mesenteric vessel. Superficial bleeding may be the result of trauma to the stoma and is usually self-limited. Heavy bleeding may relate to underlying liver disease. Bleeding may result from anticoagulant therapy or steroids as well. Identifying the cause of the bleeding is critical for treatment. Pressure should be applied to control bleeding, but surgical repair may be necessary to stop bleeding.

MUCOCUTANEOUS SEPARATION

Mucocutaneous separation is separation of the stoma from the skin at the suture line as a result of inadequate healing, increased tension, or infection. If the separation is superficial, it may be easily treated, but deeper separations pose a more difficult management problem. Additionally, the separation may be in just one area or completely around the stoma. Mucocutaneous separation is treated conservatively to allow healing unless there is a danger of contamination of the peritoneum that may result in peritonitis. In that case, the area may be resutured. For small open areas, skin barrier powder, hydrofiber, or calcium alginate can be used as absorbent material to fill open space, and appliance should be fit over this barrier. Rope packing may be used for deeper separations. If there is considerable drainage, this open draining area may need to be pouched with the stoma to prevent peristomal irritation.

RETRACTION

Retraction occurs when the stoma pulls below the skin level, caused by tension below the stoma from a variety of factors, including excessive scar formation, obesity, inadequate stoma length, recurrence of active Crohn's disease, and improper excision of skin. Management includes using a convex pouching system with a belt. Surgical revision may be needed.

STENOSIS

Stenosis is contraction and narrowing of the stoma, resulting from ischemia. A low residue diet, increased fluids, and stool softeners may prevent blockage. Stoma dilation may be used or surgical revision.

TRAUMA

Trauma is injury to the stoma mucosa usually related to pouch injury or pressure from a hard surface, such as a belt or tight clothing rubbing up against the stoma or constricting it. It is important to determine the cause of the trauma and to correct this so that it does recur. In severe cases of trauma, a transparent pouching system should be used until healing to allow visualization of the stomal circulation.

FISTULA

Fistula is an abnormal opening between the stoma and the skin. It is usually related to recurrence of disease after an ileostomy. Treatment includes using a pouching system that supports both the stoma and the fistula until surgical revision can be carried out.

PARASTOMAL HERNIA

Parastomal hernia occurs with an intestinal loop protruding through a defect in the fascia around the stoma. It can result from improper siting of the stoma outside of rectus, a too-large opening into the connective tissue of the muscle, or weak abdominal muscles. Treatment includes the use of a hernia support belt. It's important to prevent constipation and evaluate stoma size while person is sitting and reclining. Colostomy irrigations should be suspended if difficulty is encountered. Surgical repair with relocation of stoma may be necessary.

Ostomy Care: Assessment and Care Planning

Peristomal Complications

CANDIDIASIS

Candidiasis is a common fungal infection that causes inflammation with burning, itching, and red patches, related to prolonged moisture on skin, usually from secretions or leakage under pouch. **Treatment** requires identifying and eliminating the cause of the moist environment, usually a leaking pouch. The skin should be cleaned and dried and antifungal medication applied under a properly-fitted pouch that does not allow leakage.

FOLLICULITIS

Folliculitis is inflammation of the hair follicles by staphylococcus aureus. The lesions are often pustular, red, and painful. Folliculitis usually results from slight nicks in the skin from shaving with a razor, from friction, or from occlusion. **Treatment** includes shaving less frequently and clipping the hair or using an electric shaver. It can result from insufficient shaving, so hair is pulled out when the appliance is removed. Antibacterial soap such as chlorhexidine gluconate, may reduce infection by decreasing skin bacteria. The person should wash hands thoroughly after caring for the skin to avoid spreading the infection.

MUCOSAL TRANSPLANTATION

Mucosal transplantation is the "transplanting" of intestinal mucosa along the suture line and onto the peristomal area, resulting from suturing through the peristomal skin rather than the stoma during the surgical procedure, leaving areas of mucosal tissue present in the peristomal area. Because these small patches of mucosa remain moist and secrete mucous, they interfere with adhesion of the pouching system. Cauterization and barrier powders will not heal the lesions because they are essentially the wrong type of tissue and cannot be changed. Excision of mucosal tissue with stoma revision is the only effective treatment.

RADIATION TRAUMA

Radiation trauma can result in thin, friable tissue that is easily irritated and denuded by pouching systems and adhesives. Frequently the tissue is hypersensitive to chemicals in solvents or sealants, so it's best to cleanse the skin very gently with water and to avoid soaps or other irritants. Using easily removable skin barriers and pouching systems can prevent damage to skin.

CONTACT DERMATITIS

Contact dermatitis may be either irritant or allergic. Caustic secretions may erode tissue, causing irritation, or there may be a hypersensitivity reaction to a particular chemical or product in the pouching system. Skin may be red, draining, and painful. It is necessary to determine the cause of the irritation in order to eliminate the irritant. The area of the irritation usually corresponds to the area of contact with the irritant causing the dermatitis. The pouching system may need to be changed if that is the causative agent. Reducing the use of products on the skin may help. Denuded skin may be treated with triamcinolone acetonide spray, and skin barrier powder may be used to protect the irritated skin. If the cause of the irritant is not readily discerned, then the person may need referral to a dermatologist for patch tests of various products or other skin tests of product ingredients.

PYODERMA GANGRENOSUM

Pyoderma gangrenosum is a condition with ulcerations that begin as pustules that form full-thickness ulcers that become inflamed and necrotic. The condition occurs in women more than men and may result from trauma or irritation from pouch adhesive. It is associated with inflammatory bowel disease, leukemia, and multiple myeloma. Treatment must address underlying disease. Topical or systemic anti-inflammatory medications may be used. Skin must be kept clean and dry with a pouching system that lasts at least 24 hours. Hydrocolloid dressings may be placed over the ulcers to use as a base for the pouch. Skin barrier powders and foam dressings may also be used for small ulcers. Wound drainage may be extensive, and this affects how long pouching system last between changes. Healing rates vary, and even after the ulcerated areas have healed, scars and uneven skin surface may make securing the pouching system difficult. Surgical resiting of the stoma may be necessary in severe cases.

PSEUDOVERRUCOUS LESIONS

Pseudoverrucous lesions (hyperplasia, chronic papillomatous dermatitis) are lesions resulting from chronic irritation and thickening of the epithelium caused by moisture. The number and size of lesions vary, depending upon the amount of moisture and how chronic the problem has been. The lesions are raised, wart-like, and color varies from white to red to brown. The epidermis surrounding the lesions is moist. The lesions may bleed and be painful. This condition may be caused by using a pouch with an opening that is too large. It is critical to identify and correct the cause of moisture to the skin. For urinary diversions, it helps to correct urinary pH by adequate fluid intake, cranberry juice, and Vitamin C. Lesions may be treated with vinegar soaks for 5 minutes at pouch change. Occasionally cauterization with silver nitrate on large lesions may help healing. Acidic skin barriers, such as karaya or CollySeals should be used with the pouching system.

VARICES

Varices (caput medusae) are large portosystemic collateral veins that appear about the stoma, related to portal hypertension from where the portal venous system communicates with the systemic circulatory system. Varices can result from placing the stoma through the abdominal wall. Varices may result in sudden and profuse blood loss, with blood usually noted in the pouch or around the stoma when the pouch is changed. Development of varices is most common in people with liver malignancies and those with an inflammatory bowel disease treated with ileostomy and proctocolectomy. Direct pressure is used to stop bleeding, followed by cauterization, or suturing. A piece-pouching system is used to avoid pressure during application. Surgical treatment may be needed, including ligation of the portosystemic channels, creation of a portosystemic shunt to lower pressure, or liver transplantation. Person should be educated about signs of bleeding and first aid measures to stop bleeding until emergency help arrives.

SUTURE GRANULOMAS

Suture granulomas are granulation tissue at the skin-stoma base as a reaction to retained or reactive sutures. They appear as erythematous, friable lesions that bleed easily. They are usually small and round and scattered about the suture line. Remove sutures. It's important to identify any retained sutures and remove them. Silver nitrate cauterization may be needed to decrease the amount of tissue. Surgical cauterization may be necessary in severe cases.

TRAUMA

Trauma is skin injury with loss of epidermis. It usually affects small areas, but people who are sensitive to adhesive may develop sensitivity that results in sloughing of surface skin. It is often related to irritation caused by removal of tape from the skin, but it may also be caused by an insecure appliance and pressure of belt or clothes as well as incorrect shaving. It is necessary to determine the cause of the trauma and eliminate it. Skin barriers may be needed to protect skin during healing.

ATYPICAL STOMA AND PERISTOMAL COMPLICATIONS

Some atypical stomal/peristomal complications include:

- **Malignancy** at stoma site can happen as a result of implantation during surgical procedure or incomplete resection of tumor. Peristomal cancer is rare and may result from chronic skin irritation. Surgical revision with wide excision and re-siting of the stoma is treatment of choice.

Ostomy Care: Assessment and Care Planning

- **Herpes zoster and herpes simplex**, viral illnesses, remain dormant but can be triggered by illness or stress. Antiviral treatments may be used. Herpetic lesions in the peristomal area may be irritated by pouch adhesive. Hydrocolloid dressing may be used to prevent fluid from lesions from interfering with the pouching system.
- **Pemphigus** is an autoimmune skin disease causing blistering and affecting peristomal skin, requiring referral to dermatologist, who may treat with corticosteroids, dapsone, or mycophenolate mofetil. It may require temporary use of non-adhesive pouch with hydrocolloid or foam dressings as base.
- **Psoriasis** is a condition with painful crusted scaly plaques, requiring referral to dermatologist for medications to control lesions that interfere with pouch adhesion.

POSSIBLE POSTOPERATIVE COMPLICATIONS WITH FECAL AND URINARY DIVERSION PROCEDURES

Postoperative complications from a fecal/urinary diversion placement include the following:

- **Ileus** is paralysis of the bowel causing absence of bowel sounds and inability to pass flatus or stool, associated with abdominal discomfort and distention.
- **Anastomotic leak** is leakage from surgical site associated with distention and signs of infection. Leakage is most common in unstable or malnourished patients or those with fecal contamination of wound. It may be related to poor siting of stoma in a location close to bones, near old scars, or along the main incision, resulting in irritation.
- **Hemorrhage** may indicate the mesenteric vessel is open, requiring surgical intervention to repair damage.
- **Ischemia** is characterized by cyanotic discoloration of the stoma and may range from sloughing of mucosa to necrosis of tissue. It results from interruption of blood flow from numerous causes, such as too much tension on the mesentery, excessive mesentery stripping, or constrictive sutures.
- **Mucocutaneous separation** is an opening between the stoma and the skin where the sutures have separated.

REANASTOMOSIS/TAKEDOWN OF COLOSTOMY

For a reanastomosis/takedown of a colostomy, an incision is made around the stoma to separate it from the abdominal wall. Next, the proximal bowel segment is reattached to the distal segment. Finally, the abdominal wound is closed.

Complications include:

- **Anastomotic leak**: Occasionally there is a leak at the site of the anastomosis, causing fecal material to leak into the abdominal cavity and posing a danger of peritonitis.
- **Fascia dehiscence**: The fibrous tissue may split apart.
- **Wound infection**: Infection of the wound at the site of the reattachment or at the skin level can occur, especially in people who are compromised because of age or health.
- **Pulmonary complications**: Pneumonia and/or atelectasis may develop as a result of any surgery, so patients should be encouraged to stop smoking prior to surgery and to do deep-breathing/cough exercises.
- **Ileus/small bowel obstruction**: Any manipulation of the bowel may result in paralysis or obstruction of the bowel.
- **Hernia**: Post-surgical hernia may occur at surgical site.

Fistulae

FISTULA AND TERMINOLOGY RELATED TO FISTULAS

A fistula is an abnormal passage or tunnel from one internal organ to another or from an internal organ to the body surface. There may be multiple branches from a fistula rather than just one tunnel. Fistulas may be blind (only one open end), complete (openings both internally and externally), or incomplete (external skin opening with no connection to an internal organ).

- **Anorectal**: From the rectum or other anorectal area to the skin.
- **Colocutaneous**: From the colon to the skin surface.
- **Colovesical**: From the colon to the bladder.
- **Enterocolonic**: From the small intestine to the colon.
- **Enterocutaneous**: From the small intestine to the skin surface.
- **Enteroenteral**: Between two parts of the intestine.
- **Enterovaginal**: From the small intestine to the vagina.
- **Enterovesical**: From the small intestine to the bladder.
- **Rectovaginal**: From the rectum to the vagina.
- **Vesicocutaneous**: From the bladder to the skin surface.
- **Vesicovaginal**: From the bladder to the vagina.

CLASSIFICATION SYSTEMS FOR FISTULAS

Classification systems for fistulas help to characterize the fistula and assist in the management and treatment. Sometimes, more than one classification may be used. For example, a fistula may be described as "Complex, Type I with small to medium output."

SIMPLE/COMPLEX

Simple fistulas are short and direct tracts with no organ involvement or abscess. **Complex, Type I fistulas** involve multiple organs with an abscess associated. **Complex, Type II fistulas** open into the base of a disrupted wound.

VOLUME

With this classification system, the fistula is classified according to the amount of drainage from the wound in a 24-hour period. Low-output fistulas drain less than 150 mL per 24 hours. Small to medium output fistulas drain 150-500 mL per 24 hours, and high output fistulas drain more than 500 mL per 24 hours.

PSEUDOSTOMA

A pseudostoma is an unintended, nonsurgical opening on the abdominal wall that resembles a stoma. The pseudostoma most often results from a chronic enterocutaneous fistula although it can also occur at a prior stoma site. Patients with Crohn disease are especially at risk. Once a fistula forms, the channel is narrow and lined with granulation tissue, which begins to epithelialize. The drainage causes chemical irritation and maceration of surrounding tissue at the drainage site. In time, the segment of the bowel that is attached to the fistula adheres to the inner abdominal wall and the tract widens. The bowel may prolapse into the tract and through the fistula opening, where is mimics the appearance of a stoma. The tissue about the pseudostoma often becomes very inflamed and macerated, and drainage is often irregular. Management of the pseudostoma is similar to that of other fistulae: application of wound management system, peristomal skin protection, nutrition, hydration, and emotional support. A pseudostoma rarely heals spontaneously but requires surgical intervention when inflammation recedes. Preventive measures include reducing fistula output, closure of the fistula and/or wound surrounding the fistula. and protecting the skin from drainage.

ACUTE/CHRONIC FISTULAE

The differences between acute and chronic fistulae are shown below:

Acute	Chronic
• Newly-formed, less than 4–6 weeks. • Surrounding tissue inflamed, friable, necrotic. • Tract immature. • Pain intense and acute. • Etiology: surgery, trauma, infection. • High potential for spontaneous closure if underlying cause corrected. • Increased risk of abscess, sepsis, electrolyte imbalance.	• Longstanding with failure to close, more than 4–6 weeks. • Surrounding tissue fibrotic, epithelialized, scarred. • Tract mature, epithelialization present. • Pain chronic. • Etiology: Unresolved acute fistula, Crohn's disease • Low potential for spontaneous closure. • Increased risk of skin maceration, malnutrition, chronic inflammation.

Fistulae most at risk for chronicity include enterocutaneous, enterovesical, rectovaginal, and cholecystoduodenal although any type of fistula can become chronic. Fistulae are likely to become chronic if any FRIEND factors are present: **F** (foreign body), **R** (radiation-damaged tissue, **I** (infection/inflammation), **E** (epithelialization), **N** (neoplasm), and **D** (distal obstruction).

PARKS CLASSIFICATION SYSTEM FOR ANORECTAL FISTULAS

Parks classification system for anorectal fistulas classifies four different types of cryptoglandular (pertaining to the anal glands) fistulas. Anorectal fistulas are the most common type of fistula, occurring most frequently in women.

- **Intersphincteric fistulas** extend from the internal sphincter downward to the perineum, up to a high blind tract, or open into the rectum itself (70%).
- **Transsphincteric fistulas** extend from the internal and external sphincters to the ischiorectal fossa to the perineum (25%).
- **Suprasphincteric fistulas** cross the internal sphincter to the external sphincter above the puborectalis muscles and then down to the ischioanal fossa and to the skin (5%).
- **Extrasphincteric fistulas** extend from the perianal skin through the levator ani muscles and through the rectal wall (1%).

An additional classification is sometimes added to the original four:

- **Horseshoe fistulas** partially circle the anus, opening at both ends in the cutaneous tissue.

ASSESSING DRAINAGE FROM FISTULAS

Considerations when assessing the drainage from fistulas include:

- **Source of fistula**, whether it is near wound, stoma, organ, or bony prominence, helps determine the type of discharge. Enzymatic drainage, as from enterocutaneous fistula, may be corrosive to the tissue.
- **Type of drainage** includes color, consistency, and odor. Color of purulent discharge is often yellow, light brown, or slightly green. Fecal material draining through a fistula may range in color from golden (from the jejunum) or brown (from the descending colon), depending on fistula location.

- **Consistency** may range from very watery to very thick. Urinary discharge through a fistula may be combined with purulent material and mucous, and may be thin in consistency. Odor from fecal material, especially from the lower colon, is noticeable. Some types of infection have a pronounced foul odor. Odor in discharge is always a cause for concern.
- **Amount of drainage** is important for choosing the type of dressings and need for electrolyte replacement.

Percutaneous Tubes

NASOGASTRIC TUBES, SUMP TUBES, AND LEVIN TUBES

Nasogastric tubes (NG) are plastic or vinyl tubes inserted through the nose, down esophagus, and into the stomach.

Sump tubes are radiopaque with a vent lumen to prevent a vacuum from forming with high suction.

Levin tubes have no vent lumen and are used only with low suction.

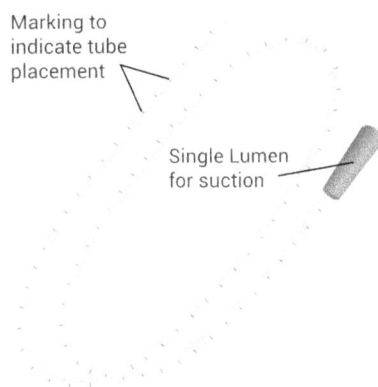

Marking to indicate tube placement

Single Lumen for suction

Levin Tube

The purpose of nasogastric tubes is to drain gastric secretions, allow sampling of secretions, or provide access to the stomach and upper gastrointestinal tract. They are used for lavage after medication overdose, for decompression, for instillation of medications or fluids. Nasogastric tubes should not be used if there is obstruction proximal to the stomach or gastric pathology, such as hemorrhage.

Management involves securing the tube at a downward angle, avoiding pressure on the nares that could lead to irritation or ulceration, providing drainage tubing and bags for gravity drainage if indicated, and monitoring drainage. Tubes attached to continuous low or intermittent high suction must be monitored frequently.

EXTENDED USE NASOGASTRIC TUBES AND INTESTINAL TUBES

Extended use nasogastric tubes or small-bore feeding tubes are flexible with weighted tips to maintain placement. These are often inserted with help of a guidewire. The purpose is to provide gastric access for temporary tube feedings. **Management** includes checking patency and flushing on a regular schedule because small lumen is easily occluded. The tube must be taped securely and angled downward, avoiding pressure on the nares that could lead to ulceration.

Intestinal tubes are longer tubes, reaching beyond the duodenum, up to 10 feet and weighted at the end with a mercury- or tungsten-filled balloon so the tube will advance through the intestine. The Cantor tube is a 10-foot single lumen tube. The Miller-Abbot tube is a double-lumen tube with an inflatable balloon that is inflated after tube is in the stomach. The purpose is decompression for bowel obstruction. **Management** includes instructing patient on positions to advance tube, securing tube, and monitoring drainage.

NEPHROSTOMY TUBES

Nephrostomy tubes are inserted into the kidney pelvis to provide drainage. The nephrostomy tube is inserted in the flank area, near the kidney, and drains through extension tubing into a bedside urinary bag or leg bag. The purpose of the tube is to provide drainage for urine and prevent hydronephrosis when there is a blockage in the urinary system. It may be used for kidney stones, cancer, strictures, stent placement, or to allow healing of a distal portion of the urinary tract. The tube may be inserted temporarily or permanently. **Management** includes irrigating with 5-10 mL of sterile water if necessary, securing the tube with sutures or attachment devices, keeping the surrounding skin dry and clean, observing for signs of complications (fever, chills, flank pain, tube leakage, blood or purulent drainage or discharge), and educating patient about the care of the tube and use and care of drainage tubes and bags.

Biliary Tubes

Biliary tubes or t-tubes are placed surgically in the liver and bile ducts to promote biliary drainage. The purpose of biliary tubes is to provide drainage, prevent blockage, serve as a stent for perforations, and allow easy access to laboratory sampling of discharge. They are used before or after surgical procedures such as liver transplants or complicated cholecystectomy. Either biliary tubes or stents may be used for decompression after common bile duct exploration. **Management** includes securing tube, measuring output, preventing backflow by maintaining gravity drainage system, keeping skin clean with normal saline and drying to prevent irritation, irrigating the drains as necessary to prevent blockage, observing for signs of infection (fever, chills, bile leakage around tube, bloody or purulent drainage or discharge), and educating the patient about the caring for the tube. Drainage after liver transplant should be observed carefully for inspissated (thickened) biliary sludge, indicating necrosis of bile duct walls.

Drains

Simple drains are latex or vinyl tubes of varying sizes and lengths inserted into a wound to provide drainage of serous material, blood, pus, or other discharge. This type of drain is usually placed through a stab wound near the area of involvement or at a surgical site. An example is a **Jackson Pratt drain**, which uses a bulb that is attached to the drainage tube to create suction. The bulb collects fluid and must be emptied when full. The suction is created by squeezing the bulb with the stopper open, then closing the stopper so there is negative pressure in the bulb and tubing.

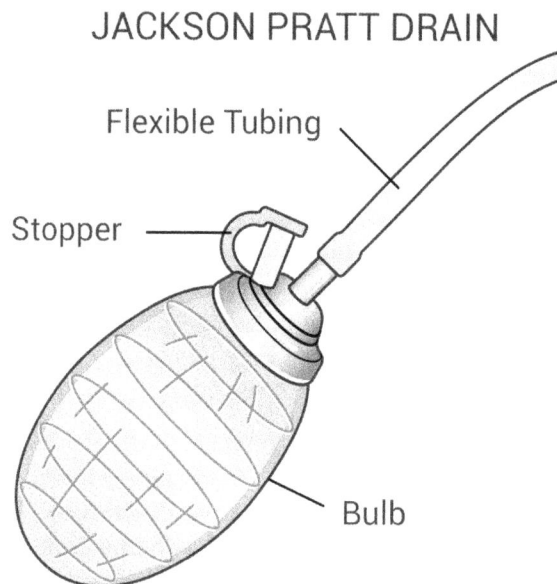

JACKSON PRATT DRAIN

Flexible Tubing

Stopper

Bulb

Penrose drains are soft rubber/latex tubes that are flat in appearance and are placed in surgical wounds to drain fluid by gravity and capillary action. They are available in various diameters and lengths.

Latex or silicone
tubing

Safety pin is attached to the end
of the tubing leaving the wound
to prevent the tube from slipping
inside of the wound

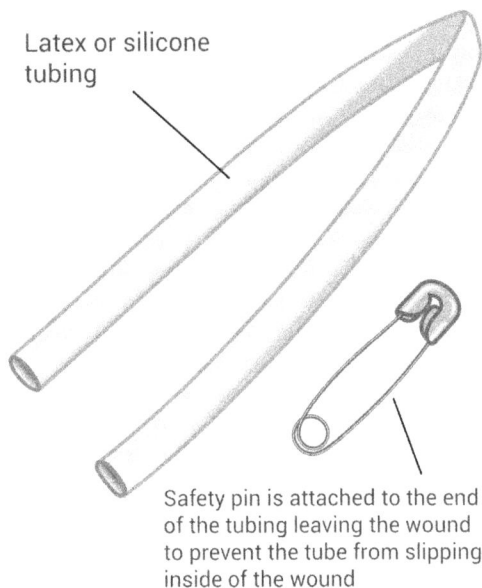

Penrose Drain

Sump drains are double-lumen or tri-lumen tubes (with a third lumen for infusions). A large outflow lumen and small inflow lumen produces venting when air enters the inflow lumen and forces drainage into the large lumen.

Percutaneous drainage catheter is inserted into wound to provide continuous drainage for infection or symptoms from collection of drainage in the wound. Irrigation of the catheter may need to be done to maintain patency. Skin barriers and pouching systems may be necessary.

SAFE PERCUTANEOUS DRAINAGE KIT

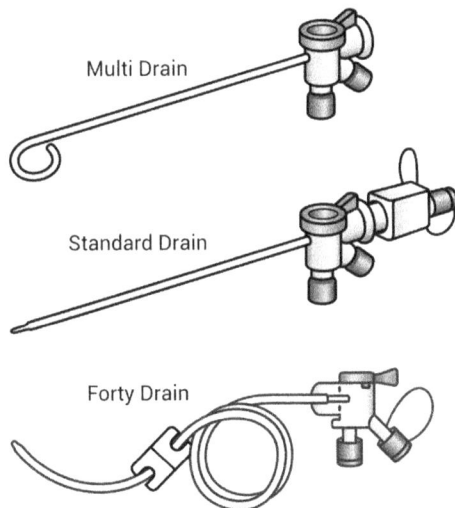

Multi Drain

Standard Drain

Forty Drain

Important Terms

Agenesis: The failure of an organ to grow or develop properly.

Atresia: Congenital absence or closure of an orifice or tubular structure.

Exstrophy: A congenital eversion (turning inside out) of an organ.

Extrusion: Protruding externally in an abnormal manner.

Fistula: An abnormal passage, tube-like structure, or opening between 2 internal structures or between an internal structure and the body surface.

Gangrene/dry gangrene: Loss of blood supply resulting in death of tissue, often allowing bacterial invasion. Dry gangrene does not involve bacterial infection of tissue, only necrosis.

Inspissation/inspissated: Condition of thickening/thick.

Ischemia: Lack of adequate blood supply to a local area due to obstruction of blood vessels, resulting in inadequate oxygen and nutrient supply to the tissue.

Necrosis: Death of cells or tissue because of insufficient blood flow, injury, disease, or other pathology.

Perforation: The condition of a hole through the wall of an organ or body structure.

Ostomy Care: Intervention and Treatment

Colostomy Management

ONE- OR TWO-PIECE POUCHING SYSTEMS

The procedures for one- and two-piece pouch systems are as follows:

1. Assemble supplies/equipment.
2. Empty pouch into toilet.
3. Gently remove pouch, working from the top down, using one hand to pull the pouch away from the skin and the other to push down on skin. Save clamp and place used pouch in a plastic bag.
4. Cleanse skin with water and examine for irritation or lesions. Dry. Shave if necessary with electric shaver.
5. Examine stoma and measure if necessary.
6. Cut appliance to fit if necessary or use precut appliance if stoma is round. Remove paper backing from appliance. Apply starting from the bottom, fitting under the stoma first and then smoothing upward so the warmth of the hands helps the appliance to adhere. If two-piece appliance, apply pouch to skin barrier.
7. Apply tape at corners of pouch if necessary.
8. Place ostomy deodorant in fecal pouch if desired and then apply clamp/close spout.

STOMA SITE LOCATION

The site of the stoma is influence by the purpose. For example, a permanent colostomy will likely be in the left ileac fossa while an ileostomy stoma will likely be in the right iliac fossa. The placement of the stoma should take into consideration what will be most convenient for the patient, collect drainage effectively, and not leak or damage the skin. There should be adequate space about the stoma for adherence of an appliance, allowing for at least 2.5 inches of flat adhesive surface for pouching. Areas that should be avoided include about the waistline and groin areas because bending would loosen the appliance and cause discomfort. Appliances will not adhere properly to skin folds, scars, bony prominences, and about the umbilicus because the surfaces are not adequately flat. When siting the stoma, the patient should be both in standing and sitting position because the abdominal contours may change. The patient should be able to see and reach the appliance easily. Additionally, the patient should wear and appliance over the chosen site for at least 24 hours to determine if it is satisfactory. Patients may need guidance in the type of clothing that helps to camouflage appliances and that allow for easy access, including loose shirts and dresses.

MARKING THE STOMA SITE

The three methods for marking the stoma site are explained below:

- **Permanent marker**: Site is marked with an X or circle, and usually covered with a transparent dressing to protect the markings. Markings will usually last for 1-3 weeks, but patients should be provided a marking pen and additional dressings in case markings fade.
- **Tattoo**: Target site is cleansed with alcohol, India ink is dropped on the site, and the skin is punctured 3 times with a small-gauge needle. The area is then cleansed and dressed. An alternate tattooing procedure is to inject a small amount of methylene blue (0.01 mL) intradermally. Tattooing is the most permanent method but is painful for the patient.
- **Laceration**: Site is marked by making circular scratches in the epidermis with a small-gauge needle. This method is not recommended because the break in the skin can lead to infection. However, some surgeons use this method prior to the surgical scrub to ensure that markings remain through scrub.

MODIFICATIONS IN PROCEDURE FOR MARKING THE STOMA SITE

Modifications in procedure for marking the stoma site in special circumstances are discussed below:

- **Thinness/cachexia**: If recent weight loss, person may regain weight, affecting stoma siting. Skin turgor may be poor.
- **Obesity/abdominal distension**: Follow nipple line down to abdomen to site stoma if rectus muscle non-palpable. If necessary, place stoma in upper quadrant to allow patient access. Evaluate females with large breasts in sitting position with and without bras to see if breasts obscure stoma site.
- **Physical considerations**:
  o Wheelchair bound should be evaluated in wheelchair.
  o Kyphosis or lordosis affects placement and people may benefit from wearing pouch for 24 hours to assure adherence.
  o Sports enthusiasts/physical laborers should be asked to go through the motions of their activities to make sure stoma is sited to avoid irritation.
- **Pediatric concerns**: avoiding umbilical cord area in newborns. Parents should be with children, and nurse should use an ostomy-teaching doll.
- **Post-radiation**: Post-radiation tissue may be damaged, so radiated area should be avoided.
- **Fecal and urinary diversions**: Both fecal and urinary diversions require that stomas be sited on different planes in case one pouch needs to be belted.

MINIMIZING ODOR FROM STOMA AND POUCH

Proper pouching is important because improper pouching is the cause of most odors:

- **Fecal diversions**: Check pouch for leaks. Check closure to verify it is clean and no fecal material has leaked around the opening. Make sure clamp is clean and secure. Avoid putting holes in appliance for release of gas as leaking gas may have a foul odor. Empty pouch regularly, using proper procedures.
- **Urinary diversions**: Wipe off end of spout to remove drops of remaining urine. Replace connecting tubing and bedside or leg bags, usually not odor proof, if odor develops.

Diet control includes avoiding gas/odor-producing foods.

- Fecal diversions:
  o **Vegetables**: cabbage, broccoli, kale, cauliflower, kohlrabi, Brussels sprouts, asparagus, onions, dried peas, rutabagas, turnips. Proteins: dried beans fish, strong cheeses, and eggs.
  o **Other**: spicy foods, chewing gum. Drinks: beer, carbonated beverages (such as sodas or juices).
- Urinary diversions:
  o Asparagus, fish, various spices.

COLOSTOMY IRRIGATION

The procedures for colostomy irrigation are as follows:

1. Gather all equipment, fill irrigating bag with lukewarm water (500-1500 mL), release air bubbles from tubing, and hang with bottom of bag at shoulder level.
2. Sit on or next to toilet and apply long irrigation sleeve, placing the end into the toilet.
3. Lubricate cone nozzle and insert into stoma (usually about 3 inches) in direction of colon.
4. Holding cone firmly in place to retain fluid, open clamp and let fluid flow into colon slowly over about 5-10 minutes. Hold cone in place for a few seconds, and then remove.

5. Drain fecal output into toilet for 10-15 minutes. Initial flow of fluids is usually followed by fecal material within 15 minutes.
6. Dry end of irrigation sleeve and clamp. Keep bag in place for up to an hour if stool continues to drain. Remove irrigation sleeve, cleanse peristomal area, and apply pouch.
7. Cleanse irrigation equipment.

MANAGEMENT OF RETAINED DISTAL SEGMENT OF BOWEL FOR COLOSTOMY PATIENTS

Management of retained distal segments depends to some degree on whether or not further surgery is planned to reattach the colon. General observations for signs of infection are especially important: fever, distention, and change in bowel habits.

- **Loop colostomy**: Loop of bowel brought to abdominal surface but not completely severed, usually with a rod holding loop above skin. Intestinal loop is cut partially open, creating two stomas—a proximal for fecal drainage and a small distal mucous fistula. Cleanse mucous fistula of discharge.
- **End-loop (double-barrel) colostomy with mucous fistula**: Portion of colon removed; both proximal and distal ends are brought through abdominal wall, creating two stomas, proximal for stool and distal for mucus.
- **Management**: Mucous fistulas should be cleansed with gauze and discharge examined for blood and/or pus or any other changes in character. Cleanse peristomal area carefully to prevent irritation. If rectum in place, check rectal area for irritation and discharge.

RELATIONSHIP BETWEEN PLACEMENT OF COLOSTOMY AND CHARACTER OF STOOL

Ascending colon: Because the stool is in liquid or semi-liquid form coming from the small intestine, it is still quite liquid or pasty in nature in the ascending colon. Diarrhea is the primary complication.

Transverse colon: With some of the fluid absorbed, the stool in the transverse colon is semi-liquid to soft, depending in part on the placement, right or left, of the stoma and the amount of transverse colon remaining. Diarrhea is the more common complication although constipation can occur, especially if much of the transverse colon is intact.

Descending colon: Much of the fluid has been reabsorbed from the stool by the time it reaches the descending colon, so the stool is semi-formed and soft. Diarrhea can occur as well as constipation.

Sigmoid colon: Reabsorption of fluids in the colon has been completed and the stool is fully formed. Diarrhea can occur, but constipation is a more common problem.

LAXATIVE AND ANTIFLATULENT AGENTS FOR THOSE WITH FECAL DIVERSION

The following are laxative and antiflatulent agents that may be helpful to those with fecal diversion:

- **Laxative agents**: Osmotic (Milk of Magnesia) and stimulant (Dulcolax) laxatives should not be taken by those with ileostomies as they can lead to increased diarrhea and electrolyte imbalance. They should be rarely used by others and only with the advice of healthcare providers. Overuse can lead to bowel dysfunction.
- **Fiber/bulk agents**: These agents dissolve or swell in the intestines, promoting peristalsis and include preparations made with methylcellulose (Citrucel), psyllium (Metamucil), and bran. These can reduce diarrhea and help with constipation.
- **Stool softeners**: These increase retention of fluid in the stool (DSS, Colace), helping to prevent constipation and impaction.

Ostomy Care: Intervention and Treatment

- **Antiflatulent agents**: These agents both disperse gas and prevent formation of gas bubbles. Simethicone (Phazyme) allows small gas bubbles to gather into larger ones, making them easier to expel by belching. The food enzyme alpha-galactosidase (Beano), which prevents gas related only to complex sugars but not sorbitol, lactose, fiber, or wheat.

Ileostomy Management

MANAGEMENT OF RETAINED DISTAL SEGMENT OF BOWEL WITH ILEOSTOMIES

Management of retained distal segments varies according to procedures completed or planned. In the case of complete proctocolectomy, the focus will simply be on healing because the distal segments have been excised. If reattachment or creation of a reservoir is planned, then distal segments must be monitored.

- **Loop ileostomy**: Loop of ileum brought to abdominal surface but not completely severed, usually with a rod holding loop above skin. Intestinal loop is cut partially open, creating two stomas—a proximal for fecal drainage and a small distal mucous fistula. Cleanse mucous discharge and check mucous fistula when pouch changed.
- **Ileostomy with ileoanal, J, S, or W pouch**: Monitor any discharge, distention, pain, fever, or other signs of infection. If anus intact, observe drainage for signs of infection. Cleanse perianal area and provide protective cream or ointment to prevent irritation. If pouch is created before closure of ileostomy, observe for pouchitis.

CONTINENT ILEOSTOMY

DRAINAGE AND MANAGEMENT OF KOCK POUCH

A **Kock pouch** uses the lower part of the small bowel to create an internal reservoir (pouch) for the collection of fecal material. This pouch is created from the small intestine and has a leak-free nipple valve inside the abdominal stoma, created by intussuscepting a portion of the ileal loop back through the ileum, to prevent leakage of stool, with an intestinal conduit leading to the pouch.

- **Draining**: Insert plastic catheter about 5 inches into stoma and lower opposite end of catheter over toilet to drain. Initially, pouch must be drained about every 3 hours because capacity is small. After about 2 months, pouch needs to be drained only 3-5 times a day.
- **Management**: Avoid eating late in the evening so pouch won't need draining during the night. Diet modification can prevent constipation or diarrhea. The stoma, about 1/2 inch in diameter, is covered with gauze or stoma cap to absorb mucus. Irrigate as directed, usually twice daily.

DRAINING

General procedures for draining the continent ileostomy in the initial postoperative phase and in later weeks and months are explained below:

- **Initial 3-4 weeks**: Prevent excessive pressure that could cause perforation or tearing by using constant drainage. If catheter plugs or falls out, replace immediately. The catheter needs to be irrigated with 1 ounce of tap water several times daily, letting liquid drain back out.
- **Next phase**: Continuous draining stops and intermittent draining begins, usually every 2 hours during the day with constant drainage at night. Pouch should be drained first thing in the morning and last thing at night. Gradually the time interval between draining increases and constant night drainage stops, but the pouch may need to be drained once or twice during the night.
- **3 months later**: The pouch should be well healed and functioning. Usual practice is to drain the pouch 4-6 times a day and irrigate 2 of these times. Any time there is a feeling of being full, bloated, or distended, the pouch should be drained as well as before physical activity.

IRRIGATING

The procedure for irrigating continent ileostomy is described below:

1. Gather supplies.
2. Remove dressing/stoma cap and discard.

Ostomy Care: Intervention and Treatment

3. Insert catheter if not in place.
4. Fill syringe with 30 mL of tap water, insert it into end of catheter, and inject with gentle pressure only.
5. Pinch the catheter to prevent drainage, remove the syringe, and then unpinch the catheter and allow it to drain into a basin or the toilet bowl.
6. The irrigation may need to be repeated until the stool flows back freely.
7. DO NOT use the syringe to pull the stool or fluid back out. Always allow it to drain back out by gravity.
8. If liquid drains back very slowly, the catheter may be blocked; remove, rinse with tap water, and reinsert.
9. DO NOT put more than 60 mL of water into pouch without ensuring the fluid is draining out.
10. Remove catheter, cleanse skin, and reapply stoma dressing.

PREVENTION FOR FLUID AND ELECTROLYTE IMBALANCE WITH AN ILEOSTOMY

Causes of fluid/electrolyte imbalance: After the large intestine is removed, the body adjusts by absorbing more fluids and nutrients in the small intestine, and the stool becomes thicker, increasing the danger of dehydration. Bouts of diarrhea with excessively watery stools can also lead to dehydration and electrolyte imbalance. With electrolyte imbalance, just increasing the oral intake of fluids is not sufficient as these fluids will be excreted through the kidneys and may not correct the electrolyte imbalance. Excessive heat can also cause dehydration and electrolyte imbalance. All types of fluid loss involve loss of electrolytes.

Signs and symptoms include:

- Mouth/tongue dry. Skin turgor poor.
- Weight loss. Diarrhea. Lethargy.

Strategies for prevention are as follows:

- Maintain adequate fluid and nutritional intake.
- Estimate/monitor intake and output.
- Monitor weight.
- Drink Gatorade or other such liquids with diarrhea or dehydration.
- If stool too liquid, increase fibrous foods; too dry, increase salty foods.
- Antidiarrheal agents may be necessary.
- Lavage.

MECHANICAL OBSTRUCTION OF AN ILEOSTOMY

Causes of mechanical obstruction: Obstruction of an ileostomy is almost always food-related. After the large intestine is removed, the body adjusts by absorbing more fluids and nutrients in the small intestine; the stool becomes thicker, increasing the danger of dehydration. Mechanical obstruction is almost always caused by high fiber foods, such as inadequately-chewed popcorn, nuts, celery, coconut, and corn. This mass causes the bowel above to become hyperactive as it contracts, trying to move the mass of fiber. As the pressure builds, the part of the intestine below the mass may collapse, causing a reverse peristalsis.

Signs and symptoms include:

- Edematous stoma. High-pitched bowel sounds.
- Obvious peristaltic waves. Nausea and vomiting.
- Abdominal pain. Distention.
- Dry mouth, loss of skin turgor. Watery diarrhea.

Strategies of prevention are as follows:

- Increase fluids and avoid dehydration.
- High fiber foods should be taken in limited quantities and chewed thoroughly.
- Warm bath may relax abdominal muscles.
- Drink warm fluids and assume the knee-chest position.

LAVAGE OF AN ILEOSTOMY TO RELIEVE BLOCKAGE

Lavage is usually done after an abdominal x-ray has determined that food is the cause of the blockage. It is NOT the same as an irrigation, which uses large volumes of fluid. Normal saline (NS) is used to prevent further dehydration, instilled with a catheter-tipped piston or bulb syringe with a 14-16 Fr catheter attached. The procedure is done to "flush" the blockage loose.

1. Gather supplies.
2. Remove pouching system and apply irrigation sleeve with end in toilet (or bedpan).
3. Do a digital exam to determine direction of intestine.
4. Lubricate the catheter and gently insert approximately 12-15 cms.
5. Slowly inject 30-50 mL of normal saline into the intestine and then slowly aspirate the entire amount with light to moderate pressure.
6. Repeat the procedure of flushing with normal saline until the blockage is relieved.
7. Measure the stoma (because of swelling) and apply the correctly-sized pouch.

ILEOSTOMY TAKEDOWN

Usually about two months after the temporary ileostomy, the ileostomy is closed and the proximal and distal segments are reattached/opened for intestinal continuity. The ileoanal reservoir is usually quite small after surgery, so 8-10 stools per day is not unusual, but the reservoir capacity will expand and stool frequency will decrease over a 6- to 12-month period. The best functional results would be 4-5 stools per day with no incontinence. Most current procedures result in 95% continence during the day and 90% during the night.

Complications are as follows:

- **Wound infection**: May be superficial at abdominal surface or at anastomosis.
- **Small bowel obstruction**: Usually corrected non-surgically.
- **Anastomotic leak**: Can lead to serious infection/peritonitis.
- **GI bleeding from peri-anastomotic ulcers**: Sometimes arises from side to side anastomosis of small bowel for pouch formation.
- **Steroids**: Can increase wound complications, so wean steroids prior to surgery.
- **Pouchitis**: Non-specific inflammation of pouch, usually in the first two years.

Ostomy Care: Intervention and Treatment

Urostomy Management

URETERAL STENT AND POST-SURGICAL MANAGEMENT

Ureteral stent: A piece of thin pliable tubing that is inserted inside of the ureter to maintain patency, during post-surgical period when edema of the ureter could cause occlusion. These tubes protrude through the stoma and are often different lengths or color-coded to differentiate which ureter they serve.

Post-surgical management: Ureteral stents are usually removed after 5 to 7 days although they may be left in for several weeks. Each protruding stent should be drained separately and clearly labeled. Stents have multiple holes along the length of the tube to promote drainage. Ensure that the stents are not dislodged or blocked. If pain, purulent discharge, or fever occurs, a chest x-ray may be taken to determine position of the stent. Patient must be advised NOT to remove the stent. The stent may be irrigated with 5-10 mL of normal saline, using care not to apply tension or pressure that may dislodge the tube.

CHANGING AND MANAGING UROSTOMY POUCH

The two main types of **urostomy pouches** are the one-piece with attached skin barrier and the two-piece with a skin barrier and pouch that detaches. The pouches have drains at the bottom for emptying and to attach a nighttime drainage tube.

- **Changing the pouch**: If possible, change pouch in the morning before eating or drinking when urine flow is decreased, or wait 2 hours after eating or drinking. Remove pouch. Stand or sit as comfortable, keeping a paper towel or gauze to absorb drops of urine. Cleanse peristomal tissue, dry skin, and apply new bag, using a mirror to guide if necessary.
- **Emptying the pouch**: Empty the pouch regularly to prevent bacteria from growing in the urine, usually every 2-4 hours during the day. Children may need more frequent draining because the pouch is smaller. Empty the pouch when it is about 1/3 full. Open the valve at the bottom and drain directly into a toilet or other container.

MODIFICATIONS AND MANAGEMENT FOR UROSTOMIES

Fluid modifications: Adequate intake of fluids is critical to prevent urinary complications, such as infections. Oral intake should be 2000-2500 mL (8-10 glasses) per day.

Nighttime management: To prevent the ostomy bag from becoming overfull during the night and pulling away from the skin, a long tube should attach a large overnight urinary drainage bag. The bag can be placed in a container on the floor or hung on the side of the bed. Overnight drainage also helps to keep the urine from constantly bathing the stoma and causing white, gritty crystals to form. Acidifying the urine by taking vitamin C can treat these crystals.

Mucus management: Mucus in urine is usually managed by increasing fluids to flush the mucus. In immediate post-surgical period, a marked increase in mucus in the urine may occur but will usually abate. Gentle irrigations will be done post-surgically to maintain patency of catheters.

PROTECTING THE PERISTOMAL TISSUE WITH A UROSTOMY

Pouching: Measure the stoma and make sure that the opening in the skin barrier is the correct size. Drain on a regular schedule to avoid leaks, and change the pouch regularly before leaks occur.

Protect skin: Remove the pouch and cleanse the skin immediately if there is pain, itching, or burning in peristomal area. Use care when removing the skin barrier so that the skin does not pull. Put pressure on the skin to push it away from the barrier. Wash peristomal skin carefully with water and mild soap if necessary or shower after the pouch is removed. Be sure that peristomal skin is thoroughly dry before applying barrier.

Observe: Check area carefully and be aware that sensitivities and allergies to adhesives, barriers, or material in pouches can develop over time. It may be necessary to try different types of barriers or to use a pouch cover to protect the skin.

Ostomy Care: Intervention and Treatment

Continent Diversion

IRRIGATING THE URINARY RESERVOIR FOR CONTINENT CUTANEOUS URINARY DIVERSIONS

Irrigation of the urinary reservoir is done frequently in the immediate post-operative period. The person with the urinary reservoir (or a care giver) should be taught irrigate in preparation for leaving the hospital.

1. Gather supplies, wash hands.
2. Remove dressing or stoma cap if one is in place.
3. Insert catheter into reservoir (unless a catheter is still in place for continuous drainage), NEVER force; drain urine.
4. Attach syringe to end of catheter and gently aspirate to make sure the reservoir is empty.
5. Draw 60 mL of sterile water/normal saline into syringe, insert syringe into catheter end, and gently inject the fluid.
6. Keep catheter elevated or pinched to prevent drainage and inject another 40 mL of water to a total of 100 mL.
7. Gently aspirate to begin flow and then allow fluid to drain by gravity.
8. Repeat irrigation if necessary until urine is clear if there is excessive mucus.

MANAGEMENT OF MUCUS FOR CONTINENT CUTANEOUS URINARY DIVERSIONS

In the immediate post-operative period, the urinary reservoir and the intestinal conduit produce large amounts of mucus, giving the urine a cloudy appearance and creating sediment or long strands of mucoid-appearing material. Mucus is usually white and can be differentiated from yellow or greenish purulent material that indicates an infection. However, any cloudiness in urine should be suspect and requires careful observation. While a catheter is in place after surgery, it may be gently irrigated maintain patency and to prevent blockage, which could put stress on the reservoir and damage the suture lines. After the catheter is removed, increasing fluid intake to 8 to 10 glasses a day can reduce the amount of mucus. Additionally, people will need to irrigate the reservoir every 4-6 hours with small amounts of sterile water for the first 3 weeks and later as directed by their physician to empty reservoir of large amounts of mucus.

SELECTION OF APPROPRIATE INTUBATION AND DRESSING SUPPLIES

Catheters: The size of the catheter used will depend to some degree on the type of nipple valve. Most people will need a 16-18 Fr straight catheter, but some tighter valves may need a 10-14 Fr catheter. Most catheters are 16 inches long, allowing for drainage into the toilet while the person is sitting on the toilet. Some catheters are latex free, some plastic, and some rubber. A clear catheter makes observation of the draining urine easier than an opaque catheter.

Irrigating syringe: A 60-70 mL injection or bulb syringe is necessary for irrigation.

Sterile water/normal saline: These solutions may be purchased or may be prepared at home.

Dressing supplies: There is a wide range of choices, including absorbent pads with hypoallergenic adhesives, and stoma caps in various shapes and sizes (look like flesh-colored adhesive bandages). Nursing pads/eye pads are inexpensive, easily available substitutions for stoma dressings.

INCONTINENCE AFTER CATHETER REMOVAL FOR THOSE WITH AN ORTHOTOPIC NEOBLADDER

Urinate on a regularly scheduled basis with straining as the bladder may not have the normal sensation of fullness:

- **First week**: Every 2 hours during the day and 3 hours during the night.
- **Second week**: Every 3 hours during the day and 4 hours during the night.
- **Third week and later**: Every 4 hours during the day and 1 time during the night.

It may take several minutes to empty the bladder completely. Men should sit initially to make sure that the bladder is emptied.

Muscles: Because the neobladder does not expel urine, the abdominal muscles must tighten, and the sphincter muscles relax, so exercises, including Kegel, should be done before surgery.

Incontinence: Some is inevitable; people must be willing and able to catheterize. Some people may never completely empty the bladder and may need to catheterize once or several times a day.

Irrigation: Rarely needed after the immediate post-operative period.

INTUBATION/CATHETERIZING THE CONTINENT CUTANEOUS URINARY DIVERSION

The procedure for intubation/catheterizing the continent cutaneous urinary diversion is explained below:

1. Gather supplies and wash hands.
2. Remove stomal covering.
3. Sit on or near toilet or with a basin beneath stoma.
4. Lubricate end of catheter with water or water-soluble lubricant.
5. Insert catheter into stoma and allow draining by gravity.
6. If catheter plugs or doesn't drain properly, remove the catheter, and rinse it with warm water under the faucet to remove mucus that may be blocking the lumen.
7. When draining is complete, remove catheter.
8. Cleanse peristomal skin and apply a clean stoma covering.
9. Cleanse reusable catheters by washing with soap and hot water; rinse thoroughly, pushing water through the catheter with a syringe.
10. Dry catheters on a paper towel; dry thoroughly inside and out before storing in a Ziploc-type bag.
11. Always keep clean catheters separate from used, and NEVER place catheters on the back of the toilet or counters in public restrooms.

Ostomy Care: Intervention and Treatment

CLEAN INTERMITTENT CATHETERIZATION (CIC) FOR MALES

CIC for males:

1. Gather supplies; wash hands.
2. Sit on toilet or chair with container near.
3. Clean end of penis and urethral opening with soap and water or individually packaged wipes containing benzalkonium chloride.
4. Lubricate catheter with water-soluble lubricant (or water).
5. Hold penis by the sides, perpendicular to the body or pointing slightly upward.
6. Gently insert catheter into meatus, guiding it through the penis. There may be resistance when the catheter passes the prostate. Deep breathing and relaxing may help to advance the catheter. Do not force past a blockage.
7. When urine flow begins, insert the catheter 1 inch more.
8. When drainage ceases, withdraw catheter incrementally, making sure bladder is empty.
9. Wash reusable catheter with soap and hot water. Rinse completely and dry. Store in a clean dry place or carrying case/Ziploc bag. Reusable catheters last about 2-4 weeks, but should be soaked in a white vinegar solution once weekly.

CLEAN INTERMITTENT CATHETERIZATION (CIC) FOR FEMALES

CIC for females:

1. Gather supplies; wash hands.
2. Sit on toilet or stand with one foot on toilet.
3. Clean vulva and urethral opening with soap and water or individually packaged wipes containing benzalkonium chloride, wiping top to bottom.
4. Lubricate catheter with water-soluble lubricant (or water).
5. Spread labia with second and fourth fingers of one hand; feel for meatus with middle finger.
6. Gently insert catheter into meatus, guiding it upward. Insert 2-3 inches until urine flow; then slowly insert another inch.
7. When drainage ceases, withdraw catheter incrementally, making sure bladder is empty.
8. Wash reusable catheter with soap and hot water. Rinse completely and dry. Store in a clean dry place or carrying case/Ziploc bag. Reusable catheters last about 2-4 weeks, but should be soaked in a white vinegar solution once weekly.
9. Observe urine flow or drain urine into a container and measure if signs of infection or incomplete emptying.

CHILDREN REQUIRING CLEAN INTERMITTENT CATHETERIZATION

The following are special considerations for children requiring clean intermittent catheterization:

- **Age/maturity**: For sense of self-worth and independence, children should become independent in catheterization. Usually, a child needs mental age of 5 and normal physical dexterity to manage catheterization. Most children can catheterize without supervision by the age of 7 or 8.
- **Physical dexterity**: Physical disabilities or lack of dexterity may delay or prevent independent catheterization.
- **Psychological readiness**: Children must be willing to do the procedure. Having the child help at a very young age, such as gathering equipment or holding supplies, can help the child to gain confidence.
- **School**: Children can manage catheterization at school. The teacher, principal, and school nurse or aide should be aware of children's needs. The school nurse or aide can assist. Careful scheduling around breaks will minimize lost class time. If possible, arrange for children to use a private bathroom if available. Make sure that extra supplies are available at school.
- **Latex**: Avoid latex products as allergies may develop.

METABOLIC ACIDOSIS AND OTHER MALABSORPTION PROBLEMS

Metabolic acidosis: The normal bladder does not reabsorb fluid or salts from urine, but the intestinal tissue, especially from the colon, used in the creation of the urinary reservoir retains its ability to secrete and absorb ions and fluids, including sodium ions, bicarbonate, and ammonium. This can result in an increase in hydrogen, chloride, and serum urea and creatinine. These problems can occur at any time so people should be monitored for metabolic acidosis. If systemic alkalization is not done, these chronic metabolic disturbances can lead to demineralization of the bones.

Malabsorption: Less transit time leads to diarrhea, malabsorption of bile salts and Vitamin B12 and sometimes fat and fat-soluble vitamins (A, D, E, K), predisposing the person to gallstones, kidney stones, and steatorrhea (fat in feces).

- **Management**: Systemic alkalization is achieved through restriction of chloride intake. Sodium bicarbonate, chlorpromazine, nicotinic acids, and vitamins may be administered.

URINARY TRACT INFECTION, URINARY RETENTION/OBSTRUCTION, AND POUCHITIS

Urinary tract infection:

- **Urine**: May be cloudy, concentrated, bloody, foul smelling, mucusy, or purulent. May have urinary leakage/incontinence.
- **Pain**: May have flank pain, low back pain, or abdominal cramping.
- **Systemic**: May develop fever with or without chills and a general feeling of malaise and lethargy.
- **Prevention**: Drink 8-10 glasses of liquid, maintain acidity of urine, catheterize on schedule and/or empty bladder completely, and avoid over-distention of reservoir.

Urinary retention/obstruction:

- **Pain**: May have pain in abdomen, lower back, flank, or pelvis.
- **Distention**: May have feeling of abdominal fullness and abdomen may appear distended.
- **Systemic**: Nausea.
- **Prevention**: Catheterize on regular schedule and irrigate as necessary to remove accumulation of mucus in reservoir. Empty bladder completely with each intubation.

Pouchitis:

- **Urine**: Increased mucus and blood urine.
- **Pain**: Pain that may be localized to area of reservoir but may be more generalized.
- **Systemic**: Fever, general malaise.
- **Preventive**: Careful follow-up care and regular monitoring of residual urine volumes.

POSTOPERATIVE COMPLICATIONS OF THE NEOBLADDER

The following are postoperative complications of the neobladder:

- **Metabolic acidosis**: Can occur at any time because of reabsorption of fluid or salts through the intestinal tissue of the neobladder and requires systemic alkalization to prevent demineralization of bones.
- **Vitamin B-12 deficiency**: Loss of a portion of the ileum can result in malabsorption.
- **Anastomotic leaks**: Can occur in the pouch or intestines.
- Urinary abnormalities:
  - **Retention**: May be a sign of tumor recurrence, stenosis, or excessive mucus.

Ostomy Care: Intervention and Treatment

- **Incontinence**: Some incontinence, especially nocturnal enuresis, is common because there is less feeling of bladder fullness. About 10% will have stress incontinence or complete incontinence after procedure.
- **Calculi**: May be related to persistent bacteriuria. May occur if the bladder is not completely emptied, resulting in urinary stasis, or if urine is exposed to staples or permanent.
- **Urinary infection**: Recurrent infections and low-grade bacteriuria are common. May have bouts of pyelonephritis.
- **Fistulas**: Gastrointestinal fistula or ureteral fistulas may occur.
- **Pouchitis**: Non-specific inflammation of neobladder reservoir.
- **Stenosis**: Ceco-urethral or ileo-urethral anastomosis stenosis may develop.

COMPLICATIONS RELATED TO ANASTOMOTIC LEAKS WITH CREATION OF NEOBLADDER

The following are complications related to anastomotic leaks with creation of the neobladder:

- **Urinary extravasation**: Urinary leaks may occur from any of the urinary anastomosed areas. Leakage around the sites of the implanted ureters can lead to leakage into the peritoneal cavity.
  - **Symptoms**: Abdominal distension and discomfort as well as urinary leakage around tubes and drains or through the incisions.
  - **Treatment**: Separation of the suture lines may require surgical repair, but surgeons may decide to insert a nephrostomy tube for urinary drainage to allow the suture lines time to heal without urinary pressure. Stents or drainage tubes may be reinserted as well. Intraperitoneal pouch leaks are more difficult to treat medically than extraperitoneal leaks.
- **Fecal leakage**: This is less common than urinary extravasation but can occur at the sites where the fecal section was removed.
  - **Symptoms**: Usually relate to acute peritonitis with fever, chills, abdominal pain, rigidity and distention and an absence of bowel sounds.
  - **Treatment**: Requires antibiotic therapy and immediate surgical intervention.

Special Populations

SIDE EFFECTS RELATED TO ADJUVANT (POSTOPERATIVE) CHEMOTHERAPY

Side effects related to adjuvant (postoperative) chemotherapy for those with ostomies are listed and explained below:

- **Myelosuppression**: People may suffer anemia but depression of the white count is a more serious problem as this compromises the immune system, leaving people susceptible to infection. People must know protective measures, such as avoiding crowds to prevent infections.
- **Mucositis**: Entire mucosa of GI tract can become inflamed, swollen, and painful. Tissue may become infected. Saline mouthwashes, topical anesthetics, and analgesics may help relieve discomfort, promote adequate intake, and prevent infection.
- **Peripheral neuropathies**: Compromised sensation in hands may make ostomy care difficult. Person may need temporary assistance.
- **Skin reactions**: Some drugs may cause photosensitivity so people need to avoid the sun. Hand and foot syndrome can cause severe pain in hands and feet, making self-care difficult.
- **Nausea/vomiting**: Bland foods and anti-emetics may help. Adequate fluid intake is necessary to avoid developing constipation or dehydration. Strong odors, such as food odors or perfume, may trigger nausea.

SIDE EFFECTS RELATED TO ADJUVANT (POSTOPERATIVE) RADIATION FOR THOSE WITH OSTOMIES

Side effects related to adjuvant (postoperative) radiation for those with ostomies are listed and explained below:

- **Injury to small bowel and rectal area**: Causes diarrhea, often treated with antidiarrheals, such as Lomotil or Imodium, which can in turn cause constipation. Mucosa of bowel becomes denuded. Bland diet with low residue and lactose may relieve symptoms. Stoma may ooze stool frequently and pouches may need to be changed more often.
- **Skin reactions**: May cause pain, burning, dryness, and irritation in radiated tissue. Irritated peristomal tissue may require non-adhesive pouch or skin barrier powder.
- **Fatigue**: People need time to rest and should schedule activities to avoid over-exertion. If fatigue severe, they may need temporary assistance with ostomy or personal care.
- **Nausea/vomiting**: Bland foods and anti-emetics may help. Adequate fluid intake is necessary to avoid developing constipation or dehydration.
- **Proctitis/cystitis**: Organs near radiated area may suffer inflammation and infection, causing pain and complications.
- **Sexual dysfunction**: Males may suffer erectile dysfunction; and females, vaginal stenosis. Open discussion and information about treatment options should be provided.

Ostomy Care: Intervention and Treatment

URINARY TRACT INFECTIONS IN UROSTOMY PATIENTS

Urinary tract infections are common in urostomy patients and often-chronic low-grade kidney infections develop over time, so observing for urinary infections and treating promptly are very important:

- **Changes in character** of urine:
  - **Appearance:** The urine may become cloudy from mucus or purulent material. Hematuria may be present.
  - **Color:** Urine usually becomes concentrated and may be dark yellow/orange or brownish in color.
  - **Odor:** Urine may have a very strong or foul odor.
  - **Output:** Urinary output may decrease markedly.
- **Pain:** There may be lower back or flank pain from inflammation of the kidneys.
- **Systemic:** Fever, chills, headache, and general malaise often accompany urine infections. Some people suffer lack of appetite as well as nausea and vomiting. Fever usually indicates that the infection has affected the kidneys. Children may develop incontinence or loose stools and cry excessively.
- **Urine specimen:** Specimen should be taken directly from the stoma after the pouch is removed and peristomal skin cleansed.

COLLECTING STERILE URINE SPECIMEN FROM ILEAL CONDUIT

Do not collect urine from the bottom of the bag as this is where bacteria will collect and the specimen can give an inaccurate result. Catheterization of the ileal urostomy should be done using aseptic technique. Clean gloves should be worn to remove the ostomy pouch and clean the stoma site with clean water. After the catheterization tray is opened, sterile gloves should be worn. Gently force urine out before inserting the catheter. Lubricate the 14 Fr catheter and insert it about 7 centimeters, or about 2 ¼ inches, into the center of the stoma. If there is resistance, do not force the catheter, but try to rotate it until it slides in easily. Place the end of the catheter into a sterile specimen cup to collect the urine. The patient may need to roll, bear down, or cough to express the urine. Once the specimen is collected, remove the catheter and replace the ostomy pouch. It is important to note on the specimen cup or lab order that the specimen was obtained via an ileal conduit.

SELECTING POUCHING SYSTEMS AND ACCESSORIES FOR NEW OSTOMIES

When selecting a pouching system and accessories, personal choice affects choice but considerations include:

- **Open or closed system:** An open system has a clamp or clip at the bottom that allows the bag to be opened and drained. The open system is most appropriate for those with continuous or liquid drainage, such as an ileostomy. A closed system is appropriate for an ostomy that is more predictable, such as those whose elimination is generally on a regular schedule or those who irrigate and have little or no discharge between irrigations.
- **One- or two-piece systems:** A one-piece system requires the entire appliance be changed each time, which increases the need for supplies and time needed to change the appliance. A two-piece system allows only the outer bag to be replaced as needed.
- **Barriers/wafers:** The type of barrier/wafer that attaches to the skin vary widely with some flat and others convex, so selection may depend on the condition of the stoma and the site. The type of adhesive varies, and some types may be more irritating to skin than others.
- **Accessories:** Various accessories are available, including ostomy belts to help secure the appliance, pouch covers, convex inserts, skin barrier pastes, tapes to secure, and adhesive remover.

Fistula Management

MANAGEMENT

Fistula management typically begins with conservative medical treatment because most close without surgical intervention. Treatment may include broad spectrum antibiotics if the area about the fistula appears infected or if the patient has fistulae associated with Crohn's disease. Infliximab may be administered to patients with Crohn's disease to decrease inflammation and promote healing of fistulae. Containment of drainage is important in order to maintain **perifistular skin** integrity, especially if the drainage contains fecal material, which has enzymes that are destructive of the skin. Continuous suction devices or stoma appliances that provide a skin barrier should be used to protect the perifistular tissue. Perifistular skin should be cleansed with a special cleaning product (such as Cavilon No-Rinse Skin Cleanser) or with tap water and a skin barrier applied. Crusting is a procedure in which a thin layer of ostomy or stoma powder is applied to wet or denuded skin about the fistula and then sprayed with an alcohol-free barrier film to form a protective "crust" to which an appliance can be attached.

NEGATIVE PRESSURE WOUND THERAPY

Negative pressure wound therapy (NPWT) uses subatmospheric (negative) pressure (-50 to -125 mm HG) with a suction unit and a semi-occlusive vapor-permeable dressing. The suction reduces periwound and interstitial edema, decompresses vessels, improves circulation, and contains effluent. NPWT stimulates production of new cells, decreases colonization of bacteria, increases the rate of granulation and re-epithelialization, reduces wound size, and increases spontaneous closure rates. The wound must be debrided of necrotic tissue prior to treatment. NPWT is contraindicated with wound malignancy, untreated osteomyelitis, exposed blood vessels, unprotected bowel in wound base, and untreated sepsis.

- **Stoma management**: Used for peristomal wound management of separation, skin breakdown, mucocutaneous dehiscence, and open abdomen with stoma.
- **Fistula management**: Used for enterocutaneous fistulae with open wounds, periwound tissue breakdown, containment of high-output effluence, and healing of open complex abdominal wounds.
- **Wound management**: Used for open surgical wounds, pressure injuries, diabetic foot ulcers, dehiscence, grafts/flaps, large cavity wounds, and burns.

Best practices include protecting exposed bowel with non-adherent layers but not applying foam directly to mucosa, using stoma paste and rings to seal edges about high-output fistulae, monitoring output volume and quality, and avoiding excessive negative pressure on bowel by using low-pressure settings.

OCTREOTIDE

Octreotide acetate (Mycapssa, Sandostatin, Sandostatin LAR) is a synthetic analog of somatostatin, a peptide hormone that inhibits several GI hormones. Within the GI tract, octreotide inhibits secretion of gastric acid, bile, pancreatic enzymes, and intestinal fluids; suppresses release of serotonin, gastrin, and vasoactive intestinal peptide; and reduces intestinal motility, splanchnic blood flow. Octreotide is available for IM, SQ, PO, or IV administration. When used for wound care, octreotide reduces effluent volume, decreases the risk of skin breakdown, and facilitates granulation. Octreotide is used as adjunctive therapy and is most effective in controlling pancreatic and small bowel (duodenal and high-output jejunal or ileal fistulae) output. Adverse effects can include confusion, dizziness, arrhythmia, bradycardia, blurred vision, hearing loss, abdominal pain, nausea, diarrhea, gallstones, hyperglycemia, hypoglycemia, anemia, arthralgia, myalgia, and alopecia. During administration of octreotide, monitoring should include electrolytes, glucose, fluid balance, output volume, and abdominal imaging to evaluate closure.

Ostomy Care: Intervention and Treatment

ADDITIONAL TREATMENT OPTIONS

Additional treatment for fistulas include:

- **Antibiotics**: Antibiotics, such as metronidazole, are first line of treatment but often combined with other therapies, such as surgical drainage or excision.
- **Corticosteroids**: Corticosteroids may be used in conjunction with antibiotics and other therapy for Crohn's disease.
- **Drains**: There is evidence that treating abscesses with antibiotics and drainage can prevent fistula formation. Drains/tubes may be left in place to ensure drainage or keep existing fistulas open.
- **Seton**: A suture is placed to hold the fistula open (draining seton). If a fistula heals at the surface and remains open underneath, the discharge will tunnel to the surface again.
- **Autologous fibrin glue**: Glue is used to close fistula.
- **Fistulotomy/fistulectomy**: Excision is often most effective treatment for a fistula. Staged repairs may be done. Surgical treatment may involve open surgery, endoscopic, or laparoscopic approaches. Conservative treatment may precede surgical therapy, but terminal or Crohn's disease patients are poor surgical candidates.

Tube and Drain Management

Securement Techniques for Percutaneous Tubes/Drains

Various types of tubes and drains, such as Penrose, may be inserted into the periwound area in order to collect fluids. The tube/drain may be open—draining directly into absorbent dressings—or closed—drainage collected in a portable suction device, such as the Hemovac or Jackson-Pratt drain. Drains should be secured, often with transparent film or tape at or near the exit site. If a portable suction device or drainage bag is attached to the tube/drain, the tubing should also be secured to the patient's clothing with a safety pin or clip below the operative site, checking to make sure that the tubing is not kinked. Drains may be lightly sutured in place in order to prevent them from inadvertently falling out. In that case, the suture and the tissue about the suture should be examined with each dressing change, but the dressing generally provides the additional securement needed.

Enteral Feeding Tube Complications

Occlusion

Prevention of occlusion involves proper administration of medications and feedings, and maintaining a regular schedule of flushing. Tubes should be flushed with 30 mL of water at least every 4 hours as well as before and after feedings and administration of medications. Medications should be in liquid form or crushed completely and enteric-coated or delayed release preparations should be avoided. Feeding solutions should be liquid consistency. Flushing of occluded tube involves first checking for kinks or obvious problems, attaching a 30-60 mL syringe and aspirating fluid. Then, 5-10 mL of water can be slowly instilled (over about a minute) and aspirated a number of times to try to loosen occlusion. After clamping for 10-15 minutes, the flushing procedure can be repeated with warm water. If the water fails, a multi-enzyme cocktail or pancrease and sodium bicarbonate solution should be attempted. If all flushing fails, the physician should be notified.

Displacement

Displacement of tube is usually the result of inadequate stabilization. Foley catheters must be marked where they exit the stoma to check for migration. Gastrostomy tubes with an internal balloon or mushroom tip, measured markings, and an external disk are easier to stabilize, but internal device should be checked daily by gently pulling until resistance is felt. External stabilizing devices can be applied to the skin to hold the tube in place. The tube may also be taped to the abdomen or secured with a binder. Sometimes surgeons suture the tube in place, especially those with no balloon, such as jejunostomy tubes, which can become easily dislodged. A solid skin barrier with the tube fed through an anchored baby nipple is an inexpensive stabilizer. Position and length of tube should be carefully documented. Balloon volume should be checked weekly to insure there are no leaks. Skin beneath disks/bumpers should be checked frequently.

Skin Irritation and Peristomal Hyperplasia Complications

Skin irritation is caused by gastric secretions or feeding solutions leaking about the tube and making contact with the skin, causing erythema, swelling, pain, and denuded areas. Control leakage can prevent skin irritation. One method is to insert a smaller tube or remove the tube for several hours to shrink the stoma. An ostomy pouching system with skin barrier may be necessary if drainage is measurable and persistent. **Treatment** includes careful cleansing of the peristomal skin and application of a skin barrier. Denuded areas require a skin barrier cream, such as zinc oxide, or skin barrier powder. Alcohol-based barrier wipes should not be used.

Peristomal hyperplasia usually results from irritation caused by latex tubes, tube migration, or moisture. Prevention must involve identifying the causative agent. **Treatment** may include cauterization with silver nitrate sticks, debridement, topical steroid creams (triamcinolone 0.5%), antifungal powder/cream, or diathermy treatments.

Ostomy Care: Intervention and Treatment

CHEMICAL CAUTERIZATION OF PERISTOMAL HYPERPLASIA

Peristomal hyperplasia involves an overgrowth of granulation tissue about the stoma of feeding tubes, resulting from irritation, tube migration, or moisture. Often, the etiology is unclear.

Hyperplasia is the result of proliferation of capillaries that form around and inside of the stoma. This tissue may cause pain, bleeding, or oozing is frequently treated with cauterization with silver nitrate sticks. Care must be taken to use silver nitrate only on the granulation tissue as it can cause painful burns if it inadvertently touches other tissue.

Chemical cauterization involves first applying a skin barrier around the tissue to be cauterized. Silver nitrate sticks usually need to be moistened with small amount of sterile water to activate. Apply silver nitrate to tissue by running the tip of the stick in a rolling manner over the tissue to be cauterized. Cauterization is usually required 2 to 3 times weekly until granulation tissue resolves.

BURIED BUMPER SYNDROME COMPLICATIONS

Buried Bumper Syndrome involves migration of the internal bumper into the gastric mucosa. The most common cause is excessive traction pulling the bumper against the gastric mucosa for extended periods, sometimes causing necrotic lesions and abscesses. Small bumpers, stiff bumpers, and malnutrition are also implicated. Symptoms include partial or complete occlusion of the tube, erythema and swelling about stoma as well as pain in the abdominal wall. The bumper may be palpable on examination. Treatment depends upon degree of injury to gastric mucosa. In all cases, the tube must be removed either by external traction or surgical excision with endoscopy. If injury to mucosa is minor, a tube can be reinserted. If there is an extensive necrosis or abscess, healing may take 4 months or longer, and the tube should be inserted in a different site. Prevention requires careful observation and leaving 1.5 cm between the external bumper and the skin to prevent excessive traction.

PREVENTING AND TREATING ASPIRATION AND IMPROPER TUBE PLACEMENT COMPLICATIONS

Aspiration is a common problem that can lead to pneumonia and poses a risk for those with multiple medical problems, such as dysphagia, decreased level of alertness, previous episodes of pneumonia or ileus. Large-bore tubes and mechanical ventilators have also been implicated. Prevention includes using a small-bore feeding tube, checking residuals every 4-6 hours, holding feedings if residual is greater than 100-150 mL, Elevating the head of the bed to 30-45 degrees, and using continuous feeding rather than bolus. Treatment may require a jejunal extension tube or replacement of gastrostomy with jejunostomy.

Improper tube placement is the result of lack of proper prevention efforts prior to tube placement. Gastrostomy tubes are usually placed in the left upper quadrant, but should avoid folds or creases that might cause leakage. General guidelines include placing the tube 3-5 cm below the costal margin. Treatment may include using skin barriers or pouching systems. In worst cases, replacement may be considered.

Important Terms

Contrast Enema: Contrast liquid, usually barium, instilled rectally to outline inside of intestines, followed by x-rays of abdomen.

Endoscopy: Procedure for minimally invasive surgical techniques using an instrument with rigid or flexible tube that can be inserted into the body, usually through an orifice or incision, to visually inspect, photograph, take biopsies, do surgical procedures, and remove foreign objects.

Intravenous Pyelogram: Imaging technique where intravenous contrast dye is given to highlight urinary structures on x-ray. Used to show path and rate of urinary flow through urinary tract.

Ultrasound: Imaging technique using high-frequency sound waves to create computer images of vessels, tissues, and organs. Used to view organs, evaluate function, and assess circulation.

Voiding Cystourethrogram (VCUG): Catheter is inserted through urethra into bladder, which is filled with liquid containing contrast dye. X-rays are taken as the bladder fills and empties, showing function and reverse flow of urine to ureters and kidneys.

Appendicostomy: Appendix brought to abdominal wall to form a stoma, usually at umbilicus, to provide open channel for insertion of catheter to irrigate bowel to prevent constipation. Procedure may be done to relieve constipation in those with myelomeningocele.

Clean Intermittent Catheterization (CIC): Procedure in which a straight catheter is inserted into the opening to the bladder, usually the urethra, to empty the bladder completely. It may be done intermittently as a temporary procedure or for long-term management of the bladder.

Cystoplasty: Surgical repair of defect in bladder. May be done as reductive procedure to reduce large distended bladder or to correct other defects.

Pyeloplasty: Incision into and repair of kidney pelvis.

Ureterostomy: The ureter is opened to abdominal wall with a stoma as a urinary diversion.

Vesicostomy: Bladder mucosa opened to lower abdominal wall with creation of stoma to allow for permanent or temporary urinary diversion.

Ostomy Care: Intervention and Treatment

Ostomy Care: Care Planning

Principles of Patient-Centered Care

SUPPORTING PATIENT AND CAREGIVER GOALS

Preventive goals: Measures to prevent disease/disability or prevent deterioration or complications of existing disorder. May include screening (BP, Pap smear, mammograms, blood glucose), disease education, fall prevention, smoking cessation, substance abuse rehabilitation, vaccinations, nutritional counseling, and exercise.

Maintenance goals: Measures to control existing disorder in order to maintain status. May include therapy (OT, PT, ST), education, ongoing lifestyle changes, supervision, ongoing assessment, medications, blood glucose management, and treatment. Maintenance therapy may follow primary therapy for some diseases, such as cancer, in order to maintain status.

Curative goals: Measures intended to cure disease rather than simply to alleviate symptoms or pain. May include medications, casting (as for broken limbs), radiotherapy, dialysis, transfusions, chemotherapy, physical therapy, rehabilitation therapy, and surgical interventions. Note: Curative treatments are also sometimes used for palliation but without intent to cure.

ACCESS TO CARE

A number of factors may affect **access to care**:

- **Proximity to medical services**: Some geographic areas have more medical services than others. For example, some rural areas lack both hospitals and physicians. Cutting edge treatments may be unavailable in some areas.
- **Socioeconomic status**: Lack of insurance or money to pay for medical services prevents many people from seeking medical care or complying with treatments. Many cannot afford to pay for prescription drugs or supplies.
- **Language differences**: Non-English speakers may not be able to communicate needs or to understand information, such as the treatment plan.
- **Health literacy**: Some may have little knowledge and understanding of anatomy, physiology, disease, and medical treatments.
- **Disability status**: Disabilities may have a profound effect of access to care or very little, depending on the type of disability and the resources available, but some disabilities impair mobility and the ability to access care.
- **Transportation**: Private and public transportation may be unavailable or the cost prohibitive.
- **Race and ethnicity**: Inequalities faced by minority populations often extend to medical services. Many live in poor neighborhoods that provide little access to medical services.

GOALS OF REHABILITATION FOR OSTOMY PATIENTS

Goals of rehabilitation include the following:

- **Independence**: Person should be able to do as much self-care as possible, with accommodations for disabilities or limitations.
- **Stoma care**: Person should be aware of complications, including signs and symptoms and should understand how to prevent complications and deal with them effectively and know when to seek medical attention.
- **Peristomal care**: Person should understand importance of regular assessment of skin and know how to avoid irritation and treat irritation if it should arise.
- **Pouching**: Person should know pouching options and how to apply, use, clean, and change pouches.
- **Ostomy function**: Person should understand normal functioning and be aware of changes that need attention or could be a sign of complications. Person should be able to irrigate if necessary.
- **Support system**: Person should be aware of support groups and agencies/organizations that provide information and should identify family and friends who can be of assistance.

ACTIVE LISTENING

Active listening requires more than simply hearing what another individual is saying. Active listening includes observing the other individual carefully for nonverbal behaviors, such as posture, eye contact, and facial expression, as well as understanding and reflecting on what the person is saying. The listener should observe carefully for inconsistencies in what the individual is saying or comments that require clarification. Feedback is critical to active listening because it shows the speaker that one is paying attention and showing interest and respect. Feedback may be as simple as nodding the head in agreement but should also include asking questions or making comments to show full engagement. Listening with empathy is especially important because it helps to build a connection with the speaker. The listener should communicate empathy with words: "You feel (emotion) because (experience)," because the speaker may not be sensitive to what the listener is comprehending.

Ostomy Care: Care Planning

Special Considerations

COUNSELING ON INTIMACY FOR THOSE WITH OSTOMIES

Emotional element validates person's anxieties and encourages expression. Sexual desire and activity can alter after surgery and affect the body image and sense of well-being and attractiveness. Provide support for both patient and partner, whose response to the ostomy can have a profound effect on the patient.

Physical element involves discussion of physical changes that may affect sexual functioning and alternative means of sexual activity. Discuss physical limitations and pain and how they relate to sexual activity. Encourage experimentation to find sexual expression rewarding to both partners.

Educational element provides practical information, such as the importance of emptying the pouch prior to sexual activity. Using smaller, low-profile pouching systems, or specially designed undergarments may help a person feel more comfortable. Pamphlets and information about sexual activity should be provided to patient.

Communicative element encourages both patient and partner to discuss fears and feelings about sexual activity. Open and honest communication is critical.

PLISSIT MODEL FOR COMMUNICATING ABOUT SEXUALITY

PLISSIT model (developed by Annon in the 1970s and still applicable in the clinical environment) for communicating about sexuality is explained below:

- Level one:
  - **Permission**: Gives the person permission to have feelings or attitudes and to do or not do something. Reassure person feelings are not abnormal. Pointing out consequences of choices is important to put patient's choices in perspective. Attempt to establish open communication by helping person to feel comfortable.
- Level two:
  - **Limited Information**: Information should help to dispel misconceptions and fears and should be specifically related to needs and concerns of patient. Information should be factual about the effects of surgery on sexuality.
- Level three:
  - **Specific Suggestions**: At this point, the person needs to take action or seek treatment with medical guidance. Some specific suggestions might include the use of lubricants, emptying pouch before sexual activity, or using pouch covers.
- Level four:
  - **Intensive Therapy**: This involves referral to an appropriate specialist as the person may, for example, need reconstructive surgery or psychotherapy beyond what the nurse is able to provide.

SUPPORTING PATIENTS THROUGH BODY IMAGE ISSUES AFTER PLACEMENT OF AN OSTOMY

Ostomy patients often develop negative body images even though their quality of life may have improved. Some may become depressed and withdrawn or even suicidal, and others may exhibit anger. Patients may go through a number of phases on the path to psychological acceptance: panic/shock, denial, acknowledgement, and acceptance. Patients may have concerns about sexuality. The nurse should practice active listening and encourage patients to express feelings and describe what is most concerning to them, such as the fear of leaks or odors, and help patients to find solutions to those concerns to give them a feeling of control. The patient may benefit from guidance about clothing options and different types of appliances as well as ostomy management and support services that are available. Actively engaging the patient in care of the ostomy can help the patient to become more accepting and confident. The patient may also benefit from assistance and practice in briefly describing or explaining the surgery to family and friends because patients often feel embarrassment or shame.

SUPPORTING PATIENTS WITH DISABILITIES

Patients often face functional, emotional, and psychosocial challenges in dealing with ostomies, diversions, and draining wounds. Special considerations must be made for patients with additional **disabilities**. These patients may need adaptive devices, such as pouching aids and mirror stands, and pouching and skin care may need to be done in seated position. If patients have a one-sided weakness or paralysis, procedures may need to be simplified or broken into short sessions. If patients are visually impaired, they may need tactile labels, verbal cues, and high-contrast materials. For cognitive impairment, step-by-step visual aids may help, and caregivers may need training.

TERMINAL CARE ISSUES FOR THOSE WITH OSTOMIES

Terminal care issues for those with ostomies include the following:

- **Curative vs. palliative**: Curative and palliative care are not mutually exclusive. Palliative care can begin during curative care to help patient and family plan and to provide services they will need to cope. The goal of palliative care is to provide the best quality of life possible.
- **Pain control**: By law, adequate pain control is the right of the terminal patient. Discussing different methods of pain control reassures the terminal patient.
- **Hospice care**: Hospice resources are invaluable to patient and caregivers, providing supplies, assistance, and respite.
- **Self-determination**: Patients have the right to self-determination regarding their care. Patients should be encouraged to complete an Advance Directive outlining their wishes.
- **Ostomy care**: Plans should be made early regarding care of the ostomy if patient unable to do so. This may entail training caregivers or making arrangements for Home Health care. Discussions about diet/fluids/constipation/diarrhea and how to manage these issues are necessary.

Ostomy Care: Care Planning

243

Additional Considerations

NEONATES

There are important considerations regarding ostomies for neonates. Most ostomies are performed for necrotizing enterocolitis, so the infant is often critically ill. Other indications include meconium ileus, intestinal atresia, Hirschsprung disease, and anorectal abnormalities. For ileostomy/colostomy, stool production is limited for the first one to two days, so petrolatum gauze is applied to protect the stoma but a bag is generally not applied. Because skin is friable, especially in preterm neonates, adhesive and skin sealant use should be limited, and adhesive remover should be avoided with adhesive loosened with a cloth dampened with warm water. Peristomal skin should be cleansed only with water or, if necessary, pH neutral soap, which is thoroughly rinsed. No skin sealant containing alcohol should be used. Likewise, skin barrier pastes should be avoided because of alcohol content, although a low-alcohol paste may be used if necessary to secure an appliance. Only appliances intended for neonates should be used. Appliances are available in various sizes and shapes. Gas production is often increased with neonates because of crying, so pouches should have a charcoal filter that allows release of gas.

PEDIATRIC PATIENTS

The following are care plan issues of long-term management of conventional colostomies in pediatric patients:

- **Activity/exercise**: Can engage in almost all activities/exercises, but should avoid rough contact sports and heavy lifting.
- **Clothing**: Should provide easy access to pouch, so children can manage care. Infants and small children may need one-piece outfits to prevent them from removing pouch.
- **Food/fluids**: Should be taught types of foods/fluids to avoid and good eating habits.
- **Bathing**: Can bathe/shower with or without a pouch. If frequent fecal leakage, a pouch can be worn during the bath.
- **Travel**: Should carry ostomy supplies for the entire trip as they may be hard to find and carry an adequate supply in carry-on luggage if flying.
- **School**: The school nurse, principal, and teacher should be aware of the child's colostomy and extra supplies and clothing should be available at school.
- **Ostomy supplies**: Can use closed-end pouches to avoid emptying appliance at school or special events. Ostomy belts and pouch covers may provide added security.

OBSTETRICS

PREGNANCY IN WOMEN WITH OSTOMIES

Implications of pregnancy in women with ostomies are as follows:

- **Nausea**: Maintain adequate fluid intake to prevent constipation/obstruction.
- **Stoma**: As abdomen becomes larger, stoma may enlarge and change shape, becoming more oval. It may recede or prolapse. Measure frequently. Stoma usually returns to normal after delivery.
- **Vaginal delivery**: If there is scar tissue from removal of the rectum, an episiotomy may be necessary. Some may not be suitable candidates for vaginal delivery. Pressure during delivery often expresses stool, so appliance should be changed after delivery. As girth increases, women may need to use a mirror to view stoma.
- **Ultrasounds**: Appliances can loosen because of oil used during procedure, so clean abdomen thoroughly and change appliance after procedure. The absence of a bladder in some women may complicate viewing and the position of the stoma may interfere with viewing of the fetus.
- **Breast-feeding**: There are usually no contraindications unless the medications the woman is taking are passed into the breast milk and considered unsafe for the child.

ILEOSTOMY CARE DURING PREGNANCY

Implications of ileostomy care during pregnancy are as follows:

- **Timing pregnancy**: If the ileostomy is for inflammatory bowel disease, it's better to be pregnant during inactive periods of disease as active disease may lead to miscarriage or premature birth. However, about 1/3 of women with inflammatory bowel disease become active during the pregnancy and receive medical treatment during pregnancy.
- **Ileostomy care**: Ileostomy may be more active during the pregnancy because of increasing pressure. As the abdomen becomes larger, the stoma often also enlarges and changes shape, becoming more oval. Measure from time to time and change sizes as necessary. Stoma usually returns to normal shortly after delivery.
- **Complications**: There is a slight chance of blockage as the fetus grows and applies pressure. Abdomen may become painful and distended. Liquid diet and rest usually suffice; intravenous fluids may be needed to rest the intestines, so close monitoring of ileostomy functioning is important.
- **Birth**: Vaginal births are possible: some need Cesareans.

BIRTH CONTROL ISSUES FOR WOMEN WITH OSTOMIES

Birth control medications: Because of absorption issues, pills may not be suitable for some women with ileostomies, depending upon how much small intestine remains. A higher dose than normal may be needed. With Crohn's disease, absorption may be so compromised that birth control pills are not effective. Injectable progesterone has been used successfully.

Intrauterine device: Generally, the IUD is not advised for women who have never had children, and is not suitable for some with ostomies, especially if uterus is fixed in a different position from usual. Fitting the coil can be a difficult.

Cervical caps/diaphragms: Some can successfully use caps or diaphragms, but if the anatomy of the uterus or vagina was altered, insertion and retention may be problematic.

Condoms: Condoms can be effective birth control if used properly and consistently.

Vasectomy: If it is important to permanently avoid pregnancy, a vasectomy for the male partner may be advisable.

BARIATRIC

There are important considerations regarding ostomies for obese patients (BMI > 35). The placement of the stoma may pose problems because of abdominal rolls, which must be avoided. The stoma should be placed if possible where it is 5 to 10 cm away from creases and folds and away from the belt line. Because subcutaneous fat may shift, the stoma site should be selected by assessing the patient in both sitting and standing position. Patients with very large breasts and protruding abdomens may have difficulty both visualizing the stoma, especially if it is placed low on the abdomen, and managing appliances. Postoperatively, bariatric patients are more likely to develop stoma necrosis because of impaired circulation. Overweight patients are especially at risk of atelectasis so they must be encouraged to practice deep breathing and coughing and early mobilization is essential. Patients may be able to manage a one-piece pouch better than one with a detachable bag if their abdomens are large. Patients who have also had bariatric surgery to lose weight and then regain the weight may develop an enlarged stoma.

Ostomy Care: Care Planning

245

Ostomy Care: Education and Referral

Principles of Education

COGNITIVE, AFFECTIVE, AND PSYCHOMOTOR LEARNING ABILITIES

Cognitive ability involves learning and gaining intellectual skills. There are 6 categories to master for effective learning, in order: knowledge, comprehension, application, analysis, synthesis, and evaluation.

Affective ability involves recognizing 5 categories of feelings and values, from simple to complex and is slower to achieve than cognitive learning.

- **Receiving phenomena**: Viewing stoma, accepting need to learn.
- **Responding to phenomena**: Taking active part in care.
- **Valuing**: Understanding value of becoming independent in care.
- **Organizing values**: Understanding how surgery has improved life.
- **Internalizing values**: Accepting condition as part of life, being consistent and self-reliant.

Psychomotor ability involves mastering 7 categories of motor skills necessary for independence, from simple to complex:

- **Perception**: Uses sensory information to learn tasks.
- **Set**: Shows willingness to perform tasks.
- **Guided response**: Follows directions.
- **Mechanism**: Does specific tasks.
- **Complex overt response**: Displays competence in self-care.
- **Adaptation**: Modifies procedures as needed.
- **Origination**: Creatively deals with problems.

EFFECTS OF SUCCESSIVE STAGES OF COGNITIVE LEARNING ON TEACHING

The effects of successive stages of cognitive learning on teaching are as follows:

- Knowledge:
  - Ask for feedback about teaching points.
  - Ask learner to identify equipment, list procedure steps and explain.
- Comprehension:
  - Ask learner to explain principles or procedures in own words: Why are things done this way?
  - Ask learner to summarize purpose of procedures.
- Application:
  - Ask learner to solve problems in different situations: What would happen if...? Or how could this problem be solved?
  - Ask learner to demonstrate procedures.
- Analysis:
  - Question learner to determine ability to distinguish fact from inference: What can happen if the opening is too large in the pouch?
  - Ask learner to troubleshoot: How do you deal with pouch leakage?
- Synthesis:
  - Ask learner to integrate knowledge to solve problems: How can odor issues be resolved?
- Evaluating knowledge:
  - Ask learner questions that demonstrate knowledge by explaining or interpreting: Why is measuring of stoma important?
  - Ask learner to choose the most effective solution to problems.

EFFECTS OF DEVELOPMENTAL STAGE OF LEARNER ON TEACHING

The effects of developmental stage of learner on teaching are discussed below:

- **Infant/toddler**: Caregivers provide care; instruction encourages bonding and acceptance.
- **Early childhood**: Children learn by participation, such as role-playing, simple explanation, and teaching dolls. Children should be independent in emptying pouch by kindergarten.
- **Childhood**: By age 6, children should be independent in care at school, but ostomy supplies should be at school and school nurse knowledgeable about ostomy care. Child should be completely independent in care by 6th grade. Parents and child should be taught together.
- **Adolescence/young adulthood**: The adolescent may be angry and resistive, extra time and guidance, including visits with other ostomy patients, may help. Parents should allow adolescent to be independent in care.
- **Middle-aged adult**: Adults may have fears about loss of income, status, sexuality, so individualized teaching that includes partners helps them to deal with these issues.
- **Elderly**: Elderly may face physiological and psychological changes. Teaching should provide coping skills and information in stages to avoid overwhelming them.

HEALTH LITERACY

Health literacy is the ability to obtain, understand, and consent to medical care, making informed healthcare decisions and must be considered when developing activities. Health literacy includes:

- Reading with comprehension, applying reason to context.
- Understanding graphs and other visual representations of information.
- Using the computer to obtain information.

Ostomy Care: Education and Referral

- Understanding the results of laboratory/radiographic studies.
- Understanding and using basic mathematical computations.
- Articulating concerns and questions.
- Understanding basic anatomy and physiology.
- Having basic knowledge of disease.
- Understanding preventive health measures.
- Knowing how to access health care and health information.

Health literacy may be impacted by a number of factors, including lack of adequate education (low reading level), illiteracy, dementia, and learning disabilities. Those most vulnerable include the elderly, ethnic minorities, immigrants, and those with low income and/or chronic medical or physical health problems. The nurse must evaluate the patient/caregiver to determine their level of health literacy and gear education to that level.

Preoperative and Postoperative Education

ELEMENTS OF PREOPERATIVE TEACHING

Elements of preoperative teaching are as follows:

- **Anatomy and physiology**: Should provide information about the gastrointestinal/urinary systems, including basic anatomy and physiology. Explain changes in function after surgery and explain how stoma will redirect fecal material or urine.
- **Stoma**: Should prepare person for mucoid appearance of stoma and explain that stoma lacks sensation so person will not feel need to pass stool/urine and thus the necessity of the pouch. Should discuss initial swelling and appearance of stoma and length of time before edema recedes.
- **Pouching concerns**: Should explain that pouching systems are odor-proof and that gas and odor can be further controlled by attention to diet. Should reassure person that pouching will be easily concealed under clothing.
- **Preoperative preparation**: Should explain all necessary preoperative bowel preparation and diet restrictions so that the bowel is adequately evacuated prior to surgery.
- **Postoperative complication**: Should explain all possible postoperative complications and answer any questions that the person may have about complications.

PREOPERATIVE COUNSELING FOR NEOBLADDER

The following are elements of preoperative counseling for those planning to have a neobladder:

- **Surgical procedure**: Detailed explanation of the procedure itself, drains, and post-operative care and expectations. If lesion is cancerous, the need for flexibility must be stressed as it may be more difficult to determine the exact surgical procedure in advance.
- **Exercises**: Kegel exercises to strengthen the muscles of the pelvic floor and well as exercises to tighten and relax the sphincter should begin prior to surgery.
- **Urinary care**: Instruction for intermittent self-catheterization should be done prior to surgery. The importance of emptying the bladder and maintenance of a schedule for urination must be stressed.
- **Dietary modifications**: Explanation of the need for fluids and foods to maintain urinary output and help avoid metabolic acidosis and diarrhea.
- **Complications**: Understanding the signs of metabolic acidosis and other complications is important.
- **Bowel care**: Loss of the ileocecal valve and part of the ileum can result in increased diarrhea, so dietary management of bowels is necessary.

DIETARY GUIDELINES FOR FIRST 6 WEEKS AFTER OSTOMY RELATED TO BOWEL SURGERY

Post-surgical swelling in the first 6 weeks after surgery causes the intestinal lumen to narrow, so **dietary modifications** are necessary to prevent obstruction:

- Ensure diet is well balanced and nutritious with at least a minimum of servings from each of the main food groups:
  - 2-3 servings of dairy products
  - 2-3 servings of protein (meats, fish, beans, eggs, & nuts)
  - 6-11 servings of breads and cereal
  - 2-4 servings of fruits
  - 3-5 servings of vegetables
- Avoid high fiber foods, which can cause obstruction.
- Eat 5-6 small meals a day, rather than 3 large meals.
- Introduce one new food at a time and evaluate response to food.
- Chew all foods thoroughly to begin digestive process.
- Cook foods until they are well cooked and tender.
- Drink 8 glasses of fluid each day and avoid using straw, which can cause gas.
- Drink caffeinated beverages in moderation as they can lead to dehydration.

PERIANAL SKIN CARE FOR ILEAL POUCH ANAL ANASTOMOSIS

After ileostomy closure, there may be seepage of fecal material and mucus from the anus, especially at night. The combination of moisture and friction from walking or wiping the area with tissue can cause severe irritation.

- **Avoid anal irritants**: Raw fruits, raw vegetables, oriental vegetables, coconut, dried fruits, spicy foods, seeds, and nuts or other foods (may be individual).
- **Careful cleansing**: Rinse the perineal area with warm water using a squirt bottle or bulb syringe or gently wipe with cotton balls, Tucks, or baby wipes. Avoid washcloths, which are too rough. Avoid soap, which may irritate because of alkalinity. Pat dry, fan, or use cool hair dryer.
- **Preventive skin care**: Apply protective skin barrier cream/ointment—A&D Ointment, Vaseline, or Desitin—in the perianal area. A soft dressing, such as a strip of cotton or a gauze dressing, may be positioned between the buttocks.
- **Clothing**: Wear cotton underwear; avoid synthetic material or restrictive clothes.

PROTECTING SKIN FROM FISTULA DRAINAGE

Providing **skin protection** is critical. Low output fistulas may need only skin barriers and easily-changed absorbent dressings. Creases, folds, and depressions may need to be filled with skin barrier paste, wafers, or powder before solid barriers applied. Solid barriers last as long as they remain intact; Liquid skin sealants, up to 24 hours; Skin powders/pastes, to 24 hours.

Containing drainage is necessary. If drainage cannot be contained with an absorbent dressing, then ostomy appliances with solid skin barriers and pouches are indicated. The barrier should extend at least 1.5 inches around perimeter of fistula. The barrier must adhere to even skin to avoid drainage getting under the barrier, so the opening may need to be enlarged. Pouching systems with barriers that can be cut to fit usually work best. If drainage is extensive, a bedside drainage bag may be used. Very large wounds (more than 4 inches) may require a custom pouching system.

POSTOPERATIVE EDUCATION FOR OSTOMY PATIENTS

Postoperative education for ostomy patients includes:

- **Pouching**: Patients need to know the types of pouching systems available (open/closed, one-piece/two-piece) and should be able to see and manipulate them to determine what they can easily handle and prefer. They must have adequate practice under supervision applying, emptying, and changing the pouching system and must understand how to assess the stoma and surrounding skin each time. Because the stoma may change in size over time, if they are using a cut-to-fit barrier, then patients must learn how to measure the stoma. They also need to understand the frequency of pouch changes.
- **Peristomal skin health**: Patients must learn how to examine, cleanse, and protect peristomal skin and need learn how to recognize and treat problems, such as skin irritation/maceration, burning, itching, odor. They must learn about crusting and various types of skin barriers and fillers, depending on their individual needs.

Educating Patients on Optimal Management

PELVIC FLOOR EXERCISES

The pelvic floor muscles cross the floor of the pelvis and attach to the pubic bone and coccyx. The urethra, rectum, and vagina all open through the pelvic floor muscles, which support the pelvic organs.

Caution: Avoid holding the breath or tightening the abdominal or buttocks muscles during pelvic floor exercises.

Procedure: Tighten and squeeze the muscles about the rectum, vagina, and urethra and try to "lift" them inside as though trying to stop from passing gas and urine. Hold. Relax. Rest a few seconds. Repeat.

Schedule: Exercises should be done at least 3 times daily. They may be done while lying down in the morning and evening and while sitting midday.

- **1-2 weeks**: Tighten 1 second, relax 5. Repeat 10 times. Then tighten 5 seconds and relax 10. Repeat 10 times.
- **3-4 weeks**: Tighten 5-10 seconds and relax 10. Repeat 20 times.
- **5-6 weeks**: Tighten 8-10 seconds and relax 10. Repeat 20 times.

PATIENT EDUCATION FOR WOUND MANAGEMENT
INFECTION CONTROL, REPOSITIONING, AND TRAUMA AVOIDANCE

Infection control: Topics include the importance of hand hygiene, methods for disposal of soiled materials, the risk of healthcare-associated infections (including asking healthcare providers to wash hands), appropriate use of antibiotics, and appropriate wound care.

Repositioning: The need for repositioning, the manner, positions, and frequency vary depending on the patient's condition, but the patient should be apprised of the importance of repositioning to prevent skin breakdown and shown how to reposition, encouraging the patient to reposition at least every 2 hours.

Trauma avoidance: Topics include fall prevention and safe driving as well as measures to improve home safety, such as removal of throw rugs and clutter, improved lighting, installation of handrails and safety bars, and use of shower chairs. Some patients may need information about avoiding choking, fire safety, and safe use of tools (such as knives and clippers).

TOBACCO CESSATION

Smoking releases carbon monoxide and hydrogen cyanide in the blood and interferes with the delivery of oxygen to the tissues, and nicotine is a vasoconstrictor, resulting in slowed healing. Smoking also increases platelet clumping, increasing risk of clotting. Patients should learn about the effects of smoking on healing and should be provided tobacco cessation aids. A number of medical treatments can assist patients through the withdrawal period, during which the person may experience anxiety, irritability, and nicotine craving. Many of the of the medications contain nicotine, but it is released in a slower manner to avoid the sudden increase in nicotine ("rush") associated with smoking: Nicotine patch, nicotine inhaler, nicotine gum, nicotine lozenge, and nicotine nasal spray. Prescription medications that are taken before quitting and then for up to 6 months include bupropion SR and varenicline. Smoking cessation programs include support groups, online forums (StopSmokingCenter.net) and informational websites (Smokefree.gov). The HHS recommends the 5A program: Ask, advise, assess, assist, and arrange followup.

ISSUES RELATED TO CAREGIVERS TO OPTIMIZE PATIENT'S ADAPTATION AND SELF-CARE

The following are issues related to caregivers to optimize patient's adaptation and self-care:

- **Paid vs. family/friends**: Paid caregivers may or may not have prior training with ostomies but will generally expect to assist with this care. Family or friends may be motivated to help or may be resentful and uncooperative. Identifying a caregiver even for the self-sufficient should be done before a need arises.
- **Knowledge**: Assessing caregiver's knowledge and ability to learn is part of the care plan. Training may need to be modified or done in small steps for some caregivers. Training of the patient and caregiver at the same time is ideal, and can provide an opportunity to discuss the impact the ostomy has on the relationship.
- **Fear/disapproval**: Caregivers who express fear, disgust, or disapproval regarding the ostomy can have a negative impact on the patient and interfere with that person's learning. Acknowledging negative feelings and openly discussing them can often lead to a positive outcome. Alternative care providers may be necessary.

Ostomy Care: Education and Referral

Supply and Information Resources

INFORMATION PATIENTS NEED TO RESUME OPTIMAL LIFESTYLE

The following is general information the patient needs to resume an optimal lifestyle:

- **Ostomy supplies**: Person needs complete list of supplies, supply numbers, and information about billing insurance or Medicare. If necessary, written prescription should be supplied and lists of local, mail order, and online suppliers. Indigent people may need referral to social services for assistance.
- **Dietary information**: Person needs information about foods to avoid, especially in first few weeks after surgery. Person should receive a list of foods that thicken or loosen stool and that cause gas or odor. Urostomy patients should be advised that asparagus, fish, and some spices cause urine odor.
- **Gas/odor management**: Person should learn common causes of gas and odor, which may include smoking, chewing gum, and swallowing air when sleeping or using a straw. Person needs help to assess individual's dietary practices that cause gas/odor. Simethicone with meals and pouch deodorants help reduce odor.
- **Contact/support information**: Person needs to know whom to call or where to go for help or support.

COMMUNITY AND INTERNET RESOURCES FOR PATIENTS AND FAMILIES

The following are types of community and internet resources that patients and their families need to know about:

- **Local agencies**: Local branches of national organizations or local agencies developed to meet particular needs may be available. Senior citizen groups may provide support and information or direct to other resources.
- **Support groups**: Agencies, hospitals, charitable foundations, hospices, and senior citizens groups are just a few that may have support groups for patients and/or caregivers. Attending a support group where patients or caregivers can meet and talk with others facing similar challenges can be very helpful from a practical as well as emotional perspective.
- **Consumer organizations**: Societies, foundations, and associations dedicated to a particular type of health problem or need can be a wealth of information, providing literature, updates on drugs and treatments, and online chat groups or message boards.
- **Product manufacturers/suppliers**: Patients should be aware of local distributors/retailers of ostomy supplies and catalog and Internet resources. In some areas, people may not have ready access to needed supplies.

RESOURCES FOR PATIENTS

Resources available to the patient include:

- **Support and advocacy**: Support groups are available through many medical centers and hospitals as well as online. Many are sponsored by national organizations and are generally free of cost and available to patients and/or families. National organizations also often provide information about clinical trials and current research.
- **Access to supplies**: Many manufacturers provides assistance programs for those unable to afford supplies, such as dressings, and some national organizations may also provide assistance. Some patients may be eligible for Medicaid, which will cover the costs of necessary supplies and equipment.
- **Post-acute care**: This level of care is less intense than that provided by an acute hospital. Post-acute care may be provided after acute hospitalization or instead of acute hospitalization. Medical treatments can be continued with post-acute care but the focus is more commonly on rehabilitation.

Ostomy Care: Education and Referral

Ostomy, Fistula, and Tube Management

MANAGEMENT PRINCIPLES FOR PATIENT TEACHING ABOUT POUCHING AND/OR CONTAINMENT STRATEGIES

Assess patient readiness and ability to learn and manage own care. Provide emotional support and allow person to express feelings.

Consider special needs as those with special needs, such as limited cognitive or physical ability, may need modifications or assistance. People who are hard of hearing, vision-impaired, or illiterate may need video or audiotapes or illustrated instructions.

Do **step-by-step instruction** of main tasks and begin with simple steps such as draining and clamping pouch and continue until person has mastered the main tasks: emptying the pouch, removing the pouch, cleansing and caring for the skin, measuring the stoma, applying a new pouch, and disposing of the old pouch.

Do **on-going assessment** over time and evaluate person's ability to manage pouching while in the hospital, after returning home, and then after one month at home and three months at home to ensure that all questions are answered and problems have been resolved.

BARRIERS TO SELF-CARE OF POUCHING AND CONTAINMENT STRATEGIES

The following are psychological, physical, and cognitive barriers to self-care of pouching and containment strategies:

- Psychological barriers:
  - **Emotional instability** may interfere with ability to learn and manage care.
  - **Sexuality issues** may cause people to be anxious about body image, sexual dysfunction, and sexual activity with a stoma appliance. Homosexual patients may need special counseling.
- Physical barriers:
  - **Vision impairment** requires that people wear glasses or any other modifiers in good light. Those who are legally blind need a tactile approach to teaching so that they can use their sense of touch. Braille text or 3-dimensional models may be helpful.
  - **Hearing impairment** requires a quiet environment or translator. Nurse should face patient to facilitate lip reading and use picture diagrams or videos.
  - **Allergies** mean require people to try different system to determine sensitivies or use non-adhesive or modified systems.
  - **Motor impairment** may necessitate simplified ostomy care and consultation with occupational therapist.
- Cognitive Barriers:
  - **Mental acuity** varies, and some may not be able to be independent in care or may need repeated step-by-step instruction over prolonged period of time.

CARE PLAN ISSUES OF LONG-TERM MANAGEMENT OF CONVENTIONAL COLOSTOMIES

The following are care plan issues of long-term management of conventional colostomies:

- **Work**: Working should pose no special problems unless it involves heavy lifting or digging, which may require a special support to prevent herniation. An ostomy belt can keep the ostomy in place for those whose jobs are very active. Extra supplies and clean clothes should be kept at the workplace, in the car, or in an easily accessible place.

- **Exercise**: An exercise program should be planned with the healthcare provider and should start slowly. For contact sports, a special support or cover for the colostomy can protect the stoma. Always empty the pouch before sports activities, especially swimming. Do not remove the pouch while swimming and secure the edges with waterproof tape.
- **Travel**: Ostomy supplies may not be available in some areas, so carry all supplies needed, including an adequate supply in carry-on bag. Keep supplies in the coolest area of the car so supplies don't melt in hot weather.
- **Bathing**: Pouch may be worn for bathing if likelihood of fecal leakage, but a shower can be taken with or without the pouch as the water will not damage the stoma and leakage will wash down the drain.
- **Relationships**: Open communication and discussion can help relieve anxiety for ostomy patient and others. The dependency involved in ostomy care can cause conflict, and this needs to be addressed.
- **Sex**: Sexual function may be impaired; information about sexual activity and alternate means of sexual expression should be provided. Pouch covers or special underwear can be utilized.
- **Constipation/irrigation**: Management strategies for constipation, prevention of impaction and irrigation should be understood. Adequate fluids, exercise, and fiber intake can help to relieve constipation.
- **Diarrhea**: People with history of diarrhea can use customary methods of control, including adequate fiber, increased carbohydrates, and sufficient fluids. An increase in diarrhea along with symptoms such as dehydration or cramping should be reported to physician.

Ostomy Care: Education and Referral

Multidisciplinary Care Collaboration

EDUCATING HEALTH CARE PROVIDERS ON OSTOMY CARE PRINCIPLES

The ostomy care nurse's role in **educating health care providers** on ostomy care includes sharing principles of ostomy care:

- Understanding that initial pouching requirements in the postoperative period may differ from maintenance requirements and usually begin with clear, drainable, cut-to-fit pouches without convexity wafers until healing takes place.
- Helping the patient to achieve a pouching system that improves the patient's quality of life and one that the patient can manage effectively.
- Achieving a predictable wear time, usually at least 3 days but no longer than 7, so ensuring that the appropriate barrier/wafer and appliance is utilized.
- Maintaining peristomal skin in optimal condition and recognizing indications of skin irritation or problems and understanding solutions.
- Helping the patient to deal emotionally with changes in body image related to the ostomy.
- Ensuring that the patient is aware of resources available for supplies/equipment and supportive services, such as support groups and online forums.

CONSULTING INFECTIOUS DISEASE AND DERMATOLOGY

The nurse has an essential role in preventing and identifying infection and dermatologic issues and making appropriate **consultations**:

- **Infectious disease**: Referral may be indicated if the patient exhibits a persistent or recurrent local infection or has systemic indications, such as elevated temperature, leukocytosis, and/or sepsis. Careful supervision is often needed to prevent and treat multi-resistant organisms. Patients who are immunocompromised (chemotherapy, transplants, HIV/AIDS) may need monitoring by an infectious disease professional. Referral is often needed for urinary diversions if UTIs are occurring and for infections related to fistulae and percutaneous tubes and drains.
- **Dermatology**: Referral may be indicated if there is skin breakdown, such as peristomal or periwound, which is unresponsive to routine care, if contact dermatitis occurs because of contact with adhesives or barrier products, and if fungal infections, such as candidiasis under a pouch, occur. Referral is often needed for ostomies, fistulae, and percutaneous tubes and drains when skin breakdown occurs.

HANDOFF/TRANSITION OF PATIENTS WITH OSTOMIES

Hand-off/transition procedures for patients with ostomies whether to another unit, another level of care, or to the home environment should be documented and adequate time allowed for communication, including questions from the receiving party. Information that must be covered may vary somewhat depending on the type of ostomy but generally includes:

- Demographic information, such as name, diagnoses, address, telephone number.
- List of current medications and treatments.
- Physical or cognitive impairments that may impact ability to manage the ostomy, such as vision impairment, impaired mobility, and dementia.
- The type of ostomy, including the site and any complications (discoloration, retraction, herniation, prolapse, stenosis, bleeding, laceration).
- History of ostomy (length of time in place, history of complications, etc.)
- Current size, condition, and appearance of stoma.
- Type of ostomy supplies and equipment needed.
- Review of education provided to the patient/family.
- Contact information for ostomy specialist.
- Dietary guidelines, including foods to avoid.
- Activity level and restrictions (such as limited lifting, avoiding strenuous exercise).
- Follow-up appointments.

Ostomy Care: Education and Referral

Continence Care: Assessment and Care Planning

Normal Micturition and Defecation

NORMAL URINATION

Normal urination: Kidneys produce urine, which flows through ureters into the bladder, which rests on pelvic floor muscles, extending from pubic bone to base of the spine. The bladder is enclosed in the **detrusor** muscle, creating a muscular reservoir. The bladder neck comprises the connection between the bladder and the urethra. Internal sphincter muscles and fibrous external sphincter muscles (urethral) encircle the bladder neck.

- **Phase 1: Filling/storing** is triggered by emptying the bladder. Neurotransmitters in the brain signal the detrusor muscle to relax and the bladder to expand, drawing urine from the kidney and ureters. When the bladder reaches capacity (8-16 ounces), nerves send a signal back to the brain. Voluntarily tightening the external sphincter muscles retains the urine.
- **Phase 2: Emptying** occurs when the nervous system signals the voiding reflex and spinal nerves contract the detrusor muscle and relax internal sphincter muscles, allowing urine to flow to the urethra. Relaxing external sphincter muscles allows urination.

BLADDER AND URETHRA

The **bladder**, a muscular reservoir in the lower pelvis, provides urinary storage. The base of the bladder, an inverted triangular region known as the Trigone, contains the sensory nerves to send and receive signals and connects both ureters. The apex of the Trigone forms the bladder neck, the connection between the bladder and the urethra with the internal sphincter muscles and fibrous external sphincter muscles, which control the flow of urine from the bladder. The bladder is composed of different layers. The **mucosa** lines and protects the bladder wall and **submucosa** contains blood vessels and nerves. The **muscularis propria**, comprises the **detrusor** muscle, whose longitudinal and circular layers allow for expansion and contraction. The female urethra averages 1.5 inches long; the lining contains epithelial cells responsive to effects of estrogen. The male urethra averages 8 inches long. The proximal portion passing through the prostate, which can cause compression, is the prostatic or sphincteric urethra.

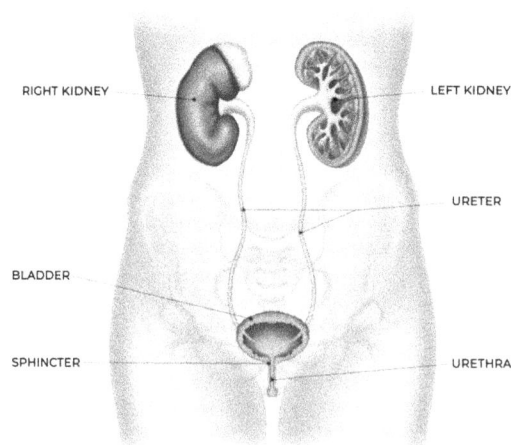

260

NORMAL DEFECATION

About 3-4 pints of liquid, including digested food, bile, and digestive enzymes, travel through the small intestine to the colon each day. The colon absorbs more than 90% of the fluid as the stool traverses the bowel. Undigested food takes only about 2 hours to reach the colon, but 2-5 days to reach the rectum, allowing time for reabsorption. The urge to defecate is caused when the stool travels from the sigmoid colon to the rectum. The rectosigmoid area provides storage. Eating stimulates contractions in the descending and rectosigmoid colon. The pelvic floor muscles of the rectum, including the **levator ani** and **puborectalis**, control both fecal retention and evacuation. When the rectum is distended with stool, the internal anal sphincter muscle relaxes. The external sphincter is voluntarily controlled, allowing continence. For defecation, the external anal sphincter and puborectalis muscle relax voluntarily and the pelvic floor muscles distend, propelling the stool through the anus.

Obtaining a Patient's Health History

PRINCIPLES OF PATIENT-CENTERED CARE
PSYCHOSOCIAL FACTORS AFFECTING CARE
Psychosocial factors affecting care include:

- **Ability to learn/perform care**: Cognitive impairment and hearing or vision deficits may interfere with the ability to learn, especially if appropriate educational materials are not available. Physical disabilities may make it difficult to patients to learn or perform some aspects of care. Language differences may result in impaired comprehension.
- **Economic implications**: Patients and families may be severely impacted if the wage earner is unable to continue to work or if they lack the resources (insurance, financial) to pay for needed care.
- **Education**: Patients may lack an adequate educational background to understand the implications of disease, to read materials, and to follow directions. Health literacy may be very low, so patients may have misconceptions about disease.
- **Mental status**: Patients often experience increased stress associated with illness, and this may interfere with functioning. Mental impairment may impact ability to participate in care. Additionally, depression is common, especially with chronic illness, and may cause patients to withdraw or fail to comply with treatment.

CULTURAL BELIEFS
Cultural beliefs may influence patients' understanding of disease, emotional response, and acceptance of treatment. It's important to ask patients about cultural preferences, to avoid making assumptions, and to respect patients' beliefs. Issues to consider include:

- **Shame**: Some may believe that wounds or drainage, especially fecal, bring shame or uncleanliness. They may have stigma about body image. Education and support are especially important to help overcome shame.
- **Traditional treatments**: Some may rely on healers or nonstandard treatments, such as poultices and herbal medications. As much as possible, these approaches should be included in the plan of care.
- **Family roles**: Decision-making may be made by someone other than the patient, such as by the eldest member of the family or the male head of the family. Showing respect for this tradition is essential for cooperation.
- **Gender**: Some cultures may resist treatment of a patient by the opposite gender. It's important to always ask permission before caring for or touching a patient.
- **Pain**: Some cultures may express pain more openly than others or may not understand the 0-10 scale often used for assessment, so the nurse should use various methods of assessment and make careful observations.

INFORMED CONSENT
The **Patient Self Determination Act** (1991) confirms the right for patients to give informed consent. Patients or family must provide informed consent for all treatment the patient receives. This includes a thorough explanation of all procedures and treatment and associated risks. Patients/family should be apprised of all options and allowed input on the type of treatments. Patients/family should be apprised of all reasonable risks and any complications that might be life threatening or increase morbidity. The American Medical Association has established guidelines for informed consent:

- Explanation of diagnosis
- Nature and reason for treatment or procedure

- Risks and benefits
- Alternative options (regardless of cost or insurance coverage)
- Risks and benefits of alternative options
- Risks and benefits of not having a treatment or procedure
- Providing informed consent is a requirement of all states

HEALTH LITERACY

Health literacy is the ability to obtain, understand, and consent to medical care, making informed healthcare decisions and must be considered when developing activities. Health literacy includes:

- Reading with comprehension, applying reason to context.
- Understanding graphs and other visual representations of information.
- Using the computer to obtain information.
- Understanding the results of laboratory/radiographic studies.
- Understanding and using basic mathematical computations.
- Articulating concerns and questions.
- Understanding basic anatomy and physiology.
- Having basic knowledge of disease.
- Understanding preventive health measures.
- Knowing how to access health care and health information.

Health literacy may be impacted by a number of factors, including lack of adequate education (low reading level), illiteracy, dementia, and learning disabilities. Those most vulnerable include the elderly, ethnic minorities, immigrants, and those with low income and/or chronic medical or physical health problems. The nurse must evaluate the patient/caregiver to determine their level of health literacy and gear education to that level.

SUPPORTING PATIENT AND CAREGIVER GOALS

Preventive goals: Measures to prevent disease/disability or prevent deterioration or complications of existing disorder. May include screening (BP, Pap smear, mammograms, blood glucose), disease education, fall prevention, smoking cessation, substance abuse rehabilitation, vaccinations, nutritional counseling, and exercise.

Maintenance goals: Measures to control existing disorder in order to maintain status. May include therapy (OT, PT, ST), education, ongoing lifestyle changes, supervision, ongoing assessment, medications, blood glucose management, and treatment. Maintenance therapy may follow primary therapy for some diseases, such as cancer, in order to maintain status.

Curative goals: Measures intended to cure disease rather than simply to alleviate symptoms or pain. May include medications, casting (as for broken limbs), radiotherapy, dialysis, transfusions, chemotherapy, physical therapy, rehabilitation therapy, and surgical interventions. Note: Curative treatments are also sometimes used for palliation but without intent to cure.

ACCESS TO CARE

A number of factors may affect **access to care**:

- **Proximity to medical services**: Some geographic areas have more medical services than others. For example, some rural areas lack both hospitals and physicians. Cutting edge treatments may be unavailable in some areas.
- **Socioeconomic status**: Lack of insurance or money to pay for medical services prevents many people from seeking medical care or complying with treatments. Many cannot afford to pay for prescription drugs or supplies.
- **Language differences**: Non-English speakers may not be able to communicate needs or to understand information, such as the treatment plan.
- **Health literacy**: Some may have little knowledge and understanding of anatomy, physiology, disease, and medical treatments.
- **Disability status**: Disabilities may have a profound effect of access to care or very little, depending on the type of disability and the resources available, but some disabilities impair mobility and the ability to access care.
- **Transportation**: Private and public transportation may be unavailable or the cost prohibitive.
- **Race and ethnicity**: Inequalities faced by minority populations often extend to medical services. Many live in poor neighborhoods that provide little access to medical services.

INTERVIEW PROCESS

The nurse should review previous medical records and have a clear idea of the purpose of the **interview** and should outline questions. If possible, the patient should be interviewed alone or should be asked if he/she wants family members present. Both verbal and nonverbal responses should be observed during an interview. Important factors include

- **Initial introductions**: Make introductions by name and explain roles and the purpose of the interview, asking how the patient wishes to be addressed and avoiding using familiar terms, such as "dear," which may be considered condescending. Stress the confidential nature of the interview and explain who will receive the information.
- **Interview structure**: The interview may be somewhat unstructured, guided by patient responses, or may be very structured with the nurse asking a list of questions, but the nurse must remain flexible while still guiding the discussion in order to accommodate different communication styles.
- **Appearance**: The nurse should be professionally dressed and wearing a clear nametag. The patient's appearance should be observed non-judgmentally for clothes (loose/tight clothes may indicate weight change), cleanliness (dirty clothes/skin/hair may indicate cognitive or physical impairment or poverty), and demeanor (calm, fidgeting, nervous).

ENVIRONMENTAL ASSESSMENT

AREAS IN HOME

Environmental assessments are very helpful when developing a care plan to provide for care and safety. Rooms should be assessed according to their function:

- **Entryway** should be free of obstacles and surfaces even. Handrails and/or ramps may be needed for those who are unsteady or wheelchair bound.
- **Stairs/steps** should have handrails, non-skid surfaces, and contrast markings for each step.
- **Living area** should be comfortable and furniture arranged for convenience. Chairs should be firm enough for people to stand from easily.

Mometrix

- **Bedrooms** should have a night light and phone near the bed. Bed should be positioned close to the nearest bathroom if possible and at the appropriate height for easy access and appropriate firmness.
- **Bathrooms** might need grab bars, hand-held shower, and elevated toilet seat, tub seat.
- **Kitchen** may need items moved for convenient access as well as a sturdy step stool. Unsafe equipment/tools should be removed.

General Elements

Some elements of environmental assessment are not specific to rooms in the house but are general needs that must be met in order for people, especially the elderly or disabled, to remain safe:

- **Environmental hazards** such as piles of papers or junk on the floors, loose carpet or rugs, and cluttered pathways can cause falls and must be cleared, organized, or repaired.
- **Lighting** should be adequate enough for reading in all rooms and stairways.
- **Heat and air conditioning** must be adequate. The young and the elderly are especially susceptible to heat and cold injury.
- **Sanitation** should ensure that health hazards do not exist, such as from rotting food or infestations of cockroaches or rodents.
- **Animals** should be cared for adequately with access to food, water, toileting, and routine veterinary care.
- **Smoke/chemicals** in the environment may pose a hazard, such as exposure to cigarette smoking or cleaning materials.

Assessing Current and Historical Environmental Factors

Environmental factors should be assessed within the actual environment if at all possible. If not, careful questioning and drawing of diagrams and approximate floor plans with the patient—or asking the patient to do drawings—can be useful, especially when showing the patient needed modifications. Family members may also assist with the assessment, providing useful information. Some patients, especially the elderly, may be reluctant to admit that the home is cluttered or that they are unable to maintain the home environment in a sanitary condition. Brochures and handouts about home safety and assistive devices should be provided to the patient as well as contact names and numbers for equipment needed in the home. A checklist should be compiled of all necessary changes or additions, with specific details, such as "Install 18-inch grab bar across from toilet." In some cases, a social worker or occupational therapist should visit the patient.

Assessing Current and Historical Functional Abilities

Functional abilities should be assessed in an active manner, with the person demonstrating the ability to sit, stand, get on and off of the toilet, walk, bend down, remove clothing and then put it on again, listen, read, and answer questions. Ideally, this should be in the home environment, but careful questioning about distances and type of facilities in the home environment can help with approximating the type of activities required. The person can walk up and down a hallway, for example, to approximate walking from the car to the front door. A careful history of functional ability can pinpoint when and if changes occurred. Again, specific questioning guides people, "When did you begin to use a cane?" "How old were you when you stopped using the tub?" "What is the biggest problem with caring for yourself?" or "When did you have a hysterectomy/prostatectomy, and how has that changed your life?"

CONSIDERING RISK FACTORS FOR INCONTINENCE

FUNCTIONAL STATUS ASSESSMENT

Functional status assessment concerns the ability to do self-care, self-maintenance, and engage in physical activities, but other factors may prevent those who should be able to function well from doing so:

- **Psychological function** assesses anxiety, worry, grief, and depression. Those with depression may be at increased risk of physical disability or may neglect self-care.
- **Social function** assesses support from family or friends, the need for a caregiver, financial resources, mistreatment or abuse, the ability to drive, and the presence of advance directives.
- **Sensory function** assesses presence of cataracts, glaucoma, myopia, presbyopia, astigmatism, macular degeneration, or eye disorders that make it difficult for people to read medication labels or do self-care. The need for audio materials or enlarged print should be assessed. Hearing is evaluated in both ears for hearing deficits and high and low frequency hearing loss as well as waxy buildup in the ear canals.

Functional status relates to the ability of people, especially the elderly, to perform social roles free of limitations or disabilities. Assessment should include basic activities of daily living:

- **Toileting** assesses the ability to adequately control urination and fecal evacuation, noting dysuria, constipation, diarrhea, the presence and degree of incontinence, and the use of protective materials.
- **Mobility** assesses the ability to transfer from bed to chair, to walk, to toilet, and to maintain balance, noting recent falls or the need for assistive devices.
- **Hygiene** assesses the ability to bathe, brush teeth, dress, and maintain basic standards of cleanliness both for the person and the environment.
- **Mental** status assesses thinking, understanding, and memory because, by age 90, about 50% of people have some dementia.
- **Nutrition** assesses basic dietary knowledge, the ability to prepare or obtain food, and adequate food and fluid intake.

PHARMACOLOGICAL AND SURGICAL HISTORY

Pharmacological history should include a complete list of all current and past medications, including over the counter or herbal medications, and people questioned about dosage to determine if they are taking medications and treatments properly. As with medical history, specific questions should be asked, "Have you taken hormone replacement therapy, such as estrogen?" rather than "What medicines have you taken?" People should also be asked specifically whether they have had chemotherapy, when, and for what?

Surgical history should include specific questions about surgical procedures rather than "Have you ever had any surgeries" because people may forget or omit surgeries in the distant past. It may be helpful to also ask people if they have any surgical scars as that may elicit more information. Men should be asked specifically if they have had a prostatectomy or vasectomy and women if they have had a hysterectomy or other gynecological or urological surgical repair.

MEDICAL HISTORY

Medical history should be assessed carefully with specific questions related to each body system rather than general questions, such as "Have you ever had a major illness?" Additionally, people should be asked if they have had any tumors, cancers, or lumps and ever had or been treated for psychological problems, such as anxiety, depression, and alcohol or drug abuse. As well as specific disorders, people should be questioned about common symptoms such as dizziness, tingling, headaches, incontinence, or weakness. Detailed questions about genitourinary history should include sexual issues, such as ejaculatory or impotence problems, painful intercourse, menstrual cycles or dysmenorrhea, menopause, and any urinary problems. A medical assessment should include radiation therapy (especially to the pelvic area), the need for or use of assistive devices, and any history of allergic reactions. General information about people's background, such as marital status, number of children, and educational status can help to formulate a care plan.

ASSESSING COGNITIVE ABILITIES

Assessment of cognitive abilities may only be officially conducted with permission of the patient or a legal representative or it can be considered an assault, so obtaining permission before beginning the assessment or documenting emergency evaluation is necessary. A medical and social history should be done before assessing cognitive abilities. During the assessment, appearance, eye contact, and affect should be documented.

The **Mini-Mental State Exam** is an assessment tool that provides a quantitative measure of cognitive status of adults. It can be used for initial assessment, to follow the patient's changes over time, and to evaluate the effectiveness of treatment. The test packet includes detachable sheets with stimuli for tasks related to comprehension, reading, writing, and drawing. The assessment tests speech, thought processes and content, hallucinations or abnormal thoughts, orientation to date, time, and place, concentration, ability to read and write, and abstract reasoning through a variety of tasks and questions.

LIFESTYLE ASSESSMENT

Lifestyle issues may change from one period of life to another, so specifically asking about current and past habits as well as changes that might have taken place is important. A non-judgmental attitude, assuring people that these questions can help to provide the best care to them, helps people be more forthcoming when providing this information.

- **Drug habits** should be assessed with specific questions about common drugs, such as marijuana, cocaine, crack, and heroin, but also prescription drugs, such as Vicodin or valium, including questions about length of use and last or current use of drugs and whether the people had treatment for addiction.
- **Alcohol intake** should be assessed with specific questions about how much and when people drink. "What time during the day do you take your first drink?" "How many drinks do you have in a normal day?" "Describe one typical drink." It's important also to ask if drinking has ever caused problems in their lives or if they have ever had treatment or attended a program to stop drinking.
- **Bowel habits** should include frequency and appearance of stools, history of constipation, diarrhea, painful evacuation, bloody stools, or incontinence.
- **Bladder habits** should include frequency of urination and appearance of urine, history of nocturia, hematuria, dysuria, and any incontinence. Men should be questioned about difficulty initiating flow or emptying bladder.
- **Diet** should include a typical day's menu, including number of meals and meal times. People should be asked specifically if they have been on any special diets, for weight loss or other health reasons. Vegetarians or vegans should be questioned about protein in their diets. Food allergies should be noted as well.
- **Hydration** should include amount and types of fluids (water and others), with specific questions, such as "What do you drink with breakfast?"
- **Smoking** assessment should include when the people first started smoking, what they smoke, and how much: "How many cigarettes do you smoke in one day?" and "How soon after you wake up do you have your first cigarette?" Assessment should include length of time people smoked, when they quit, attempts to quit, and questions about anyone living in the home or close associates who smoke.

- **Obesity** questions should avoid words like "fat" and "obese," but focus on specifics, such as "How long have you been at your current weight?" "How much did you weigh at age 20?" "How much has your weight fluctuated?" "Are you unhappy with your weight" and "Have you tried exercise or weight loss programs?"
- **Exercise** assessment should include what type of exercise people do, how often, and how long, such as "Where did you walk yesterday?" "How long did you walk?" and "What equipment do you use at the gym?"

SEXUAL HISTORY

Sexual history is an important part of any assessment for all ages and may elicit information that is helpful in diagnosing urinary or fecal incontinence. Multiple partners, certain sexual practices, or trauma may increase the risk of developing problems that can lead to urinary or fecal incontinence.

- Is the person sexually active? If so, how many partners? Are partners of the same sex, opposite sex, or both sexes?
- Is there a history of sexually transmitted diseases, such as chlamydia and gonorrhea?
- Does the person use birth control methods? What type?
- Is sexual activity painful or uncomfortable? Is there leakage of urine during sex?
- Is the woman post-menopause? If so, are there changes in sexual comfort, or urinary or fecal disorders?
- Are there erectile problems or difficulty with urination indicating an enlarged prostate?
- Is there history of sexual trauma, such as sexual abuse or surgical procedures?

VOIDING AND BOWEL DYSFUNCTION SPECIFIC TO PEDIATRIC POPULATION

ENURESIS

Enuresis is repeated involuntary urinary incontinence in children old enough to have bladder control, usually about 5-6 years old. Diabetes and other disorders should be ruled out although 95% are not associated with structural or neurological disorders. There are three types:

- **Primary**: The child has never been dry at night, and incontinence is associated with delay in maturation and small functional bladder rather than stress or psychiatric disorders.
- **Intermittent**: The child stays dry part of the time with episodes of incontinence at night.
- **Secondary**: The child has had long periods (6-12 months) staying dry and then is incontinent because of infection, stress, or sleep disorder.

Treatment includes:

- Laboratory assessment and examination to rule out primary causes.
- Fluid restriction.
- Bladder training.
- Enuresis alarms.
- Imipramine (tricyclic antidepressant) is used with many children but require close monitoring.
- Desmopressin nasal spray may be used for short-term control.
- Support and acceptance.

POSTERIOR URETHRAL VALVES

Posterior urethral valves (PUV) are a urethral abnormality in males where urethral valves have narrow slit-like openings that impede urinary flow and allow reverse flow, damaging urinary organs, which swell and become engorged with urine. Thirty percent with PUV will develop long-term kidney failure. **Symptoms** vary depending upon severity:

- **Dysuria**: Pain, weak stream, frequency.
- Hematuria. Urinary retention. Incontinence. Enlarged bladder palpable as abdominal mass. Urinary infection (most common symptom after 1 year of age). Sepsis, metabolic acidosis, and azotemia (increased blood levels of urea and other nitrogenous compounds) may develop.

Diagnosis consists of:

- Fetal ultrasound.
- Voiding cystourethrogram (VCUG): Evaluate extent of valvular abnormality and other urinary defects.
- Endoscopy: Examine inside of urinary tract/take tissue samples. Blood tests: Assess kidney function and electrolytes.

Treatment includes:

- Supportive care, antibiotics, electrolytes, Foley catheter.
- Urinary diversion: Usually closed after valve repair.
- Endoscopic ablation/resection: Examine obstruction and remove valve leaflets.

VESICOURETERAL REFLUX

Vesicoureteral reflux is an abnormality where urine flows from the bladder back up the ureter. Reflux is graded on a scale of 1-5, depending upon the degree of dilation of the ureter and renal pelvis.

- **Primary**: Congenital defect with impaired valve where ureter opens to bladder. The ureter may be too short so the valve doesn't close properly.
- **Secondary**: Caused by infection or other cause of obstruction.

Symptoms of urinary tract infection are most common:

- **Neonates**: Fever, irritability, lethargy, emesis.
- **Older infants, children**: Abdominal pain, emesis, diarrhea, fever, dysuria with enuresis, frequency, urgency, cloudy/foul urine.
- **Late symptoms**: Hypertension, dysuria with difficulty urinating, proteinuria, chronic renal insufficiency.

Diagnosis is by:

- **Ultrasound**: Evaluate appearance of urinary system.
- **Voiding cystourethrogram (VCUG)**: Identify reflux (after infection has cleared).
- **Intravenous pyelogram**: Reveal obstructions.
- **Nuclear scans**: Show urinary functioning
- **Cystoscopy**: View bladder interior.

Treatment includes:

- **Antibiotics**: For infection.
- **Surgical repair/reconstruction**: Usually involves severing ureter from bladder and reattaching at a different angle to prevent reflux.

EPISPADIAS AND HYPOSPADIAS

Epispadias is a condition in which the urethral orifice is in an abnormal position with a widened pubic bone. In boys, the urethra may open on the top (dorsum), the sides, or the complete length of the penis. In girls, the urethra, with a urethral cleft along its length, usually bifurcates the clitoris and labia but may be in the abdomen. Boys may have a short, wide penis with abnormal chordee (curvature). Epispadias is 3-5 times more common in males than females. **Hypospadias**, which occurs only in males, is a condition in which the urethral orifice opens onto the ventral surface of the penis.

Diagnosis is by physical exam and endoscopy to evaluate bladder neck and external sphincter. Intravenous pyelogram evaluates the urinary tract.

Symptoms for both conditions include urinary incontinence, infections, and reflux nephropathy (backward flow of urine to kidneys). **Treatment** is surgical repair to lengthen the urethra (and penis, in males) and reconstruct the bladder neck. Multiple surgical procedures may be required for both males and females. Urinary diversion may be necessary if incontinence cannot be corrected.

HIRSCHSPRUNG DISEASE

Hirschsprung's disease **(congenital aganglionic megacolon)** is failure of **ganglion nerve cells** to migrate to part of the bowel, usually the distal colon, so that part of the bowel lacks enervation and peristalsis, causing stool to accumulate, leading to **distention** and **megacolon**. There is a genetic predisposition to the disease that affects more males than females and is associated with trisomy 21 (Down syndrome).

Symptoms include:

- Failure to pass meconium in 24 to 48 hours
- Poor feeding
- Bilious vomitus
- Abdominal distension

Delayed diagnosis includes:

- Chronic constipation
- Failure to thrive
- Periods of diarrhea and vomiting
- With infection—severe prostration, watery diarrhea, fever, and hypotension

Treatment includes:

- Resection aganglionic section and perform colorectal anastomosis.
- There are a number of procedures, but recently, minimally invasive laparoscopic or transanal approaches have proven successful.

URETEROPELVIC JUNCTION OBSTRUCTION

Ureteropelvic junction obstruction (UPJ) is congenital obstruction at the point where the ureter connects to the renal pelvis, unilaterally or bilaterally, causing inadequate urinary flow and hydronephrosis. Some children improve markedly within the first 18 months, but others require surgery. **Symptoms** include:

- Urinary tract infections. Abdominal or flank pain
- Palpable mass from hydronephrosis. Vomiting.

Diagnosis is based on:

- **Fetal ultrasound**: in utero diagnosis.
- **Renal ultrasound**: To show dilation of renal pelvis.
- **Intravenous pyelogram (IVP)**: To identify obstruction.
- **Renal isotope scan**: To evaluate and measure kidney function.

Treatment includes:

- **Fetal urinary diversion**: Remains controversial.
- **Pyeloplasty**: Open surgical procedure where ureteropelvic junction is excised and ureter reattached to renal pelvis with wide junction, allowing adequate drainage.
- **Laparoscopic pyeloplasty**: Through abdominal wall and abdominal cavity with internal excision of ureteropelvic junction.
- **Insertion of wire through ureter**: To cut ureteropelvic junction from inside with a ureteral drain left in place for a few weeks.

MALROTATION AND VOLVULUS

Malrotation is a congenital defect in which the intestines are attached to the back of the abdominal wall by one single attachment rather than a broad band of attachments across the abdomen, essentially suspending the bowels so that they can easily twist, resulting in a **volvulus** (twisted bowel), cutting off blood supply. It may untwist but can lead to bowel infraction. Some children with malrotation have no symptoms, but most develop **symptoms** by one year:

- Cycles of cramping pain about every 15-30 minutes that cause the child to cry and pull knees to chest.
- Distended painful abdomen, diarrhea, bloody stools, or no stools.
- Vomiting (occurring soon after crying begins usually indicates small intestine obstruction; later vomiting usually indicated large intestine blockage).
- Tachycardia and tachypnea.
- Decreased urinary output.
- Fever.

Treatment includes surgical repair (Ladd procedure), which is indicated immediately if there is volvulus and most malrotations require surgical repair even with less severe symptoms.

Urinary Incontinence

CAUSES OF URINARY INCONTINENCE

The following are common causes of urinary incontinence:

- **Pregnancy/childbirth**: Childbirth weakens the pelvic floor muscles and those of the urethral sphincter. Nerve damage and bladder prolapse can also occur, further contributing to incontinence.
- **Post-menopausal changes**: Loss of estrogen causes bladder and urethral tissues to weaken.
- **Hysterectomy**: The muscles and nerves in the urinary tract may be damaged by the procedure because the urinary tract is adjacent to the uterus.
- **Interstitial cystitis**: The inflammation sometimes causes incontinence.
- **Prostate enlargement**: Constriction of the urethra as the prostate enlarges can lead to urgency or overflow incontinence.
- **Prostate cancer**: May be caused directly by the cancer or may be a response to radiation or surgical removal of prostate.
- **Bladder cancer**: Dysuria and incontinence are common symptoms.
- **Neurological deficits**: Congenital or acquired neurological damage from injury or disease can result in inability to control urination.
- **Urinary tract obstruction**: An obstruction anywhere in the urinary tract can cause overflow incontinence.

MENOPAUSE AND URINARY OR FECAL INCONTINENCE

Menopause is a major cause of urinary incontinence with about 40% of post-menopausal women developing the disorder to some degree. Estrogen maintains the lining of the bladder and the urethra and stimulates the flow of blood to the pelvic area. As levels of estrogen begin to drop with menopause, the muscles are less well-nourished and the lining of the bladder and urethra may become dry and irritated. The sphincter muscles may lose tone as well. Until recent years, many women took hormone replacement therapy (HRT), believing this protected them from the effects of aging, but subsequent studies have shown that HRT, in fact, increased the risk of urinary incontinence and did not have the same protective effect as natural estrogen, posing yet another risk factor. In addition to the loss of natural estrogen, weight gain after menopause increases the stress on the bladder and the supporting muscles, adding to the risk of urinary incontinence.

MANAGEMENT OF TRANSIENT URINARY INCONTINENCE

Transient urinary incontinence is a reversible or temporary condition caused by a number of clinical conditions. Management, therefore, is concerned with first identifying the cause, and then treating it.

- **Impaction** usually is related to chronic constipation. Bowel training and dietary modifications, including increased fiber in diet, should be instigated.
- **Dementia** may be from a disease, such as Alzheimer's, surgery, or medications. If related to Alzheimer's medications, such as Aricept, Exelon, or Namenda, may help. Scheduled toileting and absorbent pads or briefs may be necessary.
- **Urinary tract infections** require antibiotics and adequate fluid intake.
- **Vaginitis, urethritis** may respond to topical estrogen.
- **Chronic diseases** should be controlled adequately with medications and treatments as needed.
- **Chronic pain** should be assessed and a plan for pain control put in place.
- **Decreased mobility** may require assistive devices, such as elevated toilet seats, safety bars, urinals, commode chairs.
- **Medications** may need to be changed.

TRANSIENT CAUSES OF URINARY INCONTINENCE
CLINICAL CONDITIONS

Transient causes of urinary incontinence are reversible or temporary. A number of clinical conditions can affect the urinary system.

- **Impaction** may distend the rectum and anus, causing pressure on bladder neck, obstructing urinary flow, resulting in overflow incontinence.
- **Dementia** may result from illness, such as stroke, as well as surgery or medications. People may lose awareness of need to urinate or use of toilet.
- **Urinary tract infections** can cause frequency and urge incontinence.
- **Vaginitis, urethritis** with atrophic muscle changes can cause incontinence.
- **Yeast infections**, such as *Candida albicans,* result in irritation about the vagina, vulva, and urethra, resulting in burning, frequency, and urge incontinence.
- **Chronic illnesses** (diabetes mellitus or other disorders associated with polyuria and conditions with edema, such as heart failure) may cause urge incontinence.
- **Chronic pain** results in inattention to toileting needs.
- **Decreased mobility** prevents response to urge to urinate.

PSYCHOLOGICAL CONDITIONS, LIFESTYLE ISSUES, AND GENDER-SPECIFIC DISORDERS

Psychological conditions, such as severe depression, can impair the ability of a person to take care of basic needs, such as toileting.

Lifestyle issues that can cause incontinence by putting pressure on the bladder and pelvic floor muscles include obesity that weakens pelvic floor muscles, poor hygiene that causes chronic urinary tract infections, poor bowel habits that cause chronic straining for a bowel movement, and smoking, resulting in chronic cough that causes stress incontinence.

Gender-specific disorders obstruction, urinary retention, and/or incontinence. In males, an enlarged prostate may compress the urethra, causing an obstruction that results in urinary retention and overflow incontinence. Prostatectomy, on the other hand, can cause damage that result in stress incontinence. In females, a history of trauma related to childbirth, especially with multiparity, can cause stress incontinence. Pelvic radiation for both men and women can result in radiation damage to tissue that can affect bladder function.

MEDICATIONS

Medications may contribute to urinary incontinence:

- **Diuretics**, such as furosemide, hydrochlorothiazide, and caffeine can cause polyuria.
- **Sedative and hypnotics**, such as benzodiazepines and alcohol can cause confusion and depress inhibition to urinate.
- **Antihypertensives**, such as prazosin, terazosin, doxazosin, and methyldopa can cause relaxation of the urethral sphincter.
- **Narcotics**, such as morphine sulfate or meperidine can cause confusion and decrease bladder contractions, causing retention.
- **Anti-seizures**, such as thioridazine, chlorpromazine, haloperidol, and clozapine may cause enuresis because of alpha-blocker effect.
- **Anti-anxiety/muscle relaxants**, such as those of the benzodiazepine class—diazepam, alprazolam, and clonazepam--can weaken the external urethral sphincter.
- **Antidepressants/antipsychotics**, such as amitriptyline, nortriptyline and other tricyclics can decrease bladder contractions, causing retention.

- **Antihistamines**, such as chlorpheniramine and diphenhydramine, can cause decreased bladder contractions with retention.
- **Anti-Parkinson agents** cause decreased bladder contractions with retention.
- Polypharmacy can cause interactions leading to incontinence.

DIETARY FACTORS

Dietary factors can result in incontinence:

- **Caffeine** occurs naturally in coffee beans, tealeaves, and cocoa beans. Caffeine is added to many soft drinks. It is in chocolate drinks and candy. Additionally, it is also an additive in many drugs, such as Excedrin, Anacin, Darvon compounds, and Fiorinal. Caffeine can increase detrusor muscle contractions, causing increased pressure that can result in urinary urgency and frequency.
- **Artificial sweeteners** (aspartame, NutraSweet, and saccharine) are bladder irritants.
- **Citrus foods**, such as orange juice and cranberry juice are highly acidic and irritate the lining of the bladder and can worsen overactive bladder and urge incontinence.
- **Spicy foods**, such as Mexican or Chinese food, horseradish, and chili peppers irritate the bladder lining, similar to citrus foods.
- **Fluid intake** in excess of 32-48 ounces per day can worsen both stress and urge incontinence. Alcohol, especially, acts as a diuretic and acts directly on the bladder.

REVERSIBLE CAUSES OF INCONTINENCE

Reversible causes of incontinence include:

- **Delirium** is an acute sudden change in consciousness, characterized by reduced ability to focus or sustain attention, language and memory disturbance, disorientation, confusion, audiovisual hallucinations, sleep disturbance, incontinence, and psychomotor activity disorder. Delirium differs from disorders with similar symptoms in that delirium is fluctuating. Delirium occurs in 10-40% of hospitalized older adults and about 80% of patients who are terminally ill.
- **Fecal impaction** occurs when the hard stool moves into the rectum and becomes a large, dense, immovable mass that cannot be evacuated even with straining, usually as a result of chronic constipation. In addition to abdominal cramps and distention, the person may feel intense rectal pressure and pain accompanied by a sense of urgency to defecate. Nausea and vomiting may also occur. Hemorrhoids will often become engorged. Fecal incontinence, with liquid stool leaking about the impaction, is common.
- **Infection**, such as urinary tract infection or vaginal infection, may result in urinary incontinence, which usually clears once the infection is effectively treated.

RISK FACTORS FOR URINARY INCONTINENCE

The following are risk factors for urinary incontinence:

- **Age**: Bladder and sphincter muscles loosen with age, so the older a person is, the more likely to have some type of urinary incontinence, stress or chronic.
- **Contributing diseases**: Kidney diseases, among others, may make an individual prone to develop urinary incontinence if the conditions are not well controlled.
- **Obesity**: Being overweight increases pressure on the bladder and the surrounding muscles, weakening them and causing stress incontinence. This is especially true for women.
- **Sex**: Women are more likely to suffer incontinence than men because of childbirth and menopausal changes. Also, the genitourinary anatomy of women with the vagina/bladder/urethra/rectum adjacent contributes to the danger of injury to the urinary system.

- **Smoking**: The chronic cough that many smokers develop can cause stress incontinence or can aggravate stress incontinence that is already present.
- **Sports**: High impact sports with vigorous activity, such as running, can put strong pressure on the bladder during those activities.

URINARY INFECTIONS

Urinary infections can occur anywhere within the urinary tract. Cystitis, a bladder infection, is very common, especially in women because the urethra is very short and bacteria from the anal area can easily migrate to the bladder. The most common cause is the bacteria *E. coli*, which is part of the natural flora of the intestine. Untreated cystitis can result in the infection spreading to the kidneys. Urinary infections are also common in people who are elderly and dehydrated, such as those in nursing homes, and those with diabetes. Chronic bacteriuria may develop in older females, especially those with indwelling Foley catheters. *Chlamydia* and *Mycoplasma* may also cause urethral urinary infections in both males and females and is sexually transmitted. Urinary infection can cause swelling and inflammation of the mucosa and painful bladder spasms, often resulting in urinary incontinence, especially urge incontinence, in which the urge to urinate is immediately followed by involuntary urination.

PELVIC ORGAN PROLAPSE

Pelvic organ prolapse occurs when pelvic floor muscles weaken from age, trauma, or other causes and cannot support the pelvic organs, causing them to prolapse or protrude, primarily through the vaginal wall. Some types of prolapse are frequently associated with urinary incontinence.

- **Cystoceles** often result in urinary incontinence, especially during sexual intercourse when there is pressure exerted against the prolapsing bladder. Stress incontinence is also common.
- **Urethroceles** are also implicated in urinary incontinence because of impairment of function resulting from the prolapse.
- **Uterine prolapse**, depending upon the severity, may apply pressure on the bladder and urethra, preventing complete emptying of the bladder and resulting in frequent urinary tract infections with urinary frequency, urgency, and incontinence.
- **Rectoceles** are most often associated with fecal incontinence but some people may have both urinary and fecal incontinence.
- **Enteroceles** are only rarely associated with urinary incontinence usually when the enterocele is quite large.

PREDISPOSING FACTORS

There are a number of different factors that contribute to pelvic organ prolapse:

- **Trauma** related to pregnancy and childbirth is the primary cause of pelvic organ prolapse because labor and birth causes stress on the pelvic muscles and ligaments, especially if forceps are used to facilitate vaginal delivery or an episiotomy is performed.
- **Previous pelvic surgery**, especially hysterectomy or bladder repair, may damage nerves and tissues, increasing risk for prolapse.
- **Obesity** exerts pressure on the pelvic floor muscles.
- **Chronic cough/strain**, as may occur with chronic obstructive pulmonary disease or long-term smoking, may weaken the pelvic structures over prolonged periods of time.
- **Heavy lifting** can cause damage to pelvic muscles.
- **Spinal cord damage** whether congenital or acquired may cause paralysis or atrophy of the pelvic muscles, thereby weakening the support.

FISTULA

Fistulas are abnormal tunnel-like openings usually between 2 organs, or from an organ to the surface of the skin, often originating from an abscess. Fistulas involving the anus, rectum, or vagina and the perineal tissue can result in damage to intestinal and pelvic floor muscles, nerves, and sphincters.

- **Vesicovaginal** and **ureterovaginal** fistulas are common complications of female pelvic surgery, especially after a hysterectomy. The urinary incontinence that develops from these types of fistulas resembles symptoms of stress incontinence, but develops soon after surgery. Leakage occurring both during the day and night is also suggestive of vesicovaginal fistula. Surgical repair of the fistulas may, in itself, cause damage to nerves or muscles, resulting in persistent urinary incontinence.
- **Vesicouterine fistulas** are most commonly related to low segment Cesarean sections and may present with urinary incontinence. Urinary incontinence after gynecological surgery is often indication of fistula formation and should prompt urological examination.

PROSTATE DISEASE

Prostate disease is an abnormal condition of the male reproductive gland that surrounds the urethra, just below the level of the bladder.

- **Benign prostatic hypertrophy/hyperplasia** usually does not develop until after age 40 but results from the second growth phase that begins at about age 25. The prostate may slowly enlarge, but the tissue encapsulating it restrains outward growth, so the gland compresses the urethra. The bladder wall also goes through changes, becoming thicker and irritated, so that it begins to spasm, causing frequent urinations. The bladder muscle eventually weakens and the bladder fails to empty completely. People may suffer urgency, dribbling, frequency, nocturia, and urge incontinence.
- **Prostate cancer**, depending on lesion size and location, may cause similar symptoms, and resulting surgical removal or external beam radiation may result in nerve and muscle damage causing loss or compromise of bladder control although nerve-sparing techniques may minimize these complications.

CANCER

Cancer of the pelvic organs may compromise the urinary tract. Invasive cancer of the bladder may result in cystectomy and urinary diversion or bladder reconstruction, using segments of the small or large intestine to create a urinary reservoir. One complication of this type of surgery is occasional or chronic urinary incontinence. Prostate, cervical, rectal, and urethral cancers can also cause urinary incontinence because of nerve or muscle damage. Cancers outside of the pelvis may also be implicated. Lung or esophageal cancer that causes chronic cough may result in persistent stress incontinence because of weakening of pelvic floor muscles. Breast cancer may result in hormonal changes in the vaginal and urethral mucosa that cause drying and prevent the urethral sphincter from closing tightly. Treatments for cancer may also cause urinary incontinence. Radiation to the pelvic area may cause irritation of the bladder and urge incontinence. High doses of chemotherapy may cause chronic bladder irritation.

PELVIC PAIN SYNDROME

Pelvic pain syndrome is characterized by persistent or recurrent episodes of pelvic pain that is associated with urinary, sexual, bowel, or gynecological dysfunction despite lack of evident infection or other pathology and is continuous or recurrent for 6 months or more. The distribution and intensity of pain can vary considerably from one individual to another and may involve many different organs and structures. The particular aspects of pelvic pain syndrome that relate to urinary incontinence are **bladder pain syndrome, urethral pain syndrome, prostate pain syndrome, penile pain syndrome, and scrotal pain syndrome.** Prostate pain in males is often associated with a nonspecific prostatitis and may be experienced as pain at the base of the penis and around the anus. All of these manifestations may present with urological disorders, including pain on urination, failure to empty the bladder because of pain, and urinary overflow resulting in urinary incontinence.

TRAUMA

Trauma to the urinary system may involve both blunt and penetrating injuries. Blunt trauma to the abdomen may result in kidney, bladder, or ureteral damage as well as damage to the external genitalia. Vaginal injuries not related to childbirth, such as from sexual abuse or other penetrating injuries, have coexisting urological injuries in about 30% of cases. People sustaining back or flank penetrating wounds and pelvic trauma are at risk for damage to the urinary system. Injury to the bladder during automobile accidents is common because of the impact of the seat back to the lower abdomen. If the damage is severe, there may be a tear through the wall of the bladder and the vagina, causing urine to leak through the vagina. Gunshot wounds and stab injuries may cause extensive damage. Almost all trauma to the urinary system initially presents with hematuria, but untreated may develop into abscesses and fistulas and various other urinary tract symptoms, including urinary incontinence.

NEUROMUSCULAR CONDITIONS

Neuromuscular conditions include a wide range of neurodegenerative disorders, traumatic nerve injuries, toxic metabolic disorders of the peripheral nerves and muscles, and autoimmune neuromuscular disorders, many causing damage to muscles and nerves affecting urinary function, including the following:

- **Parkinson disease** is a chronic progressive neurodegenerative disease that affects both voluntary and involuntary muscles, leading to lack of urinary control and stress and urge incontinence.
- **Multiple sclerosis (MS)** is a progressive disorder in which the myelin sheath and underlying nerve fibers in the brain, eyes, and spinal cord are damaged or destroyed. About 80% of those with MS develop bladder control problems because the electrical impulses to and from the brain are interrupted.
- **Cerebrovascular accident (stroke)** results from vascular lesions of the brain causing neurological damage. About 40% of people with strokes suffer from urinary incontinence. Post-stroke incontinence may be more likely because of pre-stroke incontinence and other forms of urinary tract disorders.

ENDOCRINE Conditions

DIABETES MELLITUS

Diabetes mellitus is a disease of the pancreas that occurs when the pancreas cannot produce enough insulin to control glucose levels in the body (Type I) or where the body does not respond to the insulin that is produced (Type II), resulting in increased glucose levels in the blood and multiple associated health problems. A small percentage of people with Type I diabetes develop autonomic nervous system involvement that causes neurogenic bladder. About 6.5% of all women with urinary incontinence also have diabetes. As neurogenic bladder progresses there may be mild loss of the sensation of the bladder being full to complete bladder paralysis. In order to urinate, the person must strain to void and often dribbles urine. They may have urge, stress, or mixed incontinence, which worsens if the diabetes is not well controlled and the person suffers from thirst and the frequent need to urinate.

> **Review Video: Diet, Exercise, and Medications for Diabetes**
> Visit mometrix.com/academy and enter code: 774388

CUSHING'S DISEASE

Cushing's disease is a condition that results in over-production of corticosteroids from a neoplasm of the adrenal glands or of the anterior pituitary gland. In rare cases, some types of lung cancers may produce corticosteroids. Cushing's syndrome may result from medical use of corticosteroids. Cushing's disease/syndrome has many negative effects, including hypertension, obesity, weakness, glucose intolerance, and persistent polydipsia and polyuria. The constant thirst and need to urinate, coupled with weakness and other health problems, often lead to urinary incontinence.

DIABETES INSIPIDUS

Diabetes insipidus is triggered by lack of antidiuretic hormone (ADH), which is stored in and released from the pituitary gland, or the inability of the kidneys to respond to ADH so that they are unable to conserve water as they filter the blood, resulting in excessive urination and extreme thirst. Patients drink copious amounts of water to compensate for fluid loss, often leading to the need to urinate every 1-2 hours and resulting urinary incontinence.

OBSTRUCTION

Obstruction within the bladder outlet is a frequent cause of overflow incontinence. The obstruction may be related to an enlarged prostate or a prolapse that compresses the urethra or interferes with the contraction of the detrusor muscle. Calculi, cancerous lesions, and strictures may also cause obstruction. Urethral trauma or sexually transmitted diseases may result in obstructive strictures of the urethra. When obstruction occurs, the part of the urinary tract proximal to the obstruction becomes distended and pressure builds, forcing the urine past the obstruction and often resulting in urinary stasis and infection. Chronic obstruction can cause permanent urinary tract damage. Upper urinary tract obstruction within the ureters or kidneys often causes pain and systemic reactions as hydronephrosis develops and the kidneys fail, but lower urinary tract obstruction of the bladder and/or urethra is more likely to present as urinary dysfunction with frequency, dribbling, hematuria, inadequate emptying, nocturia, and incontinence.

PREGNANCY AND CHILDBIRTH

Pregnancy and childbirth increase the risk of urinary and fecal incontinence, both during pregnancy from increased pressure exerted by the fetus and weakening of the pelvic floor muscles and after childbirth with a vaginal delivery, especially if forceps were used to aid in the delivery or if an episiotomy was done. Cesarean sections do not appear to result in post-partal incontinence. Older and multiparous women, especially after high-risk deliveries, are more likely to develop both urinary and fecal incontinence because of nerve damage sustained during childbirth as well as damage to the anal sphincter. The first vaginal delivery a woman has usually accounts for most of the damage to the anal sphincter, but subsequent births increase damage to the pudendal nerve, making fecal incontinence more common as the maternal age increases. Weakening of the vaginal walls and pelvic muscles can lead to prolapse, further causing urinary incontinence.

EFFECTS OF INCONTINENCE ON MALES

Incontinence in males is much less prevalent than in females with only 3-11% of males affected, but this still means that 5 million men in the United States suffer from incontinence. Males have about half the rate of incontinence as women. Urge incontinence (40-80%) is the most common type, followed by mixed incontinence (10-30%), and only rare occurrences of stress incontinence (<10%), primarily because of the longer urethra in males. Stress incontinence, when it does occur, is usually the result of neurological injury or trauma, especially after surgery on the prostate. Urge incontinence is often related to bladder outlet obstruction causing bladder overactivity. It is also common with men who have Parkinson's disease, diabetes mellitus, stroke, or dementia. Overflow incontinence, often transient, is caused by blockage or weak contractions of the detrusor muscle. It is usually a result of prostatic hypertrophy or urethral stenosis related to scarring.

NORMAL CHANGES OF AGING THAT CAN CONTRIBUTE TO INCONTINENCE

Normal changes of aging are physiological changes that take place, as people grow older. Most changes do not impact normal functioning although they may become more apparent under stress caused by physical exertion or illness. Some physiological changes can impact the urinary system:

- **Renal filtration** decreases, and the urine becomes less concentrated, so pH may be low even if dehydration is present. There is a loss of about 30-40% of functional nephrons in the kidney, decreasing the size of the kidneys and resulting in a decrease in the ability to concentrate urine. Excess potassium may be secreted, leading to dehydration.
- **Neurological changes due to degeneration** in the nerves or reflex arcs that control the bladder and sphincter muscles can cause frequency and urgency, leading to a decreased bladder capacity.
- **Muscle deterioration** can cause detrusor muscle of the bladder to lose contractibility, decreasing bladder capacity and preventing complete emptying of the bladder. Pelvic floor and sphincter muscles may atrophy, resulting in incontinence.
- **Prostatic hypertrophy** may cause obstruction of urinary flow and overflow incontinence.
- **Nocturnal urine production** increases, and this may result in nocturia and enuresis.

STRESS INCONTINENCE

ETIOLOGY

Stress incontinence is the leakage of urine during activities that apply pressure to a full bladder. When the stress on the bladder ends, the leakage ends. If the leakage continues after the pressure has been relieved, then the patient more likely has urge incontinence.

Stress incontinence is most often the result of urethral sphincter incompetence caused by weakened pelvic floor muscles and ligaments. This weakening causes the urethra, sphincters, and bladder neck to lose support and muscle tone and the urethra to rotate downward during episodes of stress, such as coughing or sneezing, overloading the urethral sphincters. When there is an increase in intra-abdominal pressure, it forces urine past the sphincters. The most common causes of this type of problem are related to trauma of childbirth causing damage to the sphincters or the pelvic floor muscles, loss of estrogen after menopause resulting in atrophy and loss of pliability of the urethra, and obesity, which causes chronic pressure to the pelvic floor muscles. Some muscle changes are common in the elderly, especially women. Stress incontinence in men is usually caused by neurological injury or trauma to the urethral sphincters, usually related to surgery on the prostate.

Having a **chronic cough** forces the patient to perform a bearing down type of activity, which applies pressure to the bladder and can cause some urine leakage.

Urethral hypermobility occurs when the urethra does not close properly, resulting in the leakage of urine. This is one of the main causes of stress incontinence. It is due to a weakening of the muscles in the pelvic floor, which occurs after vaginal deliveries. Urethral hypermobility may also occur after menopause when estrogen levels are low, causing the lining of the urethra to thin and not close properly. Treatment of stress incontinence involves performing exercises to help strengthen the muscles of the pelvic floor and the urethral sphincter.

PHYSICAL CAUSES

Physical causes of stress incontinence varies between females and males. In females, it results from one or more of the following:

- **Urethral hypermobility** is failure of urethral sphincter to close completely and the urethra being too mobile and out of normal position, related to weakening of the pelvic floor muscles. Urethral hypermobility is classified as Type I with incomplete closure of the bladder neck and urethra. With Type II, the bladder neck shifts position and a cystocele may develop.
- **Intrinsic sphincteric deficiency** is weakening of muscles around the bladder neck so the urethral sphincter cannot maintain adequate resistance for urinary continence. The bladder neck stays open when the bladder fills.
- **Denervation** related to trauma of childbirth, chronic cough, or lifting.

In males, stress incontinence is usually the result of trauma from surgical or radiation treatments for cancer of the prostate.

FUNCTIONAL INCONTINENCE

Functional incontinence is characterized by leakage of urine because of the inability of the person to manage toileting or remove clothing for a variety of reasons. Management depends upon the cause.

- **Pain** may prevent people from attending to body functions, so adequate pain assessment and pain control must be initiated.
- **Dementia** may, in some cases, respond to medications. In other cases, the person may need the assistance of a caregiver to set up a program of scheduled, prompted voiding.
- **Inaccessibility** issues in the home may require modifications of bathrooms, including elevated toilet seats and safety bars. Bedside commodes or urinals may make toileting easier. Outside the home, accessible toileting facilities may need to be identified in advance.
- **Motor disability** must be dealt with according to disability. Sometimes assistive devices may be used. Clothes that are easy to remove, without buttons or zippers, may make toileting easier.

ENVIRONMENTAL CAUSES

Environmental factors can have an impact on the ability of people, especially the elderly or disabled, to remain continent, resulting in functional incontinence:

- **Decreased mobility** may prevent people from being independent in toileting, and lack of assistance from caregivers can lead to inability to use toilet when needed.
- **Inaccessibility of toilet facilities**, such as no wheelchair accessible toilets or no assistive devices, including elevated toilet seats and safety bars, may be a barrier to toileting. Poor lighting may also be a factor for those who are visually impaired.
- **Restraints** can include clothes that are too tight or difficult to remove or physical restraints that preclude toileting. Restraining chairs or other types of restraints in nursing homes without adequately scheduled toileting can lead to incontinence.
- **Social attitudes** may prevent people from asking for the assistance that they need because some people feel ashamed or embarrassed, recognizing negative attitudes toward incontinence.

URGE INCONTINENCE

Urge incontinence is usually the result of over-activity of the detrusor muscle of the bladder and hyperreflexia, resulting in inappropriate contractions of the detrusor muscle during the urinary storage stage. Usually, the bladder stretches to hold up to 550 mL of urine, with the urge to urinate occurring at about 200 mL, at which point, voluntary contraction of the bladder results in relaxation of the external sphincters and urination. With urge incontinence, contractions are unrelated to the amount of urine in the bladder. These premature contractions cause increased pressure in the bladder accompanied by an intense urge to urinate. When bladder pressure exceeds urethral pressure, urge incontinence occurs. This condition may be caused by lesions of the upper motor neurons, stroke, spinal cord tumors, neuromuscular disorders (Parkinson's disease, multiple sclerosis), and transverse myelitis. Urinary infections may also cause urge incontinence although infrequently. The cause for most urge incontinence is idiopathic.

PHYSICAL CAUSES

Urge incontinence occurs when bladder pressure exceeds urethral sphincter pressure. People feel the urge to urinate followed by immediate urination before they are able to reach a toilet. Causes relate to the detrusor muscle.

- **Detrusor hyperactivity with hyperreflexia** involves the detrusor muscle contracting involuntarily during the storage phase, causing a sensory perception of urgency, and forcing urine past the sphincters, leading to decreased bladder volume. The cause may relate to strokes, cervical stenosis, Parkinson's disease, urinary infection, or neoplasms.
- **Detrusor hyperactivity with impaired contractile function (DHIC)** results from involuntary contractions that may be ineffective to empty the bladder. This condition is characterized by overactive detrusor contractions during the storage phase but underactive contractions during urination, resulting in both frequency and residual urine in bladder. It is common with neurological impairment from trauma or disease, such as Parkinson's or multiple sclerosis.
- **Urinary infection** or other conditions that irritate the bladder may trigger contractions.

REFLEX INCONTINENCE

Reflex incontinence is a type of urge incontinence related to impairment of the neurological system. The transmission that is necessary in the spinal and brainstem reflex loops is impaired, so sensations of bladder fullness, sphincter control, and coordination of detrusor muscle and sphincter muscles are also impaired. Bladder emptying is impaired and usually incomplete. Reflex incontinence is common in patients with stroke, brain tumors, Parkinson's disease, multiple sclerosis, advanced dementia, and those with suprapontine or suprasacral spinal cord injuries. Physiologically, there are primarily two conditions that result from the neurological damage:

- **Detrusor hyperreflexia** involves aberrant contractions of the detrusor muscle without the sensation of needing to urinate. This can cause incontinence at unpredictable times and with no warning.
- **Dyssynergic contractions of the urethral sphincter muscle** are often present as well, resulting in urinary obstruction, which in turn causes a distended bladder with large residual urine volumes.

OVERFLOW INCONTINENCE

Overflow incontinence is the leakage of small amounts of urine both day and night from a distended bladder overflowing. The bladder fills normally, but cannot properly empty, leading to frequency and dribbling. Overflow incontinence is usually the result of bladder neuropathy with diabetes mellitus being a common cause of a neurogenic bladder. Tumors of the spine, meningomyelocele, and disk disorder may also result in bladder neuropathy. Overflow incontinence occurs when there is either a nonfunctioning detrusor or outlet obstruction from prostatic hypertrophy, urethral stricture, neoplasm, or urethral obstruction resulting post-operatively from a pubovaginal sling. A non-functioning detrusor may be the result of an underlying neurologic disease, such as Parkinson's disease, that essentially paralyzes the muscle. It may also result from an atonic bladder caused by chronic over-distention that has made the bladder lose muscle tone. Obstruction may be caused by a cystocele as well. Some medications also may interfere with bladder contractibility. With overflow incontinence, the bladder fills normally, but does not properly empty until the pressure becomes sufficient to force urine from the bladder or past an obstruction.

PHYSICAL CAUSES

Physical causes of overflow incontinence include:

- **Detrusor underactivity** results in a bladder that cannot adequately contract. Diabetes Mellitus is a common cause of nerve damage, resulting in a neurogenic bladder. Other causes are tumors of the spine, meningomyelocele, and disk disorders. Underactivity may also be the result of a neurological disorder, such as Parkinson's disease. Anticholinergics and opioids are also a cause.
- **Bladder outlet obstruction** may be caused by a cystocele, prostatic hypertrophy, urethral stricture, trauma from a sling procedure, or a fecal impaction.
- **Detrusor-sphincter dyssynergia** is a loss of coordination resulting in the sphincter contracting when the detrusor muscle contracts, creating an outlet obstruction. This condition often results from spinal cord lesions that interrupt neurological pathways and reflex arcs.

POST-PROSTATECTOMY INCONTINENCE

Post-prostatectomy incontinence is common with some studies showing that 30-47% reported some incontinence, ranging from dribbling to full emptying of the bladder. There are a number of reasons, and more than one may contribute to a person's incontinence:

- **Trauma to urethral sphincter** during the surgical procedure may result in transient or permanent stress incontinence with coughing, straining, or physical activity that increases intra-abdominal pressure.
- **Detrusor hypertrophy** occurs preoperatively as the bladder tries to compensate for urinary blockage with increasing muscle mass and pressure during contractions. After surgery, the bladder continues to contract with too much pressure for the urethra to prevent urination, resulting in urge incontinence. Hypertrophy may also cause frequency and sometimes enuresis. If this condition occurs with urethral trauma, it results in mixed incontinence,
- **Nerve damage** may affect the ability of the bladder to store low volumes of urine, resulting in dribbling.

NOCTURNAL ENURESIS

Nocturnal enuresis is involuntary urination during sleep after the age of 5 while remaining continent during the daytime. In **primary enuresis**, the person may never have consistently stayed dry at night from childhood, sometimes lasting throughout adulthood. There appears to be a genetic factor involved in some cases. With primary enuresis, urinary output increases during the night. **Secondary enuresis** is adult onset, and there are a variety of causes:

- Chronic urinary retention with urethral obstruction causes overflow incontinence.
- Urinary tract infections may cause bladder spasms.
- Congestive heart failure may result in peripheral edema that resolves at night with an increase in urinary output.
- Neurological disorders, such as Parkinson's disease, may cause bladder spasms and chronic retention with overflow.
- Prostatic hypertrophy or cancer may cause obstruction
- Abnormalities of anatomy.
- Sleep apnea

People who suffer from urge or overflow incontinence during the daytime often also suffer from nocturnal enuresis.

Continence Care: Assessment and Care Planning

Bowel Dysfunction

COLON MOTILITY DISORDERS AND INTRACTABLE CONSTIPATION

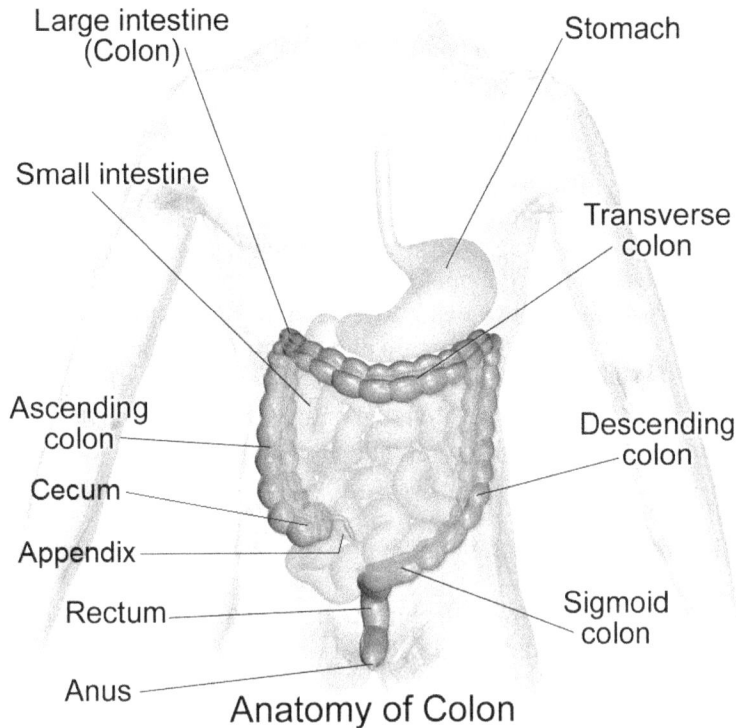

Large intestine (Colon)

Small intestine

Ascending colon

Cecum

Appendix

Rectum

Anus

Stomach

Transverse colon

Descending colon

Sigmoid colon

Anatomy of Colon

Colon motility disorders may involve the colon, pelvic floor muscles, and anal sphincter muscles. Many of these disorders so impair functioning that intractable constipation results. These disorders may include:

- **Abnormal contractions of the colon** may be spastic and ineffectual in pushing the stool through the bowel so that the stool becomes increasing dry and impacted.
- **Dysfunction of nerves or muscles of the colon** because of a neuromuscular disorder may cause an absence of contraction that delays movement of stool through the colon or allows only incomplete bowel movements. Severe constipation and impaction may result.
- **Functional obstruction of anal sphincters** results in the stool becoming trapped in the rectum because the anal sphincters partially or completely fail to relax to allow defecation.
- **Dyssynergia of pelvic floor muscles** prevents coordination of relaxation and contraction that propel stool from the rectum and through the anus, preventing normal fecal evacuation.

CONTRIBUTING FACTORS TO BOWEL DYSFUNCTION

Contributing factors to bowel dysfunction range from those things that can be corrected and others that require compensation:

- **Dietary factors** include insufficient fiber and fluids as well as foods that cause diarrhea, constipation, and gas.
- **Clinical conditions** such as hemorrhoids may cause pain that delays defecation. Surgical treatment of hemorrhoids, fistulas, or the rectum may create trauma and injury to the sphincters. Chronic diseases, such as irritable bowel syndrome and multiple sclerosis may be associated with bowel dysfunction. Dementia may result in the inability to manage toileting.

- **Delaying defecation**, often because of functional disability or dementia, is the leading cause of constipation, impaction, and fecal incontinence.
- **Pregnancy** can result in damage to anal sphincters, causing incontinence.
- **Medications** frequently cause constipation, but some, including antacids and antibiotics, may cause diarrhea. Laxative abuse causes laxative tolerance to develop.
- **Physical inactivity** decreases bowel motility and increases constipation.

CAUSES OF FECAL INCONTINENCE

Common causes of fecal incontinence include:

- **Constipation**: Chronic constipation causes stretching and weakening of intestinal and anal muscles. Weakened intestinal muscles slow down the passage of fecal material that forms impactions, and the weakened anal muscles prevent the rectal sphincter from closing. Chronic constipation may create a cycle of constipation/diarrhea, and stool leaks around impactions.
- **Chronic or severe diarrhea**: Inflammation and irritation from severe diarrhea with urgency can make it difficult to be continent of watery stools.
- **Injury to anal sphincter**: Usually related to damage during childbirth.
- **Neurological abnormalities/ injuries**: Congenital defects, such as myelomeningocele, can damage nerves and paralyze intestinal or anal muscles. Spinal cord injuries may also damage nerves.
- **Chronic laxative abuse**: Laxatives stimulate bowels to contract, causing irritation and cycles of constipation/diarrhea.
- **Surgical/radiation complications**: Rectal, prostate, or gynecological surgery may damage nerves or muscles controlling defecation. Radiation may cause scarring, inflammation, and stenosis.
- **Psychological/ psychiatric disturbances**: Severe mental or emotional problems may interfere with control of bodily functions.

CAUSES OF CONSTIPATION AND IMPACTION

Causes of constipation and impaction include:

- **Insufficient fiber** in the diet reduces bulk of stool, making it move more slowly through the colon.
- **Insufficient liquids** can make stools too dry and compact.
- **Lack of exercise** may decrease motility of bowel, slowing down the passage of stool and allowing more fluid to be absorbed.
- **Medications**, such as narcotic analgesics (codeine, meperidine, hydrocodone-containing drugs), antacids (Maalox, Mylanta), anticholinergics (tolterodine, oxybutynin, Donnatal), beta-blockers, (atenolol, propanolol), tricyclic antidepressants, iron supplements, calcium supplements, anticonvulsants (phenytoin), Antidiarrheals (diphenoxylate/atropine, bismuth subsalicylate) and diuretics (chlorothiazide, furosemide) can all result in constipation. Overuse of laxatives can result in a cycle of diarrhea and increasing constipation.
- **Irritable bowel syndrome** may be characterized by diarrhea, constipation, and impaction.
- **Pregnancy** with hormonal changes and pressure on the colon may lead to constipation.
- **Delayed toileting** for any reason, such as inaccessible toilets, travel, or pain about anus can cause people to delay defecation.

RISK FACTORS FOR FECAL INCONTINENCE

Common risk factors for fecal incontinence include:

- **Age**: Fecal incontinence is most common among people who are elderly and may suffer from other health problems, including urinary incontinence.
- **Sex**: Women suffer more from fecal incontinence than men because women often suffer damage to the sphincter after childbirth, especially as scar tissue forms after episiotomies or muscles weaken after multiple childbirths.
- **Neurological damage**: Congenital or acquired neurological defects are frequently associated with fecal incontinence. Additionally, people with chronic disorders, such as diabetes mellitus or multiple sclerosis may lose the ability to control defecation because of progressive neuropathy.
- **Dementia/Alzheimer disease**: Late-stage Alzheimer disease is characterized by both fecal and urinary incontinence.
- **Physical disability**: Congenital or acquired physical disabilities may lead to fecal incontinence for many reasons. People confined to wheelchairs might find toilet access difficult. People may not be able to express the need to defecate. Others may not be able to physically manage toileting without assistance.

RECTOCELES AND ENTEROCELES

Rectoceles **(rectal prolapses)** occur when the muscles between the wall of the vagina and rectum weaken and the rectum prolapses or protrudes into the back wall of the vagina. **Enteroceles** occur similarly when the small bowel protrudes into the upper vaginal wall. Both can result from damage to the lower pelvic muscles from childbirth-related trauma, pelvic surgery, or muscle weakness attributed to aging. Rectoceles and enteroceles may occur together after hysterectomy. They can be felt as a bulging mass in the vagina. Enteroceles rarely after bowel habits, but rectoceles can cause chronic constipation and difficulty in passing stool because of weakening of the muscles, contributing to fecal incontinence. Untreated, rectoceles can cause inflammation, ulcerations, and fistula formation. Pessaries may reduce the prolapse. Surgical repair may not correct all symptoms, especially underlying damage to muscles, and can result in surgical trauma to the rectum or sphincters, adding to the risk of incontinence.

INTESTINAL INFECTIONS

Intestinal infections may be caused by numerous varieties of bacteria (*E. coli, Campylobacter, Clostridioides difficile, Shigella),* viruses (*Rotavirus, Cytomegalovirus)*, fungal parasites (*Microsporidia)*, protozoan parasites (*Giardia intestinalis, Entamoeba histolytica), and* helminth parasites (*Strongyloides stercoralis, Angiostrongylus costaricensis*). While the pathogens may be different, most result in acute or chronic enteritis and/or colitis. Diarrhea is a common finding with almost all infections of the intestine, and in about 40% of cases, the etiologic agent cannot be identified. Infections can result in inflammation and ulceration of the mucosal lining as well as damage to the muscular layer. Recent studies have indicated that some individual with acute enteritis will develop chronic abdominal pain and altered bowel habits, a condition now referred to as **postinfectious irritable bowel syndrome (IBS)**. Some enteric infections will result in long-term effects on the neurological and muscular functions of the bowels, sometimes resulting in alterations of bowel habits, reduced sensation, and incontinence.

FISTULAS

Fistulas are abnormal tunnel-like openings usually between two organs, or from an organ to the surface of the skin. Fistulas involving the anus, rectum, or vagina and the perineal tissue can result in damage to intestinal and pelvic floor muscles, nerves, and sphincters. Anorectal fistulas, the most common type, usually result from an abscess and may have one or more tunnels connecting the rectum and the skin around the anus. Fistulas may also result from trauma, disease, or radiation. Fecal incontinence is common with fistulas because of the extensive inflammation and tissue involvement. Fecal material may leak from the fistula as well as the anus. Surgical repair may require much dissection, especially if there are multiple tracts and the origin is high in the rectum, and can lead to cutting the muscles of the anus as well as the formation of scar tissue, further contributing to fecal incontinence.

NEUROMUSCULAR CONDITIONS

Neuromuscular conditions may include a wide range of neurodegenerative disorders, traumatic nerve injuries, toxic metabolic disorders of the peripheral nerves and muscles, and autoimmune neuromuscular disorders, many of which result in damage to muscles and nerves, affecting bowel function, including the following:

- **Parkinson disease**, a chronic progressive neurodegenerative disease, affects movement. Both voluntary and involuntary muscle control may be compromised, sometimes resulting in loss of sphincter control and fecal incontinence.
- **Multiple sclerosis (MS)** is a progressive disorder in which the myelin sheath and underlying nerve fibers in the brain, eyes, and spinal cord are damaged or destroyed. The nerves that control bowel movements can be affected, causing constipation and fecal incontinence.
- **Muscular dystrophy (MD)** is a term designating a group of genetic disorders that cause progressive weakening and atrophy of muscles. Any level of the gastrointestinal tract may be involved, and fecal incontinence is a frequent problem with some types of MD.

CANCER

Several kinds of cancer are associated with fecal incontinence with the treatment rather than the cancer often being the precipitating factor. Colon and rectal cancer may remove or damage the muscles or nerves that control defecation. **Radiation therapy** may further cause weakening of the intestinal muscles or damage to the nerves. This damage may result in temporary fecal incontinence, but in some cases, the damage may be so severe that the fecal incontinence remains permanent. In some cases, cancer outside of the gastrointestinal tract may precipitate fecal incontinence. **Cancerous lesions** of the brain or spinal cord may both be related to bowel dysfunction and loss of bowel control because of cognitive defects or neurological damage. Because the nerves carry impulses from the brain to the spinal cord to the bowels, lesions involving these nerves or parts of the brain that controls these nerves can lead to incontinence.

BOWEL OBSTRUCTION

Bowel obstruction is a mechanical blockage at any level of the small or large intestines. Bowel obstruction can be the result of a disease process, such as Crohn's disease, a cancerous lesion, herniation, foreign bodies, or a fecal impaction. Obstruction may be caused by something inside the lumen of the intestine, which is creating a blockage; within the wall of the intestine, which is narrowing the lumen; or outside of the intestine (such as a volvulus), which is causing a compression blockage. Complete or incomplete obstruction can result in ileus, cramping, distention, constipation and paradoxical or overflow diarrhea. Chronic constipation with impaction is a common cause of obstruction in the elderly or those who are bedridden and unable to manage their own toileting. Distention of the intestine brought on by the impaction can interfere with peristalsis, worsening the condition, and increasing the incidence of fecal incontinence.

BOWEL TRAUMA

Bowel trauma comprises both blunt and penetrating abdominal wounds.

- **Blunt** trauma is usually the result of accidents or assaults and can result in intestinal injury through compression or deceleration. Compression of the lumen can stretch or perforate the bowel wall. Blunt injuries to the transverse colon, sigmoid colon, or cecum are common. Deceleration forces can tear the bowel and result in ischemia.

Continence Care: Assessment and Care Planning

- **Penetrating** trauma is usually secondary to knife, shrapnel, or gunshot wounds and can involve minor to catastrophic injury. War injuries such as bomb and grenade trauma can involve both blunt and penetrating trauma. Small bowel wounds are easily misdiagnosed but can result in peritonitis and ileus. Bowel dysfunction, including fecal incontinence can result from both blunt and penetrating wounds, depending upon the degree, type, location of injury, and medical or surgical intervention. Bowel trauma may also be caused by laparoscopic injury during surgical procedures, especially gynecological endoscopy.

ENCOPRESIS

Encopresis is the voluntary or involuntary passage of stool in places or manners that are inappropriate for a child, 80% of whom are male, 4 years or older. There are two types: **retentive encopresis**, which accounts for about 80% of those affected, and **non-retentive**, which accounts for the other 20%.

- **Retentive encopresis** is characterized by a history of long term, painful constipation and the development of overflow diarrhea. The chronic constipation causes distention of the rectum and stretching of both the internal and external anal sphincters; as a result, the child may no longer feel the urge to defecate, so stool eventually leaks from the rectum, causing chronic fecal incontinence.
- **Non-retentive encopresis**, usually involving passage of normally formed stools on a daily basis, does not involve constipation or bowel abnormalities, except in a small subset that may have irritable bowel syndrome, but is generally a behavioral/psychological problem.

ENDOCRINE CONDITIONS

Endocrine conditions are those related to endocrine glands, which are glands that secrete hormones into the blood stream, through which the hormones reach the cells of the body.

- The **thyroid gland**, in the neck, regulates body metabolism. Hypothyroidism occurs when the gland does not produce enough hormones, causing multiple symptoms, including chronic constipation. Hyperthyroidism, on the other hand, causes increased bowel movements. Both conditions can lead to fecal incontinence, especially in the elderly and weak.
- The **adrenal glands**, located on top of the kidneys, produce adrenaline and cortisol. Addison's disease occurs with inadequate production of cortisol, affecting almost every body system. One symptom is chronic diarrhea, which coupled with weakness and vomiting, can lead to fecal incontinence.
- The **pancreas** produces insulin. Insufficient insulin leads to Type I diabetes mellitus, for which diabetic neuropathy is a complication causing autonomic and peripheral nerve changes, resulting in poor rectal tone, perianal hypoesthesia, and fecal incontinence.

PELVIC PAIN SYNDROME AND FECAL INCONTINENCE

Pelvic pain syndrome is characterized by persistent or recurrent episodes of pelvic pain that is associated with urinary, sexual, bowel, or gynecological dysfunction despite lack of evident infection or other pathology. The pain must be continuous or recurrent for 6 months or more. In males, it is often associated with perineal (including anal) and penile pain (often referred to as chronic prostatitis). The distribution and intensity of pain can vary considerably from one individual to another and may involve many different organs and structures. The particular aspects of pelvic pain syndrome that relate to fecal incontinence are the anorectal pain syndrome, which relates to bowel dysfunction and **anismus**, which is pain related to defecation. Because the pain is so severe, people afflicted with the disorder may retain stool because of the pain associated with defecation, leading to chronic constipation, which further aggravates the condition and is a factor in fecal incontinence.

TYPES OF PELVIC ORGAN PROLAPSE

Pelvic organ prolapse occurs when pelvic floor muscles weaken with age or trauma and cannot support the pelvic organs. The uterus is the only organ that can fall into the vagina. Other organs can push against and cause a protrusion in the wall of the vagina.

- **Cystocele** is the bladder falling toward the vagina, causing an anterior vaginal wall protrusion.
- **Urethrocele** is the urethra pushing against the anterior vaginal wall, near the vaginal orifice, often occurring with a cystocele and called a cystourethrocele.
- **Enterocele** is part of the small intestine falling into the space between the rectum and posterior vaginal wall.
- **Rectocele** is the rectum protruding into the posterior vaginal wall while a rectal prolapse is the rectum falling through the anus.
- **Uterine prolapse** is the uterus falling into the vagina.
- **Vaginal vault prolapse** is the top of the vagina falling in on itself after hysterectomy.

COLONIC INERTIA AND CONSTIPATION

Colonic inertia is a condition resulting from neuromuscular disorders of the colon causing a marked delay in the movement of fecal material through the colon. Stool often remains in the ascending or transverse colon rather than progressing to the rectosigmoid area. There may also be a lack of urgency even when the stool in the rectum. Three or more bowel movements weekly are average, but, because of delay in passage of stool, the person with colonic inertia may defecate only about every 7-10 days. Other abnormalities may occur, such as delayed emptying of the stomach and a condition calls pseudo-obstruction of the small intestine with no blockage but symptoms of blockage. The cause of colonic inertia is not always clear, but sometimes the nerves and muscles are diseased. It can also be caused by chronic use of stimulant laxatives. Colonic transit studies help to diagnose the condition. Complete colonic inertia may require ileostomy.

PELVIC FLOOR DYSFUNCTION AND CONSTIPATION

Pelvic floor dysfunction is also referred to as functional outlet obstruction or outlet delay, occurs when the pelvic floor muscles that surround the rectum cannot contract properly or loose muscle tone. Essentially the pelvic floor muscles act as a sling for the rectum. With pelvic floor dysfunction, there is a non-neurogenic lack of coordination of the muscles. The muscles may not relax properly to allow the anal sphincter to open, so stool remains in the rectal vault. Even if colonic motility is normal and there is no delay in transit, chronic constipation and impaction can result. Stool in the rectal area presses on the bladder and urethra and increases urinary problems, so constipation needs to be managed carefully. Pelvic floor dysfunction can occur in both males and females, and in men it is usually called prostatodynia. Ano-rectal motility studies may be done to help with diagnosis.

COMPLICATIONS OF INCONTINENCE

Moisture-associated skin damage, a common complication of incontinence, is inflammation of the skin from frequent and prolonged exposure to liquid, such as urine or feces, resulting in erosion of the tissue. Irritation most commonly occurs in the perineal region and up the gluteal fold and down the inner thighs. Treatment includes controlling incontinence, use of barrier creams, and avoidance of alkaline skin cleansers or detergents.

Intertriginous dermatitis occurs when moisture develops or accumulates in folds of skin, such as under abdominal rolls, in the axillae, or under breasts. The tissue may become erythematous, itching, painful, and denuded. The skin must be kept clean and dry and exposed to air. Powder may help prevent moisture.

Fungal skin infection occurs when the irritation and moisture results in alterations of normal skin flora and overgrowth of fungi, such as *Candida.* The skin becomes red, weepy, and itching. Treatment includes identifying and treating underlying cause and topical antifungal.

Continence Care: Assessment and Care Planning

Screening

ROUTINE URINARY SCREENING

Routine urinary screening measures several components of urine to determine if there is an abnormality:

- **Color** should be pale amber. Concentrated urine is often dark. Blood in the urine will discolor urine red or brownish. Some medications change color of the urine.
- **Clarity** assesses the cloudiness of the urine. Normal urine should be clear. Other material in the blood, such as pus, blood, sperm, and mucous, can increase opacity.
- **Odor** should be faint. A foul odor may indicate infection, and concentrated urine may have a strong odor. Some foods, such as asparagus or fish, change the odor.
- **Specific gravity** should range from 1.005 to 1.035. Higher levels can indicate concentrated urine. Low levels may indicate dilute urine, diuretic use, or kidney disease.
- **Protein** should not be found in the urine. Its presence is a sign of kidney disease, heart failure, leukemia, mercury or lead poisoning, or preeclampsia.
- **pH** should range from 4.5 to 8.0. An alkaline (high) pH can be caused by urinary tract infections, diarrhea, or kidney infection. An acidic (low) pH may reflect lung disease, severe diabetes, diarrhea with dehydration, excessive alcohol intake, or starvation.
- **Glucose** should not be found in the urine and may indicate uncontrolled diabetes mellitus but may also indicate liver damage, brain injury, and some kinds of kidney disease.
- **Nitrites** in the urine are indicative of a urinary tract infection.
- **Leukocyte esterase** indicates that there are white blood cells in the urine, probably from a urinary tract infection.
- **Ketones** should not be found in urine and can indicate uncontrolled diabetes, a low carbohydrate diet, anorexia or bulimia, excessive alcohol intake, or fasting for 18 hours or more.

MICROSCOPIC ANALYSES

Microscopic analysis of urine involves placing the urine specimen in a centrifuge to separate out the sediment, which is then examined under a microscope:

- **Erythrocytes** should not be in the urine and may indicate inflammation, injury, or slight bleeding from strenuous exercise.
- **Leukocytes** in the urine usually are indicative of infection, cancer, or kidney disorders.
- **Casts** are caused from kidney disease that causes tiny tube-like plugs of material (red or white cells, protein, and fatty substances) to be flushed from the kidneys to the urine. The type of cast may help with diagnosis.
- **Crystals** should appear in small numbers. Some types of crystals or large numbers of crystals may be a sign of kidney stones or a metabolic disorder.
- **Bacteria** in the urine indicate an infection.
- **Fungi** in the urine indicate a yeast infection
- **Parasites** may migrate to the urinary system in some types of infestation.

Continence Care: Assessment and Care Planning

Diagnostic Tests

ENDOANAL ULTRASOUND AND RECTAL ULTRASOUND

Endoanal ultrasound uses high frequency sound waves and a computer to visualize to a depth of 5 cm the structure of the sphincter muscles and surrounding tissue. It is used to diagnose perianal fistulas and abscesses and to assess sphincter damage related to fecal incontinence and for staging and follow-up of malignant infiltrations of sphincters with anal neoplasms.

The **procedure** is as follows:

- With the patient lying on the left side, a narrow, wand-like endoscopic probe with a transducer and a lubricated rigid plastic cone covering the end is inserted into the anal canal and pictures are viewed on a computer screen. The cone has a uniform diameter to prevent anatomical distortion.
- Patients may feel vibration during procedure.

Rectal ultrasound is a similar procedure in which an ultrasound probe with an inflatable balloon is inserted through a scope to the rectum. The balloon is inflated and images are taken. This test is used to evaluate rectal masses.

RENAL AND BLADDER ULTRASOUND

Renal ultrasound uses high frequency sound waves and a computer to visualize the location, size, and shape of the kidneys and other urinary structures, such as the ureters. It is used to diagnose tumors, cysts, calculi, and abscesses as well as for placement of drainage tubes.

The **procedure** is as follows:

- Patient is placed in prone position on table.
- Clear gel lubricant is placed on skin over kidney area.
- The transducer is pressed against the skin and moved about the kidney area for scans.

Bladder ultrasound is often done at the same time as the renal ultrasound and the procedure is similar.

The **procedure** is as follows:

- Patient is given fluids prior to the test to ensure full bladder.
- Patient is placed in the supine position on the table.
- Scans are taken of full bladder as for kidney scans.
- Patient empties bladder.
- Additional scans of bladder area are done.
- Gel wiped from skin.

ANAL SPHINCTER ELECTROMYOGRAPHY

Anal sphincter electromyography (EMG) assesses muscle contractions to determine if the sphincter muscles are contracting properly. A normal EMG reading with manometry findings of low anal pressure can indicate a torn sphincter muscle. If the pelvic floor muscles and sphincter muscles are contracting paradoxically rather than in concert, electrical activity increases during simulated defecation rather than decreases. Drugs such as muscle relaxants, cholinergic and anti-cholinergic preparations can affect the outcome of the test and may need to be stopped prior to having the EMG.

The **procedure** is as follows:

- With patient lying on the left side, a small lubricated sponge or plug electrode is inserted into the anal canal. Alternately, needle electrodes may be used.
- Patient must lie still during the procedure or results will be affected.
- Electrical activity of the anal sphincter muscles is recorded on a computer screen while the patient tightens the sphincter muscles, relaxes, and pushes.

BALLOON EXPULSION TEST AND PUDENDAL NERVE TERMINAL MOTOR LATENCY TEST

Balloon expulsion test assess the length of time it takes to expel an inflated balloon. A dysfunction in the anorectal area may result in prolonged expulsion time.

The **procedure** is as follows:

- With patient lying on the left side, a balloon is inserted into the rectum and inflated with water.
- The patient sits on the toilet and tries to expel the balloon as though defecating.
- The time needed to expel the balloon is recorded.

Pudendal nerve terminal motor latency test assesses the pudendal nerve and the delay between an electrical impulse and the corresponding muscle contraction. It is used to evaluate incontinence, rectal prolapse, and constipation.

The **procedure** is as follows:

- With the patient lying on the left side, a gloved finger is inserted into the anus. The glove contains a stimulating electrode. With the finger serving as a guiding probe, several electrical impulses are delivered and nerve conduction assessed.
- Mild discomfort may be felt with stimulation.

CYSTOMETROGRAM

Cystometrogram (CMG) assesses bladder capacity and pressure and is used to diagnose incontinence, dysuria, or neurological disorders affecting bladder function.

The **procedure** (may vary) is as follows:

- After emptying bladder, patient is placed in supine position.
- A very small thin catheter is inserted into the bladder. It has a tiny filament inside that is connected to a computerized device or a cystometer.
- Sterile saline at room temperature is instilled into the bladder followed by instillation of warm water to evaluate thermal sensation.
- The fluid is drained and then water or carbon dioxide gas is instilled into the bladder in a slow controlled manner while patient reports first need to urinate.
- The patient coughs or performs other activities while bladder is full, and pressure readings are obtained.
- The patient urinates with sensor in place to record pressures for voiding cystometrogram.
- Another catheter may be placed in rectum to record pressures.
- Catheter(s) removed.

Continence Care: Assessment and Care Planning

URODYNAMIC TESTING

Urodynamic testing assesses bladder and sphincter muscles and the ability of the bladder and urethra to store and release urine. It diagnoses problems with urination, such as frequency, incontinence, dysuria, recurrent infections, frequent urge to urinate, and difficulty initiating stream of urine or emptying bladder.

- **Uroflowmetry** measures the flow rate of urine, including the speed of urination and the volume.
- **Post-void residual measurement** shows how much urine is left in the bladder after urination is completed.
- **Cystometry** assesses bladder capacity and pressure, including how full the bladder is when the urge to urinate is felt.
- **Leak point pressure** measures the bladder pressure at the point where leakage of urine occurs.
- **Pressure flow study** measures bladder pressure that is needed to urinate and the flow rate at different pressures.
- **Electromyography** measures activity of muscles in and around the urethral sphincter.
- **Video** with fluoroscopy shows filling and emptying of bladder.

VLLP

Valsalva Leak point pressure (VLPP) measures the pressure at which bladder pressure overcomes urethral resistance without contraction of the detrusor muscle of the bladder wall. A decreased leak point pressure suggests stress urinary incontinence.

The **procedure** (may vary) is as follows:

- Position patient in supine position.
- A 6-10 Fr. Microtip pressure transducer catheter is inserted into the bladder. There may be a urinary sensor that slides over the catheter and up to the urethral meatus to measure any drops of urine.
- A rectal probe monitors intra-abdominal pressure.
- The patient sits or stands during the testing.
- The bladder is instilled with saline or contrast material at 50 mL/min to a total of 200 mL.
- Patient asked to make a progressive Valsalva motion, bearing down with a closed glottis, until incontinence. Patient may also be asked to cough.
- Procedure repeated for comparison measurements and catheters removed.

URETHRAL PRESSURE PROFILE

Urethral pressure profile is a graph recording the intraluminal pressure of the entire length of the urethra. The profile assesses the function of the urethra during filling cystometry.

- **Urethral pressure**: The pressure of fluid needed to open a urethra.
- **Maximum urethral closure pressure**: The maximum pressure exerted by the urethra as indicated on the profile.
- **Functional profile length**: The length of the urethra (in females) where the pressure is greater in the urethra than the pressure inside the bladder.
- **Pressure transmission ratio**: The relationship (in percentage) between an increase in urethral pressure as a response to stress and the simultaneous increase in bladder pressure.
- **Abnormal leak point pressure**: The pressure at which bladder pressure overcomes urethral resistance without contraction of the detrusor muscle.
- **Detrusor leak point pressure**: The lowest pressure of the detrusor muscle at which urinary incontinence occurs without contraction of detrusor muscle or increased abdominal pressure.

CYSTOGRAPHY

Cystography is a urinary diagnostic test that uses x-rays or fluoroscopy to examine the bladder. The test may be used to determine how well the bladder empties and whether there is a vesicoureteral reflux (backflow of urine to the kidneys). It can assess the cause of hematuria, chronic urinary tract infections, obstructions, and urinary incontinence.

The **procedure** is as follows:

- Patient may be given laxatives or enema before cystography.
- Patient will empty bladder before procedure.
- Patient is placed in supine position on x-ray table.
- Catheter is inserted into bladder and contrast dye is injected through the catheter, which is then clamped.
- X-rays or fluoroscopy are done.
- Patient may have to change positions for different views.
- Catheter removed.
- For **voiding cystography**, x-ray or fluoroscopy will be done while the patient urinates. The patient may be allowed to sit up if unable to urinate in supine position.

UROFLOWMETRY AND PAD TEST

Uroflowmetry is a non-invasive test that plots the flow rate of urination over time and is used to assess function of the bladder and sphincters. During normal urination, the first stream starts slowly, speeds up and then slows down again as the bladder nears empty. This pattern may alter with urinary tract obstruction.

The **procedure** is as follows:

- Patient urinates into special funnel attached to a measuring instrument.
- The instrument calculates rate of flow in seconds, amount of urine, and time of urination.
- The uroflowmeter converts the information into a graph.

Pad test is a non-invasive method of assessing frequency and severity of urinary incontinence.

The **procedure** is as follows:

- Patient is asked to keep a bladder diary.
- Pre-weighed absorbent pads are provided to patient.
- The pad is worn until leakage occurs, and then removed, sealed in a Ziploc-type bag, labeled with date and time.
- Pads are weighed and urine output estimated according to weight.

INTRAVENOUS PYELOGRAM

Intravenous pyelogram is an x-ray of the kidneys and ureters after injection of a contrast dye used to diagnose kidney disease or disorders of the urinary tract. This test may be completed with a CT scan of the kidneys. IVP helps to evaluate kidney function and diagnose bladder or ureteral stones, injury, trauma, and tumors.

The **procedure** is as follows:

- The patient may be given a laxative and enema or suppository before test.
- An intravenous line will be inserted.
- The patient is positioned in supine position on x-ray table.

Continence Care: Assessment
and Care Planning

- A KUB x-ray is taken.
- Contrast dye is injected into the IV.
- To help with visualization, a band may be placed around the waist.
- X-rays are taken at timed-intervals over about 30 minutes as dye progresses through the urinary tract.
- Patient may be asked to change positions.
- Patient empties bladder.
- A final x-ray is taken.
- Intravenous line is removed.

ANTEGRADE PYELOGRAM

Antegrade pyelogram is an x-ray used for the diagnosis of obstruction in the kidneys and ureters. Fluoroscopy or ultrasound may be used to locate kidney and ureters.

The **procedure** is as follows:

- Patient may be given prophylactic antibiotics before or after procedure.
- An intravenous line may be inserted for emergencies.
- Patient lies prone on the x-ray table.
- Area of lower back will be cleansed and sterile drapes applied.
- A local anesthetic is injected at dye injection site.
- Under ultrasound or fluoroscopy, a needle is inserted into the renal pelvis. A wire may be fed through the needle to allow for placement of catheters or tubes.
- Contrast dye is injected into the renal pelvis.
- A number of x-rays are taken at timed intervals as the dye progresses from the kidney through the ureters.
- Needle removed or tubes placed.
- Urine is monitored for volume and hematuria.

RETROGRADE PYELOGRAM

Retrograde pyelogram is an x-ray with contrast dye that provides visualization of the organs of the urinary tract. It is usually performed during a cystoscopy. The retrograde pyelogram is done to diagnose a suspected obstruction of the upper urinary tract or for placement of ureteral stents or catheters.

The **procedure** is as follows:

- Patient may be asked to fast for a number of hours.
- Laxatives or cleansing enemas may be done as preparation.
- The patient may receive a sedative.
- An intravenous line may be inserted for emergencies.
- Patient will be positioned in supine position on the x-ray table with feet in stirrups.
- An endoscope is inserted through the urethra and into the bladder to examine the bladder.
- Catheters may be inserted into ureters and contrast dye injected through catheters. Endoscope is removed.
- X-rays are taken at timed intervals.
- Catheter is removed.

KIDNEY SCAN

Kidney scan is done after administration of a radioactive substance (radionuclide), usually technetium or iodine, which is absorbed by normal kidney tissue. The radioactive substance emits gamma radiation that is detected by a special scanner that converts the information into computerized pictures. Areas with uptake of the radioactive material are called "hot spots," and areas with fewer uptakes are "cold spots," indicating abnormal tissue. The scan is used to diagnose tumorous lesions, hematomas, abscesses, cysts, or enlargement of the kidney and to assess renal function and circulation.

Frontal section through the Kidney

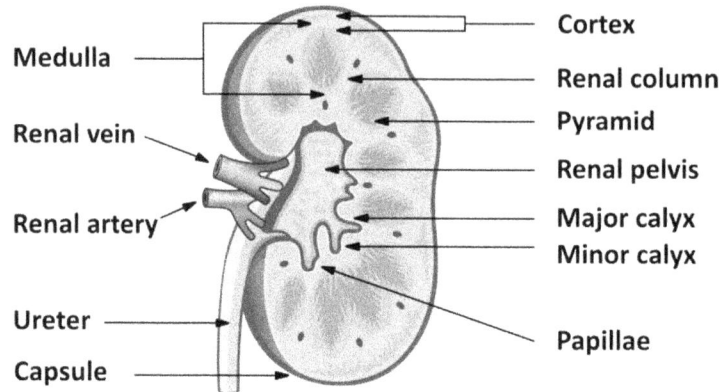

The **procedure** is as follows:

- Patient may be asked to drink fluids prior to scan.
- An intravenous line is started.
- The radioactive material (radionuclide) is injected into the IV.
- Patient may be asked to lie or sit without moving during the scan.
- Patient may receive other medications, such as a diuretic or ACE inhibitor during procedure.
- IV is removed on completion of scan.

KIDNEY, URETER, AND BLADDER (KUB) X-RAYS AND POST-VOID RESIDUAL URINE MEASUREMENT

Kidney, ureter, bladder (KUB) x-rays assess the urinary system as well as other structures of the abdominal area. They may be done to diagnose tumorous lesions, obstructions, and obstruction.

The **procedure** is as follows:

- No special preparation is needed.
- Depending upon the type of equipment, the x-rays may be taken standing or lying down, and from various positions.

Post-void residual urine measurement measures the amount of urine remaining in the bladder after the patient urinates and attempts to empty the bladder. It is used for diagnosis of neurogenic bladder, incontinence, bladder retention, and other urinary problems.

The **procedure** is as follows:

- The patient is placed in supine position and women usually with feet in stirrups.
- A small straight catheter is inserted into bladder to drain residual urine.
- Alternately, a bladder ultrasound with a B-mode (grayscale) sector scan may be done to estimate urine volume. Studies have shown that trans-vaginal ultrasounds are less accurate.

CYSTOSCOPY

Cystoscopy assesses the urethra, bladder, and associated structures using an endoscope. It is used to diagnose urinary problems, such as cancer, retention, infections, obstruction, strictures, and bleeding. Tissue biopsy as well as irrigations or instillations may be done through the endoscope.

The **procedure** is as follows:

- Patient may be asked to fast or have a special diet before test.
- Patient may need to stop anticoagulants or aspirin therapy before test.
- The procedure may be done under a local anesthesia or with conscious sedation.
- An intravenous line is inserted.
- Patient is positioned in supine position with feet in stirrups.
- A topical anesthetic gel is placed in urethral meatus with a catheter.
- The cystoscope is inserted through the urethra into the bladder.
- Sterile water or saline may be instilled in the bladder to allow better visualization.
- A biopsy or urine specimen may be obtained.
- Cystoscope is removed.

PROSTATE/RECTAL SONOGRAM

Prostate/rectal sonogram uses ultrasound technology with sound waves and computers to assess the size, shape, and location of the prostate, rectum, and surrounding structures. A transducer with a Doppler probe may be used to assess circulation of the prostate. This sonogram is used to diagnose prostatic cancer, especially after blood tests that show an elevated prostate-specific antigen (PSA). It may also be used to diagnose or stage rectal cancer.

The **procedure** is as follows:

- Patient may be given a small cleansing enema to clear rectum of fecal material prior to sonogram.
- Patient lies on examining table on the left side with knees drawn toward chest.
- A digital rectal exam may be performed.
- The transducer wand is lubricated and inserted into rectum and then rotated for visualization of the rectum and the prostate.
- A whooshing sound may be heard while Doppler is used. Wand is removed and gel wiped from skin.

Q-TIP TEST AND PROVOKED STRESS TEST

Q-tip test measures mobility and axis position of the urethra to assess urinary incontinence in women.

The **procedure** is as follows:

- Patient lies in supine position.
- Cotton swab (Q-tip), sterile and lubricated with anesthetic gel, is inserted through the urethra to the bladder and then pulled back to the bladder neck.
- Supine, patient strains as though urinating, and straining and resting angles of the swab are measured.
- Standing, the patient again strains and angles are measured.
- A positive result is a Q-tip angle of 30 degrees or more at maximal straining, indicating urethral hypermobility.

Provocative stress test is a cough test of urinary incontinence for women.

The **procedure** is as follows:

- Patient with full bladder in supine position with legs apart coughs, and leakage of urine confirms stress incontinence.
- Patient then stands with one leg on stool and holds pad or paper towel over perineum and coughs. A wet stain confirms stress incontinence.

ELECTROMYOGRAM OF THE BLADDER

Electromyogram (EMG) measures activity of muscles in and around the urethral sphincters and measures coordination between the bladder and the urethra. EMG is used for spinal cord injuries and neurogenic bladder.

The procedure is as follows:

- The patient is in supine position.
- A catheter may be inserted into the bladder.
- Electrodes are placed. There are 3 types: Skin electrodes require skin clean and shaved; electrodes are taped in place around the urethra for females or on the lower abdomen, and between the scrotum and anus for males. Needle electrodes are inserted directly around and into the sphincter muscles for females and through the skin in the perineal area for males. Anal plug electrodes are inserted into the rectum.
- Patient is asked to contract and relax muscles, and electrical activity is recorded on a graph.
- Normal saline or water may be instilled into bladder and patient asked to urinate.
- Catheter and electrodes are removed.

COLONIC AND NUCLEAR TRANSIT STUDIES

Colonic transit studies are x-rays showing how long food takes to go through the intestines. For 1-2 days, the patient ingests gelatin capsules containing small plastic radiopaque markers that can be visualized on x-ray. The gelatin dissolves and the plastic passes, with digested food, through the intestine. After 5-7 days, an abdominal x-ray is taken and the plastic markers are counted in different parts of the intestine. The counts show if there is a delay. In normal evacuation, all markers are expelled. If there is colon inertia, the markers may remain scattered about the colon, suggesting neuromuscular problems. With pelvic floor dysfunction, the markers may accumulate in the rectum.

Nuclear transit studies are similar but a small amount of radioactive material is dissolved in milk or fruit juice and ingested. Images are taken after 6 hours and daily for 4 days, 10 minutes from a large camera scan overhead and 10 minutes from below.

ANAL MANOMETRY

Anal manometry is an assessment of anal sphincter function, often used to evaluate the reason for chronic constipation or fecal incontinence. The test measures the pressure of the sphincter muscles, the degree of sensation in the rectum, and whether the neural reflexes that control normal bowel movements are intact.

The procedure (about 30 minutes) is as follows:

- The lower bowel is cleansed, usually with Fleet enemas about 2 hours before the assessment and food is restricted during this time.
- With patient lying on left side, a balloon catheter is inserted into the rectum. A machine connects to the catheter to measure pressure.

- The balloon is inflated in the rectum to simulate a feeling of fullness and the need to defecate to test neurological response of the reflex pathways.
- Pressure measurements are taken while the patient tightens, relaxes, and pushes with the anal sphincter muscles, simulating holding stool and expelling stool.

ANO-RECTAL MANOMETRY

Ano-rectal manometry is motility studies to evaluate the function of the nerves and muscles of the anus and rectum. In order to perform measurements of pressure, a small flexible tube with sensors is inserted through the anus into the rectum. A balloon may be inflated in the rectum to test pressures. The person is asked to do such things as tightening or relaxing the anal sphincter muscles while the sensors measure the changes in pressure generated by the muscles. These studies can assess whether the muscles of the anus and muscles are working normally or are impaired. With impairment, the muscles cannot coordinate to effect defecation, causing obstruction with resulting constipation. This condition is similar to pelvic floor dysfunction. Tests may show an inadequate sphincter response to rectal distention. Ano-rectal motility defects are common after radiotherapy for pelvic malignancies. Manometry may also be done to assess Hirschsprung's disease and idiopathic megacolon.

DEFECOGRAPHY AND COLONIC MOTILITY STUDIES

Defecography is a type of barium enema, with some modifications. It assesses the process of defecation and shows abnormalities in the anatomy of the rectum and pelvic floor muscles. A thick barium paste is inserted rectally, and then x-rays are taken as the person defecates. The barium outlines the physical structures and shows changes that occur in the pelvic floor muscles during evacuation.

Colonic motility studies measure the contraction pressures of the muscles of the colon. The procedure is done with colonoscopy. Sensors in the long 1/8-inch diameter manometry tube that is passed through the colon measure the pressure. Abnormal activity of the nerves and muscles will result in a pattern of abnormal colonic pressures. This test is useful for diagnosing colonic inertia and determining both cause and treatment for chronic constipation. Excessive contractions may be treated with medications, but complete colonic inertia may require colectomy and ileostomy.

MEDICAL PROCEDURES TO EVALUATE CAUSES OF CONSTIPATION

Medical procedures to evaluate causes of constipation should be preceded by a careful history as this may help to define the type of diarrhea and guide the choice of diagnostic procedures. Most tests are necessary only for severe constipation that does not respond to treatment. Medical diagnostic procedures may include the following:

- **Physical exam** should include rectal exam and abdominal palpation to assess for obvious hard stool or impaction.
- **Blood tests** can identify hypothyroidism and excess parathyroid hormone.
- **Abdominal x-ray** may show large amounts of stool in the colon.
- **Barium enema** can indicate tumors or strictures causing obstruction.
- **Colonic transit studies** can show defects of the neuromuscular system.
- **Defecography** shows defecation process and abnormalities of anatomy.
- **Ano-rectal manometry studies** show malfunction of anorectal muscles.
- **Colonic motility studies** measure the pattern of colonic pressure.
- **Colonoscope** allows direct visualization of the lumen of the rectum and colon.

Physical Assessment and Tools

EXTERNAL UROGENITAL EXAM

The external urogenital exam for males requires examination of the scrotum, testes, spermatic cords, and penis.

Inspect for any obvious abnormality, such as difference in size of testes, curvature of penis, discolorations, lesions, or mites. The scrotum is often slightly asymmetric with the left testicle lower than right. Note circumcision or intact prepuce. Check for inguinal hernias.

Palpate the scrotal skin for sebaceous cysts or other lesions. Gently palpate each testis between thumb and first 2 fingers for enlargement, masses, or tenderness. Testes should feel smooth and rubbery. The epididymis at the top of each testis should be smooth and nontender. Palpate each spermatic cord beside the penis and above each testis and note swelling or nodules. Slight tenderness is normal. Palpate the penis shaft for lesions or tenderness. Check the external urethral meatus for signs of inflammation or discharge and milk for discharge if necessary. Probe the inguinal ring around base of penis.

PHYSICAL EXAMINATION OF THE SKIN

The skin, the largest organ in the body, is composed of 3 layers (epidermis, dermis, and subcutaneous tissue) and contains nerves, vessels, glands, and hair follicles. Some changes are normal signs of aging and don't represent pathology: diminished hair, liver spots, seborrheic keratoses, wrinkles, and spider angiomas.

Inspect by observing skin color for rashes, erythema, discoloration (hypopigmentation or hyperpigmentation), or cyanosis. Observe for plaques, ecchymosis, urticaria, nodules, nevi, macular spots, or chances. Note the size, shape, color, and character of any lesions as well as any discharge, odor, or necrosis.

Palpate the skin to feel the temperature for signs of inflammation (warm) or decreased circulation (cool). If rash is present, gently stretch the skin and palpate rim of lesions. Gently run fingers across skin to assess texture, dryness, or moistness. Pinch skin gently to observe for skin turgor and elasticity. Apply both light and heavier pressure to skin to check for sensory deficits.

RECTAL EXAM

The rectal exam is approached differently for males and females. Males usually stand for the exam and may lean slightly against the examining table. Females usually have the exam while on the examining table with feet in stirrups or lying on their side. The exam in done with a lubricated gloved finger inserted into the rectum while the other hand may press against the abdomen. Having the person bear down during the exam relaxes the external sphincter.

Inspect the perianal area, noting any internal or external hemorrhoids, fissures, skin tags, perianal fistulas.

Palpate upward, to both sides, and posteriorly to feel for masses or prolapse of the rectum. For examination of males, palpate anteriorly to examine for enlargement or nodules of the prostate. For females, a combined rectovaginal exam may be done to examine the uterus, cervix, and ovaries.

Usually, the stool on the glove is examined and may be tested for occult blood.

PELVIC EXAM

The pelvic exam is done with the woman on the exam table and feet in stirrups.

Inspect vulva with a bright light, and check pubic hair for nits or lice. Separate labia to inspect for swelling or lesions, such as venereal warts. Examine skin folds for ulcerative lesions, and retract clitoral hood to look for periclitoral lesions. Note if hymen is intact. Check position of the urethra and note any redness, swelling, or discharge. Check the Skene's glands next to the urethra.

Palpate the labia majora for masses. Bartholin cysts are felt in the middle or lower part of the labia majora.

Digital exam is done with 1 or 2 fingers in the vagina, palm upward, and the other hand compressing downward externally. Press the urethra upward against the pubic bone and note any tenderness that could indicate urethritis. Then insert finger(s) deeper and press bladder against pubic bone. Note pain that can indicate cystitis.

ANAL WINK AND BULBOCAVERNOSUS REFLEX

Anal wink **(anocutaneous reflex)** is the reflexive contraction of the anus in response to gentle stroking or stimulation of the skin around the rectum. It occurs in both females and males. Pulling the penis elicits the response in males as well; at one time, this response was believed indicative of sexual abuse, but that has been disproved. Failure of this response indicates that there in an interruption in the reflex arc in the sensory or motor nerves.

Bulbocavernosus reflex is the reflexive contraction of the anus in response to natural or electrical stimulation of the bulbocavernosus muscle of the penis. Both the bulbocavernosus and the ischiocavernosus contract during the rigid stage of erection, resulting in a suprasystolic pressure within the penis and causing the anal sphincter to contract, presumably to prevent leak of flatus or fecal material during coitus. Failure of the reflex is indicative of an interruption or defect in the reflex arc.

EVALUATING ODOR AND OTHER ABNORMAL STOOL CHARACTERISTICS

Odor and other abnormal stool characteristics should be noted as part of an evaluation of diarrhea or other bowel dysfunction:

- **Foul-smelling light grey, oily or frothy stool** may relate to malabsorption problems, such as decrease in bile, resulting in undigested fat (steatorrhea).
- **Heavy stools with high fat content** may to relate malabsorption, intestinal, or pancreatic disorders.
- **Floating stools** are related to malabsorption or excessive flatus as stools float because of increased air or gas in the stool.
- **Excessively foul-smelling stool** may be related to food intake or bacteria in the bowel.
- **Ammonia smelling stool** may be related to bacteria in stool or insufficiently digested nitrogen in foods.
- **Sulfur smelling stool** may be related to foods high in sulfur (cabbage, broccoli)
- **Mucus in stool** indicates irritation of the intestinal lining, such as from irritable bowel syndrome and ulcerative colitis. Bacterial infections, such as *Campylobacter* and *Shigella* may also produce mucus.

STOOL COLOR

Stool color is directly affected by disease, foods, fluids, and amount of bile in the stool. Stools may normally vary in color, including all shades of brown and green-tinged:

- **Green stool** may be caused by leafy vegetables or green dye in foods. If stools are diarrhea, the bile may not have broken down as the stool moved quickly through the colon, causing green color.
- **Clay-colored stool** may indicate lack of sufficient bile or use of antidiarrheals, such as Kaopectate.
- **Black tarry stool** is often a sign of digested blood from upper gastrointestinal tract or from iron supplements, black dye (licorice), or Pepto-Bismol.
- **Red or bloody stool** may be a sign of bleeding in colon or rectum or caused by red dye in foods, beets, or tomato products.
- **Orange stool** may be caused by medications (rifampin) or beta-carotene in pills or foods, such as apricots, carrots, sweet potatoes, pumpkin, and mangoes.
- **Bright yellow stool** may indicate bile obstruction.

INCONTINENCE SYMPTOM PROFILE

An incontinence symptom profile helps to confirm the severity and pattern of incontinence. It also includes management strategies. The following factors are assessed:

- **Amount of leakage** may range from small amounts to full emptying of bladder.
- **Frequency** may range from normal (about 6 x daily) to every 1 or 2 hours.
- **Nocturia** may be present or absent.
- **Enuresis** may be present or absent.
- **Stream** may be normal, weak, difficult to start, or intermittent.
- **Sensation** of incontinence may be missing or related to strong urge.
- **Bladder emptying** may be complete or incomplete. Post urination dribbling may occur.
- **Mobility impairment** may interfere with toileting.
- **Medications** may impair awareness or bladder control.
- **Depression/dementia** can affect ability to control body functions.
- **Pain** may interfere with toileting or prevent people from emptying bladder.
- **Management** may include incontinence pads, disposable underwear, pessaries, dietary modifications, environmental modifications, and scheduled urination.

STRESS INCONTINENCE, URGE INCONTINENCE, AND MIXED INCONTINENCE

Stress incontinence is characterized by small involuntary amounts of urinary leakage, usually without sensation. It occurs during the daytime, especially during physical activity that increases intra-abdominal pressure, such as coughing, laughing, bending, heavy lifting, exercising, or sneezing. Bladder capacity is normal and bladder usually empties completely on urination. There is generally no nocturia.

Urge incontinence is characterized by moderate to large amounts of involuntary urinary leakage caused by the sudden urge to urinate and the inability to hold the urine until able to reach a toilet. It is associated with frequency and nocturia more than two times nightly as well as small bladder capacity. Enuresis may occur.

Mixed incontinence is usually a combination of stress and urge incontinence with both small involuntary amounts of urinary leakage during activities as well as moderate to large amounts with the urge to urinate. Bladder capacity may be small and there is usually nocturia and possibly enuresis.

Overflow Incontinence and Functional Incontinence

Overflow incontinence is characterized by usually small leakages of urine, similar to stress incontinence, but resulting from pressure on an overdistended ladder. There is often difficulty initiating flow, requiring straining with a weak urinary stream so that urination can take longer than normal. There may also be dribbling after urination because bladder has not emptied. The person may feel the frequent need to urinate because the bladder feels full.

Functional incontinence is characterized by leakage of urine because of inability of the person to manage toileting or remove clothing for a variety of reasons. Some people may be constrained by pain. Some people with dementia, or those taking medications that cause sensory impairment, are not aware of the need to urinate. Sometimes, barriers, such as no wheelchair accessible toilets, may be the cause. Generally, bladder and urinary functions are normal for the person's age and condition.

Diarrhea

Diarrhea is passing liquid or semi-formed stool more frequently than is normal for an individual, often accompanied by abdominal cramping, distention, and sense of urgency to defecate. Severe diarrhea may occur hourly. Diarrhea should be characterized according to color, odor, consistency, and frequency. Diarrhea may be acute or chronic.

- **Acute diarrhea** generally has a sudden onset and may be related to medications such as chemotherapy, irritating foods, gastrointestinal organisms, and stress. Diarrhea may be very watery or bloody and may be accompanied by flatus. Acute diarrhea usually responds to Antidiarrheals or is self-limiting within a few days.
- **Chronic diarrhea** lasts longer than 3 days and is usually the result of a long-term disease process, such as Crohn's disease, or trauma, such as from radiation therapy. It may also result from dietary irritation or from overuse of constipation, in which case there may be a cycle of constipation followed by diarrhea.

Constipation and Impaction

Constipation is a condition with bowel movements less frequent than normal for a person, or hard, small stool that is evacuated fewer than 3 times weekly. Food moves through the gastrointestinal from the small intestine to the colon in semi-liquid form. Constipation results from the colon, where fluid is absorbed. If too much fluid is absorbed, the stool can become too dry. People may have Abdominal distension and cramps and need to strain for defecation.

Fecal impaction occurs when the hard stool moves into the rectum and becomes a large, dense, immovable mass that cannot be evacuated even with straining, usually as a result of chronic constipation. In addition to abdominal cramps and distention, the person may feel intense rectal pressure and pain accompanied by a sense of urgency to defecate. Nausea and vomiting may also occur. Hemorrhoids will often become engorged. Fecal incontinence, with liquid stool leaking about the impaction is common.

IAD

Incontinence-associated dermatitis (IAD), also known as perineal dermatitis, is the breakdown of skin expressed as inflammation, redness, or erosion, and causes a painful, itching, or burning sensation. This breakdown is due to the skin's continual contact with urine or stool. In some cases, IAD can lead to a secondary bacterial skin infection. Fungal infections can also occur from incontinence associated dermatitis. To prevent this, it is important that the patient or their caregiver keep the skin clean and dry. The use of thick barrier creams should be avoided. If the condition worsens, it can lead to total skin breakdown and the development of pressure ulcers as the skin becomes macerated from exposure to urine. If necessary, absorbent briefs or pads should be used to wick moisture away from the skin and prevent the development of incontinence associated dermatitis. Seams and rough edges from these products should also be kept from the skin to prevent chafing or further irritation from rubbing. Patients should be educated to contact their physician if they should develop any signs of skin breakdown.

ASSESSMENT TOOLS RELEVANT TO CONTINENCE AND ASSOCIATED RISK FACTORS
URINARY INCONTINENCE SEVERITY INDEX AND TIMED UP AND GO

Assessment tools available to support the continence care nurse include:

- **Urinary Incontinence Severity Index**: This simple two-question screening tool is used to screen for urinary incontinence, track symptoms, triage patients, and document severity:

Q1 How often do you experience urinary leakage?	Q2 How much urine do you lose each time?
0 = Never	1 = drops or very little
1 = less than once per month	2 = small splashes
2 = one to several times per month	3 = more
3 = one to several times per week	
4 = every day	
Scoring: 1-2 slight; 3-6 moderate; 8-0 severe; 12 very severe.	

- **Timed up and go (TUG)**: This procedure is used to evaluate functional mobility, screen for risk of falls, assess balance and gait, and monitor progress. The patient stands from a chair with armrests, walks 3 meters, and turns, walks back, and sits back down. Those requiring >13.5 seconds indicates some risk for falls: Scoring: 7-10 seconds is normal for young, healthy adults, 10-19 seconds is typical of independent mobile older adults, 20-29 seconds indicates some functional limitations, and ≥30 indicates high risk of falls.

FECAL INCONTINENCE SEVERITY INDEX

The Fecal Incontinence Severity Index is a matrix that provides information about the type of incontinence and the frequency, helping with evaluation and treatment. Types include:

- **Flatus** incontinence is characterized by uncontrolled flatulence often exacerbated by activity that increases bowel motility.
- **Mucus** incontinence occurs in inflammatory bowel disease in response to irritation of the mucous lining of the bowel. Mucus may also be produced in response to fecal impaction. Mucus may be thick or watery.
- **Liquid stool** in the form of diarrhea can be difficult to contain, especially chronic diarrhea or leakage around impaction. Liquid stool may be watery, bloody, or purulent, depending upon the cause.
- **Formed stool** may be expelled, especially with neurological damage or damage the anal sphincter.

Patients are asked to indicate the frequency of these incidents by selecting one of the following:

- 2 or more times a day
- Once daily
- 2 or more times weekly
- Once weekly
- 1-3 times monthly
- Never

BRISTOL STOOL FORM

The Bristol Stool Form is named for Bristol University in England, where it was designed as a general description of stool constancy or form. The form is often given to people when they do a bowel diary so that they can more clearly identify for healthcare providers what types of stools they are passing.

The scale has descriptions and pictures to help people identify the correct type of stool:

- **Type 1** is separate small hard lumps of stool that are difficult to pass.
- **Type 2** is sausage-shaped lumpy stool.
- **Type 3** is sausage-shaped and lumpy but with cracks on the surface.
- **Type 4** is long, smooth, soft, snake-like stool.
- **Type 5** is soft blobs of stool that are easily passed and have clear-cut edges.
- **Type 6** is mushy, fluffy pieces of stool with uneven ragged edges.
- **Type 7** is watery stool that is entirely liquid with no solid pieces.

Continence Care: Intervention and Treatment

Stress, Functional, and Urge Incontinence Management

MANAGEMENT STRATEGIES FOR STRESS INCONTINENCE

There are a number of management strategies for dealing with stress incontinence, and the starting procedure depends on the level of incontinence and the motivation the person has to deal with the problem. Exercise alone may be enough for some people to control incontinence; others may need surgery:

- **Kegel exercises** can be used to strengthen the pelvic floor muscles and the "knack" to prevent incontinence.
- **Absorbent pads** may be used to contain leakage.
- **Urethral plugs** can be inserted into the urethra to block the urethra or **urethral patches** can be applied to seal the urethra externally.
- **Pessary** may relieve symptoms by elevating the angle of the urethral sphincter.
- **Weight loss** to relieve pressure on pelvic floor muscles may help.
- **Medications**, such as estrogens and adrenergic agents may increase control.
- **Surgical procedures** include the sling procedures, needle suspensions, and retropubic colposuspension, and injectable bulking implants.

THE KNACK

The knack is the use of precisely-timed muscle contractions to prevent stress incontinence. It is the practice of squeezing up before bearing down. The knack is a preventive use of Kegel exercises. Women are taught to contract the pelvic floor muscles right before and during events that usually cause stress incontinence. For example, if a woman feels a cough or sneeze coming, she immediately contracts the pelvic floor muscles and holds until the stress event is over. This contraction augments support of the proximal urethra, reducing the amount of displacement that usually takes place with compromised muscle support, thereby preventing incontinence. It is particularly useful if used before and during stress events, such as coughing, sneezing, lifting, standing, swinging a golf club, or laughing. Studies have shown that women who are taught this technique for mild to moderate urinary incontinence and use it consistently are able to decrease incontinence by 73-98%.

VAGINAL WEIGHTS/CONES FOR REHABILITATION OF PELVIC FLOOR MUSCLES

Vaginal weights are tampon-sizes cones that are inserted into the vagina during Kegel exercises to provide weight training and resistance for the pelvic floor muscles for stress incontinence. The stainless-steel cones come in sets of 5 in several weights (20-70 grams). They are usually coated with plastic and have a retrieval cord, like a tampon. Another type cone unscrews so that different weights can be placed inside. A test to determine correct size is to start with the weight that can be held for one minute. In the beginning, usually the lightest weight cone is inserted into the vagina, requiring the pelvic muscles to tighten to hold it in place. When the person can hold the lightest cone in comfortably, she moves up to the next size. Exercise with the vaginal weights is usually done two times a day for 15 minutes until the heaviest weight can be held.

PESSARIES

Pessaries are plastic or silicone removable prosthetic devices that are placed in the vagina for management of pelvic muscle support defects, such as cystocele and rectocele. They are also frequently

Copyright © Mometrix Media. You have been licensed one copy of this document for personal use only. Any other reproduction or redistribution is strictly prohibited. All rights reserved.
This content is provided for test preparation purposes only and does not imply an endorsement by Mometrix of any particular political, scientific, or religious point of view.

used for stress incontinence. There are a wide variety of pessaries, and they are fitted to the individual. A pelvic exam is done prior to fitting a person for a pessary. Fitting sets are available to help the healthcare provider pick the right size, as the correct fit is crucial if the pessary is to be comfortable and provide needed support. Some pessaries are intended for self-care, and can be removed daily, weekly, monthly, (depending upon the type) washed with soap and water, and reinserted. Others are removed, cleansed, and reinserted periodically by a healthcare provider. In general, pessaries should not be left in place for more than 4 months at a time to ensure that there are no complications.

TYPES

Types of pessaries range from simple rings to inflatable balls. Different types are used for different disorders.

- **Ring/ring with support** is for 1st and 2nd degree uterine prolapse and cystocele.
- **Donut** is for 3rd and 4th degree uterine prolapse and vaginal vault prolapse.
- **Gehrung (arched U-shaped)** is for 2nd, 3rd, and 4th degree cystocele and rectocele.
- **Gellhorn (rigid and flexible)** is for 3rd and 4th grade uterine prolapse and must be removed prior to sexual intercourse.
- **Cube** is for 3rd degree uterine prolapse and must be removed daily.
- **Hodge** (with/without knob) is for mild cystocele.
- **Inflato-ball** supports prolapsing vaginal structures, is inflatable, and must be removed daily.
- **Shaatz** is for mild cystocele and uterine prolapse.
- **Incontinence dish and ring (with/without support)** is placed at base of bladder to support bladder neck and compress urethra to prevent stress incontinence.

PROCEDURE FOR FITTING

Fitting a pessary may require trial and error to arrive at the correct size and style. The type of pessary is determined by the problem the pessary is intended to correct and the type of muscle weakness or prolapse present.

- Pelvic exam performed.
- Average size pessary, usually in a simple style, inserted and checked for fit and effectiveness.
- A smaller or larger pessary may be inserted until the correct fit obtained, with the largest comfortable pessary the optimum choice for effectiveness.
- A finger must pass easily between the vaginal wall and the pessary.
- If treatment is for stress incontinence, the person coughs to test for urinary leakage.
- Person stands, sit, performs Valsalva maneuvers, and squats to make sure that the pessary remains in place.
- Person urinates to ensure there is no pressure that prevents urination.
- Person instructed regarding care and return visit to check placement.

CONTRAINDICATIONS AND COMPLICATIONS

Contraindications for a pessary include infection, such as vaginitis. Because most pessaries are made of silicone or latex, some people may have allergic response, especially to latex. Patients should not be fitted with a pessary if they are noncompliant and may not do follow up care.

Complications may occur, especially if the pessary is not cared for properly:

- **Vaginal discharge and odor** may be treated with acidic vaginal gel (Trimo-San) or vinegar douche.
- **Vaginal ulceration** may occur in post-menopausal women with atrophic vaginal mucosa. Estrogen cream can be used with pessary.

Continence Care: Intervention and Treatment

- **Embedding of pessary** may occur with a neglected pessary. Estrogen cream may help to decrease inflammation and allow removal, but surgical removal may be necessary. Fistulas may develop in severe cases.
- **Herniation of cervix and lower uterus with incarceration** can happen if a ring pessary is not fitted properly, causing herniation through the open center. Surgical repair may be needed.

MEDICAL DEVICES FOR WOMEN FOR INCONTINENCE

Medical devices that are available for women to use to control incontinence stop the flow of urine by blocking the urethra. They are quite effective for many women.

- **Urethral plugs** are available in different types, but all are inserted into the urethral meatus. One type is inflatable with a balloon that prevents leakage. FemSoft is a typical one-use disposable plug. It looks like a tiny tampon but is a fluid-filled insert that seals the urethra. It is removed to urinate, and then a new plug is inserted. Plugs are fitted to the individual and may cause infection.
- **Urethral patches** are small multiple-use foam pads with gel adhesive. They are placed over the urethra to create a watertight seal and absorb small leakages if necessary.
- **Tampons** are intended for menstrual flow, but some women find that tampons provide pressure against the urethra, preventing mild incontinence.

PROMPTED VOIDING TO PROMOTE CONTINENCE

Prompted voiding is a communication protocol for people with mild to moderate cognitive impairment. It uses positive reinforcement for recognizing being wet or dry, staying dry, urinating, and drinking liquids.

- Ask people every 2 hours (8 am to 8 pm) whether they are wet or dry.
- Verify if they are correct and give feedback, "You are right, Mrs. Brown, you are dry."
- Prompt people, whether wet or dry, to use the toilet or urinal. **If yes**, assist them, record results, and give positive reinforcement by praising and visiting for a short time. **If no**, repeat the request again once or twice. If they are wet, and decline toileting, change and tell them you will return in two hours and ask them to try to wait to urinate until then.
- Offer liquids and record amount.
- Record results of each attempt to urinate or wet check.

URGE INCONTINENCE

Management strategies for urge incontinence are primarily conservative because surgical treatment has a high rate of morbidity:

- **Bladder training**, a behavioral therapy, has an improvement rate of about 75%. Scheduled urination should be done, gradually increasing time between urinations, along with strategies to delay urination. People who have dementia or caregivers may need prompted urination in order to maintain a schedule.
- **Fluid management** involves maintaining adequate fluid intake but decreasing fluids in the evening.
- **Reducing caffeine** and other bladder irritants may reduce contractions.
- **Medications** that cause bladder contractions should be reviewed as these may need to be discontinued or changed in order to control the incontinence.
- **Medications** include anticholinergics, such as tolterodine and oxybutynin and bladder relaxants, such tri-cyclic antidepressants, such as imipramine and dicyclomine. Medications are usually given only if behavioral therapy is unsuccessful. Medications with about a 46% rate of improvement have proven less effective than behavioral modifications

REFLEX INCONTINENCE

Management strategies for reflex incontinence are similar to those for urge incontinence, often with medication and catheterization:

- **Behavioral therapy** with scheduled urination to prevent distention and frequency, double voiding to prevent residual urine, use of the Credé maneuver to stimulate contraction of the bladder, and "trigger" voiding.
- **Absorbent pads or briefs** may be necessary to contain leakage.
- **External catheters** may be used by males instead of absorbent protective materials.
- **Intermittent clean catheterization** or long-term catheterization may be needed in order to empty the bladder if other methods fail.
- **Medications** such as tolterodine and Ditropan are used to control the overactive bladder and decrease contractions.
- **Neuromodulation/sacral nerve stimulation** with implantable neural prosthesis suppresses detrusor hyperreflexia through electrical stimulation of the sacral nerves.
- **Botulinum toxin** injections may be used to paralyze the bladder and sphincter muscles, but they must be repeated as the results are not long lasting.

BLADDER TRAINING

Bladder training usually requires the person to keep a toileting diary for at least 3 days so patterns can be assessed. There are a number of different approaches:

- **Scheduled toileting** is toileting or a regular schedule, usually every 2 to 4 hours during the daytime.
- **Habit training** involves an attempt to match the scheduled toileting to a person's individual voiding habits, based on the toileting diary. This is useful for people who have a natural and fairly consistent voiding pattern. Toileting is done every 2-4 hours.
- **Prompted voiding** is often used in nursing homes and attempts to teach people to assess their own incontinence status and prompts them to ask for toileting.
- **Bladder retraining** is a behavioral modification program that teaches people to inhibit the urge to urinate and to urinate according to an established schedule, restoring normal bladder function as much as possible. Bladder training can improve incontinence in 80% of cases.

BLADDER RETRAINING TO PROMOTE CONTINENCE

Bladder retraining usually takes about 3 months to rehabilitate a bladder muscle weakened from frequent urination, causing a decreased urinary capacity. A short urination interval is gradually lengthened to every 2-4 hours during the daytime as the person suppresses bladder urges and stays dry.

- The person keeps urination diary for a week.
- An individual program is established with scheduled voiding times and goals. For example, if a person is urinating every hour, the goal might be every 80 minutes with increased output.
- The person is taught techniques to withhold urination: sitting on a hard seat or on a tightly rolled towel to put pressure on pelvic floor muscles, doing 5 squeezes of pelvic floor muscles, deep breathing, counting backward from 50.
- When the person consistently meets the goal, a new goal is established.
- The person maintains the use of a urination diary.

BIOFEEDBACK FOR REHABILITATION OF PELVIC FLOOR MUSCLES

Biofeedback uses electronic or mechanical instruments to measure, process, and give feedback to people about neuromuscular activity. The perineometer, a pressure-sensitive vaginal probe, is the biofeedback device that helps women identify, train, and rehabilitate the pelvic floor muscles. A smaller device can be inserted into the rectum of men or women. The probes sense muscular activity. Occasionally, surface electrodes are placed around the rectum rather than using a probe. The therapy provides immediate visual or auditory feedback about the status of the muscle contractions. The biofeedback machine for pelvic floor muscles uses computer graphs or lights to indicate when the correct muscle is flexed. Some systems have both pressure and electromyograph channels, which allow various muscles to be monitored at the same time. Treatments are usually 20-30 minutes long and the average number of treatments is 6. Once a person has the ability to flex the correct muscles, Kegel exercises can be done.

Urge Suppression Techniques for Urinary Incontinence

Urge suppression techniques help suppress the urge to urinate, decrease frequency, and improve bladder tone and capacity:

- **Deep breathing** requires people to sit or lie down and take slow deep breaths in through the nose. Then exhalation is done through the mouth. The person is encouraged to concentrate, as in meditation, only on the breathing and to repeat the cycle 10 times.
- **Distraction** involves thinking of something else, such as counting backward or reciting out loud. Some people might keep a music player close at hand and listen to music.
- **Applying pressure** by sitting on a firm surface or on a rolled towel may apply pressure to the pelvic floor muscles and control urge.
- **Quick flicks** are the use of Kegel exercises. The person remains still, usually sitting or lying, and quickly tightens and relaxes the pelvic floor muscles about 10 times, in "flicks."

Other Incontinence Management Strategies

OVERFLOW INCONTINENCE

Management strategies for overflow incontinence include:

- **Behavioral therapy** with scheduled urination to prevent distention and frequency, double voiding to prevent residual urine, and use of the Credé maneuver to stimulate contraction of the bladder.
- **Absorbent pads or briefs** may be necessary to contain leakage.
- **External catheters** may be used by males instead of absorbent protective materials.
- **Intermittent clean catheterization** or long-term catheterization may be needed in order to empty the bladder if other methods fail.
- **Medications** for detrusor underactivity include cholinergic agonists, such as bethanechol. Males may get relief from outlet obstruction with alpha adrenergic blockers, such as doxazosin, prazosin, tamsulosin, and terazosin.
- **Treatment of prostatic hypertrophy** with surgery or medication, such as finasteride, which reduces the size of the prostate and relieves obstruction.
- **Bowel training**, including dietary interventions, to prevent chronic constipation and impaction will reduce associated overflow leakage.

POST-PROSTATECTOMY INCONTINENCE

Management of post-prostatectomy incontinence depends upon the reason for the incontinence.

- **Medications**, such as tolterodine and oxybutynin, relax bladder pressure with detrusor hypertrophy but are contraindicated in those with narrow angle glaucoma or with residual volume after urination. The Oxytrol patch (oxybutynin) may be used, usually with fewer side effects.
- External catheter, penile clamp, absorbent pads manage leakage.
- **Pelvic floor muscle exercises** may be helpful for mild stress incontinence.
- **Bladder pacemaker**, such as Interstim, requires a 2-stage surgical procedure where an electrode is placed by the main nerve controlling the bladder.
- **Artificial urinary sphincter** may be surgically implanted, with an inflatable cuff to control incontinence.
- **Male sling procedure** is done through a scrotal incision. Screws are placed in the pubic bone, to which the sling graft material (donor or synthetic) is attached with sutures that tighten the urethra. Studies show the failure rate is 20%, but 80% stay dry or improve.

Continence Care: Intervention and Treatment

MIXED INCONTINENCE

Mixed incontinence includes both stress incontinence with impaired external sphincter control and urge incontinence with detrusor pressure exceeding sphincter pressure. Treatment deals with both problems and is primarily aimed at the most prominent type of incontinence:

- **Kegel exercises** strengthen the pelvic floor muscles and the "knack" may prevent stress incontinence.
- **Bladder training** with scheduled urination should be done, gradually increasing time between urinations, along with strategies to delay urination.
- **Fluid management** involves maintaining adequate fluid intake but decreasing fluids in the evening.
- **Reducing caffeine** and other bladder irritants may reduce bladder contractions.
- **Medications** that may cause bladder contractions should be reviewed as these may need to be discontinued or changed.
- **Absorbent pads** may be used to contain leakage.
- **Pessary** may relieve symptoms by elevating the angle of the urethral sphincter.
- **Weight loss** to relieve pressure on pelvic floor muscles may help.

NOCTURNAL ENURESIS

Nocturnal enuresis may be managed in a number of different ways, depending upon whether the enuresis is primary or secondary, the severity, and whether there is also incontinence during the daytime.

- **Behavior modifications** such as bladder training, scheduled urination, fluid restriction, and dietary modifications as well as conditioning therapy with enuresis alarms may be helpful, especially for primary nocturnal enuresis.
- **Medications** such as antidepressants (imipramine) relax the bladder and tighten the urethral sphincter, desmopressin at bedtime reduces urinary production for 5-6 hours, and anticholinergics reduce instability of the detrusor muscle.
- **Neuromodulation** by sacral nerve stimulation may help voiding dysfunction.
- **Botulinum toxin** is a neuromuscular blocking agent that reduces detrusor overactivity.
- **Surgical treatment** includes clam cystoplasty, bladder augmentation to increase bladder capacity, and detrusor myectomy, which is removal of part of the outer muscle of the bladder to reduce the overactive contractions.

NOCTURIA

Nocturia is waking up one or more times during the night with the need to urinate. Some authorities believe that one event at night is within normal limits. Some people have to urinate 5 or 6 times at night. About 70% of cases of nocturia are related to over-production of urine at night. Nocturia is one of the most common causes of sleep deprivation. It affects about two-thirds of those aged 50-59. Studies have shown that nocturia more than 2 times nightly is strongly linked with depression. Treatment aims at reducing urination during the night:

- **Desmopressin** acts as an antidiuretic hormone that reduces volume of urine by increasing concentration and allows for about 5 hours of undisturbed sleep. It increases the first period of sleep by about 2 hours. Desmopressin is the primary treatment for nocturia.
- **Fluid management** by reducing fluids in the evening can help some people.

Overactive Bladder (Urgency/Frequency) Without Incontinence

Overactive bladder is a condition with urgency, frequency, and nocturia but without incontinence. The urge to urinate may be as frequent as every 20-30 minutes in extreme cases and, if nocturia is present, people may become sleep-deprived. If overactive bladder includes incontinence, it is known as urge incontinence, and the treatment is similar for both:

- **Anticholinergics (antimuscarinics)**, such as tolterodine and oxybutynin relax the bladder muscle and relieve the symptoms.
- **Pelvic floor muscle exercises**, such as Kegel exercises, vaginal weight training, as well as biofeedback or pelvic floor electrical stimulation done with the Kegel exercise program.
- **Behavioral modification** with bladder training that includes scheduled voiding with increasing time between urination and strategies to delay urination. Prompted urination may be needed for some people, especially those with dementia.
- **Fluid management** involves maintaining adequate fluid intake but decreasing fluids in the evening.
- **Reducing caffeine** and other bladder irritants may reduce contractions.

Obsessive Toileting

Obsessive toileting, as frequently as every 20-30 minutes, may occur with neurogenic bladder when people develop the fear that they will be incontinent. The goal is to stop the behavior and institute successful retraining.

- **Educate** person about bladder capacity, the normal capacity and the amount of urine in the bladder after repeated urinations (usually about 50-75 mL).
- An **ultrasound** scan may be used to check volume of urine in the bladder when person wants to urinate to show actual need.
- If bladder volume is under 100-150 mL, encourage person to **extend toileting time**. If the person has some dementia, it is important to stay with the person, giving assurance and support, until the urge to urinate eases.
- Try to **distract** the person by talking, playing music, engaging in activities.
- **Monitor fluids** as people may be drinking less in the mistaken belief it will reduce incontinence.

Detrusor Hyperactivity with Impaired Contractile Function

Detrusor hyperactivity with impaired contractile function (DHIC) results from involuntary contractions that may be ineffective to empty the bladder. This condition is characterized by overactive detrusor contractions during the storage phase but underactive contractions during urination, resulting in both frequency and residual urine in bladder. It is common with neurological impairment from trauma or disease, such as Parkinson's or multiple sclerosis. Some medications commonly used for hyperactivity (tolterodine and oxybutynin) can make DHIC, so treatment can be challenging. Conservative treatment is the most common:

- **Behavioral modification** with bladder training that includes scheduled urination, prompted urination if necessary, Credé maneuver, and double voiding may help with emptying bladder and reducing frequency. Diet modifications to eliminate bladder irritants and to control fluid intake may help control incontinence.
- **Clean intermittent catheterization** to completely empty bladder on a regular schedule can decrease or eliminate incontinence and is often necessary to prevent bladder distention.

DETRUSOR SPHINCTER DYSSYNERGIA

Detrusor sphincter dyssynergia is a loss of coordination resulting in the sphincter contracting when the detrusor muscle contracts, creating an outlet obstruction. This condition results from spinal cord lesions interrupting neurological pathways and reflex arcs. Some treatments result in constant leakage and are not done for females because of the risk of skin irritation:

- **External catheters or penile clamps** may be used by males.
- **Intermittent clean catheterization** or long-term catheterization is often needed, especially for females, in order to empty the bladder.
- **Insertion of urethral stent**, such as UroLume, which is a mesh tube that holds the urethra open (for males), resulting in incontinence requiring external catheter.
- **Pudendal nerve block with 5% phenol** may be effective.
- **Intraurethral botulinum injections** help but must be repeated.
- **External sphincterotomy** enlarges the urethral sphincter in males, resulting in incontinence requiring external catheter.
- **Muscle relaxants** may be used to relax urethra.

Device Management and Absorptive Products

ENVIRONMENTAL MODIFICATIONS TO HELP PREVENT URINARY INCONTINENCE

Environmental modifications are those changes that make it easier for people to toilet and to prevent incontinence.

- **Bedside commodes** are useful at night if the bathroom is not near the bed. They can also be used during the daytime to make toilet access easier especially if there is no toilet on the same floor. They should be adjusted for height and easy to empty.
- **Urinals** are available for both men and women although male urinals are easier to use and generally more successful. They can be kept within arm's length.
- **Bedpans** can be used, if there are care providers. They are very difficult to use without assistance because they spill easily.
- **Doorknobs** may be replaced with levers to facilitate opening doors.
- **Elevated toilet seats** and **safety bars** in the bathroom may help people to get on and off of the toilet more easily.

CATHETERIZATION FOR URINARY INCONTINENCE

Catheterization for control of urinary incontinence can be done in 3 different manners.

- **Clean intermittent catheterization** is used for spinal cord injuries and urinary retention. Catheterization is done several times per day, usually on a regular schedule about every 4 hours, using clean catheters. Sterile catheters may be advised for impaired immunity. Catheters must be cleansed properly and replaced as needed.
- **Indwelling Foley catheters** provide a closed, sterile system that is useful for urinary incontinence related to obstruction or urinary retention. Foley catheters may be inserted if people are too ill to care for themselves or to protect the skin. The catheters are usually changed monthly or as needed.
- **Suprapubic catheters** are inserted through a surgical opening in the lower abdomen. They are used for those who need long-term catheterization as they are more comfortable and have fewer problems than Foleys. The catheters are changed at least every month.

EXTERNAL CATHETERS AND PENILE CLAMPS FOR MEN FOR URINARY INCONTINENCE

External catheter systems are condom catheters that are available for men. They are usually made of latex or silicone and are attached to the penis shaft by adhesive, inflatable cuffs, or straps. They come in different sizes, and proper sizing is important to prevent constriction. They are disposable and usually only used for 24-49 hours. A drainage tube and leg bag or overnight bag is attached to the external catheter. Many men prefer these to disposable adult diapers.

Penile clamp is a device that is clamped on the penis to prevent incontinence. It is clamped about halfway down the penis shaft and has soft foam on the inside of the clamp. The clamp is released every 1-2 hours to prevent circulatory restriction and to allow for urination. It is very important that the clamp not be placed too tightly as it can cause strictures or skin breakdown, even necrosis.

INDWELLING CATHETERS

Indwelling catheters are left in place for continuous urinary drainage either through the urethra or a suprapubic opening into the bladder. Foley catheters have double lumens, a larger for urinary drainage and a smaller leading to an inflatable balloon near the end of the catheter. There are various types:

- **Antibiotic coated catheters** are expensive catheters impregnated with antibiotics to discourage infection.
- **Coudé catheters** have a 45-degree angled tip, especially useful with enlarged prostate.

315

- **Silicone catheters** are thin walled, resulting in a larger lumen for drainage. They discourage protein and mucus buildup, preventing obstruction.
- **Silicone/Teflon coated latex catheters** have a coating to protect urethra from contact with latex.
- **Silver-coated catheters** have a bacteriostatic effect that decreases inflammatory response to catheter.

The smallest catheter that allows drainage is preferred; usually 12-18 Fr. Larger sizes can cause urethral irritation. Balloon size is usually 5 mL; 10-30 mL sizes are available but can interfere with urinary drainage and increase inflammation.

PROBLEMS RELATED TO CATHETERS

Catheters are invasive devices that can result in a number of problems:

- **Spasms** are a normal reaction to the catheter and may cause some urinary leakage. Some burning may be felt as well.
- **Catheter loss** may occur because of strong spasms that expel it or it can be pulled out accidentally or intentionally. People with confusion often pull at the catheter.
- **Urinary leakage** may happen for a variety of reasons: spasms, infection, bladder irritation, over-inflated balloon, or catheter size too large.
- **Obstruction** may be caused by encrustations from mucus, crystallizations, or purulent material. The tip may become plugged with calculous material, especially if the urine is alkaline. Increasing fluid intake and acidifying the urine with 500-1000 mg per day may help.
- **Infection** is common because bacteria usually develop in 2-4 weeks after insertion. Bacteria may migrate up the catheter so hygiene is very important.

CONTAINMENT PRODUCTS FOR INCONTINENCE

ABSORBENT PADS

Containment products vary in quality and type. Depends and Poise are brands that are widely available. The product needed relates to the degree of incontinence.

Absorbent pads are rated for size and degree of absorbency, light to heavy. Some women use panty liners, but these are less absorbent than urinary products and need to be changed frequently. Absorbent pads have fill, such as wood pulp or polymer, which binds with urine and changes it to a gel. The surface area wicks the urine to the absorbent layer so that the skin can stay dry, decreasing skin irritation. Absorbent pads usually have a plastic layer to prevent leaks and an adhesive strip on the back so that they can be placed inside panties or shorts and secured into position. There are pouch-type absorbent pads that fit over the male penis. Absorbent pads are most useful for stress incontinence or those with light to moderate incontinence.

REUSABLE UNDERGARMENTS AND DISPOSABLE BRIEFS

Containment products for moderate heavy urinary or fecal leakage vary, but all are intended to protect clothing and furniture as well as to give the user a feeling of confidence that incontinence will be contained.

- **Reusable undergarments/brief** are made with a fiber core of rayon or polyester and can be washed and reused. They may have a plastic covering on the outside. They are less expensive but also less convenient than disposables.

- **Disposable adult undergarments** include open-sided products with a belt around that can be worn alone or under panties or shorts. There are a number of different types of briefs. Most are paper products with elastic around the hips to accommodate different sizes, an absorbent center, and elastic gathering at the legs. Some are simple pull-ups. Overnight briefs may have an outside plastic lining for more absorbency. Some briefs are refastenable, which is useful for people who are bedridden.

Surgical Interventions

SURGICAL PROCEDURES FOR URINARY INCONTINENCE

Common surgical interventions in the treatment of urinary incontinence include the following:

- **Anterior bladder repair** releases the anterior vaginal wall from the bladder, folds the supportive tissue, and secures it to tighten the vaginal wall and repair prolapses.
- **Artificial sphincter** is a balloon reservoir, pump, and cuff encircling the urethra to manually inflate and deflate.
- **Injectable bulking implants** include collagen or silicone injected into tissue about the urethra, increasing bulk of the surrounding tissue and compressing the urethra.
- **Needle suspension** places stitches on side of bladder and attaches them to muscle tissue or pubic bone for support.
- **Percutaneous sling procedure** uses a piece of ligament, muscle tendon, or synthetic material to create a sling about the urethra to lift it to normal position.
- **Retropubic colposuspension** lifts the bladder neck and urethra by attaching bladder and urethra or the vaginal wall to other pelvic structures.
- **Tension-free vaginal tape procedure** uses a mesh-like synthetic tape under urethra to form a sling to lift it to normal position.

ARTIFICIAL SPHINCTER

Artificial sphincter is a balloon reservoir and pump with a cuff encircling the urethra to manually inflate and deflate. The 3 components are filled with normal saline. This procedure is done when the urethral sphincters are non-functioning, and is used for both men, especially after radical prostatectomy, and women. For males, the pump is installed in the scrotum, the reservoir in the lower abdomen, and the cuff around the urethra near the bladder neck. For women, pump and reservoir are installed in the labia. The pump activates by squeezing or pressing on a button. When the cuff is deflated, the saline drains into the reservoir and then returns to the cuff after button is re-pressed. The procedure is done under a general or spinal anesthesia. A Foley catheter is inserted during surgery and is left in for a few days. The artificial sphincter is not inflated for about 6 weeks, giving the tissue time to heal.

ANTERIOR BLADDER REPAIR

Anterior bladder repair Is a procedure that releases the anterior vaginal wall from the bladder, folds the supportive tissue, and secures it to tighten the vaginal wall and repair urethroceles or cystoceles. Different techniques are employed, depending upon the degree of prolapse. This procedure is not specifically done for control of urinary incontinence, but repairing the prolapse may resolve the incontinence.

Surgical procedure involves either a general or spinal anesthesia. The procedure is performed through a vaginal incision. Usually a Foley catheter is inserted into the bladder and left for the first day or two until the swelling recedes. Then, urination about every 2 hours is needed to prevent pressure on the bladder. A liquid diet is followed by a low residue diet when normal bowel function occurs. Stool softeners or laxatives are used to prevent constipation. The "knack" maneuver should be done when coughing, sneezing, or doing activities that induce abdominal stress.

Needle Suspension

Needle suspension places stitches through the pubic skin or an incision on both sides of the bladder neck and attaches them to muscle tissue or the pubic bone for support. Surgery may be done with general or spinal anesthetic.

- The **Stamey procedure** is done vaginally or suprapubically with nylon sutures suspending the urethra.
- The **Raz procedure** uses a vaginal incision and releases fibroid bands around the bladder neck and urethra. Suspending sutures lift the anterior vagina and urethra.
- The **Gittes procedure** is done suprapubically through a small puncture. A needle is inserted through the puncture and the vaginal wall and then the suture is pulled back through the opening and secured with another suture, suspending the anterior vagina. A second puncture and suspending suture is placed about 2 cm from the first site.

A Foley catheter is usually in place for about 10 days after surgery. Difficulty urinating may result from overcorrection.

Injectable Bulking Implants

Injectable bulking implants include collagen or silicone injected into the tissue about the urethra, increasing bulk of the surrounding tissue and compressing the urethra. This procedure, for both men and women, is done through a cystoscope with regional, general, or local anesthetic. The bulking material is injected through the cystoscope or, in some cases, into the skin around the sphincter. The procedure usually takes only 20-40 minutes and may be done as an outpatient. Often 2 or 3 additional implants need to be done to achieve continence. There may be urinary retention postoperative, but it is generally transient. Usually clean intermittent catheterization is done for a few days after the treatment until swelling recedes. There is usually initial improvement followed a relapse of incontinence about a week or so later and then gradual improvement again. It takes about 1 month to determine the effectiveness of the procedure.

Retropubic Colposuspension

Retropubic colposuspension lifts the bladder neck and urethra by attaching bladder and urethra or the vaginal wall to other pelvic structures. Surgery is done under general or spinal anesthetic with an open suprapubic incision or through laparoscopy. The **Burch procedure** is most common and requires a wide abdominal incision. The urethra and bladder neck are secured with lateral sutures through the muscles along the pubic bones. **Marshall-Marchetti-Krantz** is a similar procedure that anchors the urethra and bladder neck to cartilage; however, it poses more risk of scarring than the Burch procedure. A suprapubic catheter is left in place for about 5 days and there may be difficulty urinating initially. If this persists, corrective surgery is done to release the urethra to a more normal position. Person must refrain from strenuous activities for 3 months after surgery. Urethral kinking may occur after the Burch procedure. People have less bleeding and less pain after laparoscopy.

Percutaneous Sling Procedure

Percutaneous sling procedure uses a piece of ligament or muscle tendon, usually from the thigh or abdomen, or synthetic material to create a sling under the urethra and bladder neck to lift it to normal position. The graft is then secured to the abdominal wall and pelvic bone. The sling compresses the urethra, pushing it back into normal position. There are a number of different procedures. **Surgery** may be done under general anesthesia through a vaginal or suprapubic incision, or both. It may also be done with laparoscopy. A Foley catheter and vaginal packing are inserted during surgery and a suprapubic catheter may also be inserted. The catheters are usually removed shortly after surgery. Serious complications from this procedure are not common, but urethral obstruction can occur if the sling is too tight. If this occurs, revision may be necessary. If the sling is too loose, a suprapubic revision is usually tried.

Continence Care: Intervention and Treatment

319

TENSION FREE VAGINAL TAPE PROCEDURE

Tension-free vaginal tape procedure uses a mesh-like synthetic tape under urethra to form a sling to lift it to normal position. The tape is inserted through the vagina and attached to both sides of the urethra to support the bladder neck. Within a few weeks, tissue forms about the tape and holds it in place.

Surgery is done with a local anesthesia and conscious sedation. Usually a small incision is made in the vagina, and occasionally in the suprapubic area, depending upon the procedure used. Once the tape is in place, the person is asked to cough to test the tape's support of the urethra. The procedure takes only about 30 minutes and causes only mild pain. A Foley catheter or intermittent catheterization may be used temporarily. The person is asked not to drive for 2 weeks and to avoid sexual intercourse or strenuous activities, such as sports, for 6 weeks.

Bowel Dysfunction and Fecal Incontinence Management

MANAGEMENT STRATEGIES FOR CONSTIPATION AND FECAL IMPACTION

Management strategies for constipation and impaction include:

- **Add fiber** with bran, fresh/dried fruits, and whole grains, to 20-35 grams per day.
- **Increase fluids** to 64 ounces each day.
- **Exercise** program should include walking if possible, and exercises on a daily basis.
- **Change in medications** causing constipation can relieve constipation. Additionally, use of stool softeners, such as Colace, or bulk formers, such as Metamucil, may decrease fluid absorption and move stool through the colon more quickly. Overuse of laxatives can cause constipation.
- **Irritable bowel syndrome** requires careful monitoring of diet, fluids and medical treatment.
- **Pregnancy-related** constipation may be controlled through dietary and fluid modifications and regular exercise.
- **Delayed toileting** should be avoided and bowel training regimen done to promote evacuation at the same time each day. During travel, stool softeners, increased fluid, and exercise may alleviate constipation.
- Enemas and manual removal of impaction may be necessary initially.

REMOVAL OF FECAL IMPACTION

The procedure for removal of fecal impaction is explained below:

- Gather equipment and supplies.
- Position person on left side in bed with plastic bed protection, or sitting on the toilet and leaning forward onto a pillow-covered stool or chair.
- Insert lubricated gloved finger into rectum, gently encircling mass to assess size and hardness.
- Administer oil retention enema to soften stool, guiding nozzle to side of mass. Encourage person to breathe deeply and walk about or move from side to side, while retaining enema for 30 minutes, if possible.
- Break up impaction after oil has passed or after 30-60 minutes if oil retained. Gently break up and remove stool, pulling pieces through the rectum.
- Encourage evacuation without undue straining.
- Enema, usually soapsuds, should follow even if rectal vault empty because stool may be impacted higher.
- Laxative and/or stool softener may be needed.
- Institute bowel training with diet and fluid modifications as needed.

MANAGEMENT OF DIARRHEA

Management of diarrhea includes the following:

- Institute dietary modification includes limiting alcohol and caffeine, which can cause loose stools. Artificial sugar substitutes, such as sorbitol and mannitol, should be avoided. People with lactose intolerance should use Lactaid with dairy products. Yogurt helps control diarrhea from antibiotic use. Increase foods that thicken stool, such as bananas, and soluble fiber.
- Rule-out bacterial, viral, and parasitic infections and treat as needed.
- Avoid foods or additives that trigger diarrhea.
- Stop medications that are causing diarrhea. Antibiotics frequently cause diarrhea.
- Restore fluid and electrolyte imbalance through diet, adequate fluids, or supplements, Gatorade.
- Use antidiarrheals including anti-motilities, such as Lomotil (diphenoxylate and atropine) and loperamide; Bismuth compounds, such as Pepto-Bismol; and absorbents may be used to get diarrhea under control.

Continence Care: Intervention and Treatment

- Treat underlying disease process, such as inflammatory bowel disease or Crohn's disease.
- Treat laxative abuse resulting in cycle of constipation and diarrhea.

SECCA PROCEDURE FOR CONTROL OF FECAL INCONTINENCE

The Secca procedure is done as a non-surgical procedure, on an outpatient basis with conscious sedation and a local pudendal and perianal nerve block. It takes only about 45 minutes. It involves using radiofrequency energy delivered by a small generator to a hand piece with one end that is inserted into the anal canal. When triggered, small needle electrodes pierce the mucosa and radiofrequency energy causes small thermal lesions that result in shrinkage of the tissue and tightening of the anal sphincters as collagen deposits and the tissue begins to contract about the lesions. It may take several months for complete healing, but it improves fecal continence and perception of the urge to defecate in most people. This procedure is used if conservative treatment is ineffective or if sphincter repair fails. There is little pain involved with the procedure and complications are rare. Studies have shown about a 70% decrease in fecal incontinence after 6 months.

PROCEDURE FOR SACRAL NERVE STIMULATION FOR FECAL INCONTINENCE

Sacral nerve stimulation **(sacral neuromodulation)** involves stimulating the nerves that travel from the spine to enervate the rectum and anal sphincters. It is useful when there are functional defects but not structural ones. This procedure assists with neurological control of the sphincter. Nerve evaluation is done percutaneously with temporary electrodes places in the lower spine with an external stimulator for about two weeks to make sure that the nerves are intact and there is adequate response of the pelvic floor muscles. If this is successful, a permanent electrode is implanted and attached to a neurostimulator in the lower abdomen. The electrical impulse can be adjusted post-surgically by use of an external programmer. The implanted neurotransmitter lasts 5-10 years after which it needs to be replaced. This procedure has been especially helpful for those with spinal cord trauma and those with urge fecal incontinence. This treatment is less invasive than other surgical treatments.

MEDICATIONS AND TREATMENTS FOR FECAL INCONTINENCE

The following are medications for fecal incontinence:

- **Antidiarrheals**: to decrease diarrhea, increase tone of rectal muscle, decrease fluid content, and protect the lining of the intestine from irritation.
- **Cholinergic medications**: Decrease intestinal motility and secretions.
- **Opium derivatives**: Increase intestinal muscle tone and decrease motility.
- **Laxatives**: Treat constipation, useful with neurological deficits.
- **Stool softeners**: Increase fluid in stool.
- **Rectal stimulants**: Increase contractions to evacuate stool.
- **Hormones**: For post-menopausal women.

Additional **treatment** consists of the following:

- Diet:
  - High fiber products: Absorb fluid/add bulk. Add slowly to diet.
  - Food allergies or intolerances: need evaluation. Removing items from diet and reintroducing one at a time helps identify foods to avoid.
- Bowel training: Combines medication/diet/enemas for evacuation. It is useful for neurological deficits.
- Biofeedback: Trains people to respond to rectal distention by contracting pelvic floor and external sphincter muscles.
- Procon incontinence device: Catheter with sensor inserted into rectum with inflatable balloon to prevent leakage.

CONTAINMENT DEVICES FOR FECAL INCONTINENCE AND PREVENTIVE SKIN CARE

Absorbent pads, briefs, disposable underwear used for fecal incontinence are the same products used for urinary leakage. Briefs usually can be refastened and often have a plastic liner on the outside, giving added protection but are noisier and bulkier than disposable underwear, which pull on like panties or shorts. Refastenable briefs are useful for the person who is bed bound or not independent in care.

The **anal bag** protects the anus and perianal area from contamination and irritation caused by fecal incontinence. It is a plastic pouch that attaches around the anus with adhesive for a secure fit and is removed and disposed of as needed.

Preventive skin care includes scrupulous hygiene, washing the soiled area with water or disposable wipes, drying thoroughly, and applying a skin barrier cream, such as Desitin or A & D ointment as needed. Soiled containment devices should be removed as soon as possible to prevent skin irritation.

INDWELLING FECAL DIVERSION SYSTEM

Indwelling fecal diversion systems are used for incontinent clients with loose or watery stools in order to prevent skin breakdown, discomfort, odor, and contamination of wounds, and to control the spread of organisms, such as *Clostridioides difficile,* in bedridden or immobile clients. A number of different devices, such as the Flexi-Seal FMS, are available and work similarly. A typical management system includes:

- silicone catheter
- silicone retention balloon at end of catheter
- 45-mL syringe
- lubricant
- charcoal filter collection bags.

The application of the fecal management system (FMS)is relatively simple: The balloon portion of the catheter is lubricated and the catheter is inserted into the rectum and balloon inflated with water or saline (using the 45 mL syringe) to hold it in place and to block fecal leakage. Some systems, such as Flexi-Seal FMS, have a pop-up button to indicate when the balloon is adequately filled for the size of the rectum. The catheter contains an irrigation port so that irrigating fluid can be instilled if necessary. The charcoal filter collection bag is attached to the end of the silicone catheter to contain fecal material.

BOWEL RETRAINING

Bowel retraining is a behavioral modification program that helps people establish control over bowel disorders. It teaches strategies to develop a routine schedule for defecation.

- The person keeps a bowel diary for a week.
- Diet and fluid intake are modified to assure normal stool consistency. This may include increased fiber and fluids, eating meals at scheduled times, and avoiding foods that increase bowel dysfunction.
- A schedule for defecation is established, preferably at the same time each day and about 20-30 minutes after a meal, which stimulates the gastrocolic reflex that propels fecal material through the colon.
- The person is taught Kegel exercises to strengthen muscles.
- A stimulus is used to promote defecation. This may be enemas, suppositories, or laxatives in the beginning, but the goal is to decrease such use. Digital stimulation or hot drinks may be used.
- The person keeps a record of stool consistency and evacuation.

Continence Care: Intervention and Treatment

EXERCISE AS PART OF A BOWEL PROGRAM

Exercise increases the motility of the bowel by stimulating muscle contractions. Walking is one of the best exercises for this purpose, and the person should try to walk one or two miles a day. If the person is unable to walk, then other activities, such as chair exercises that involve the arms and legs and bending can be very effective. Those who are bed bound need to turn from side to side frequently and change position.

Kegel exercises increase strength of the pelvic floor muscles. Kegel exercises for urinary incontinence and fecal incontinence are essentially the same, but the person tries to pull in the muscles around the anus, as though trying to prevent the release of stool or flatus. The person should feel the muscles tightening while holding for 2 seconds and then relaxing for 2, gradually building the time holding time to 10 seconds or more. Exercises should be done 4 times a day.

SUPPOSITORIES

Suppositories are used to stimulate defecation for those with spinal injuries or with normal stools but tight sphincter.

1. Insert suppository rectally, guiding with gloved finger high into the rectum to the side of the rectal wall rather than in the middle of stool.
2. Sit on toilet or commode as sitting allows gravity to bring stool down.
3. Massage abdomen along the colon, from lower right abdomen, up to ribs, across abdomen, and down left side. Repeat the sequence about 10 times with 30 seconds rest in between for a total of 5-10 minutes.
4. Wait 10-15 minutes for bowel movement.
5. If no bowel movement after 15 minutes, digitally stimulate rectum. Insert lubricated gloved finger 2-3 inches inside the anus, moving finger around the walls of the rectum to stimulate the inner sphincter.
6. After evacuation, repeat digital stimulation 2 or 3 times with 5-10 minutes wait time between to ensure empty bowel.

LAXATIVES

STIMULANTS

Stimulants increase intestinal motility, moving the stool through the bowel faster and reducing the absorption of fluids so that the stool remains softer. Common ingredients include cascara in Castor oil, senna in Senokot and sennosides in Ex-lax. Stimulants work quickly and are effective but can result in electrolyte imbalance, Abdominal distension, and cramping. Chronic use may cause a cycle of constipation and diarrhea. Stimulant suppositories, such as Dulcolax are also available. Lubiprostone, marketed as Amitiza (by prescription) taken twice daily increases chloride, sodium, and water secretion from the intestinal lining, and is a treatment that softens stools and increases frequency of defecation. The FDA approved the drug in February 2006 for treatment of chronic idiopathic constipation. Prucalopride (Motegrity) enhances colonic peristalsis to promote bowel motility and was approved by the FDA for the treatment of chronic idiopathic constipation in 2018. Plecanatide (Trulance) once daily was approved in 2017 to treat the same condition by stimulating the upper GI tract to secrete fluids to support bowel function.

BULK FORMERS, LUBRICANTS, AND SALINE

Bulk formers have high fiber content and both soften stool and create more formed stools. These include products such as Metamucil, Citrucel, and FiberCon, which are usually added to liquids because without adequate fluids, they can increase constipation.

Lubricants include both oral mineral oil and glycerin suppositories. They coat the stool, preventing fluid absorption and keeping the stool soft. Mineral oil absorbs fat soluble vitamins and should be used only temporarily

Saline, such as Milk of Magnesia and Epsom Salt, contain ions, such as magnesium phosphate, magnesium hydroxide, and citrate, which are not absorbed through the intestines and draw more fluid into the stool. The magnesium in the preparations also stimulates the bowel. People with impairment of kidney function should avoid magnesium products, and saline laxatives should be used infrequently to avoid dependence. Epsom Salt often has a purging effect and is rarely used.

STOOL SOFTENERS, HYPEROSMOTICS, AND COMBINATION

Stool softeners (emollients) such as Colace, and Phillip's Liqui-Gels use wetting agents, such as docusate sodium, to increase liquid in the stool, thereby softening it. They should not be used with mineral oil because of increased absorption of the oil through the intestines.

Hyperosmotics (available by prescription) contain materials that are not digestible and serve to retain fluid in the stool. Products, such as Kristalose and MiraLAX soften the stool but may result in increased Abdominal distension and flatus, especially initially. There are 3 types of hyperosmolar laxatives: lactulose, polymer, and saline. Lactulose types use a form of sugar and work similarly to saline laxatives, but more slowly, and may be used for long-term treatment. The salines empty the bowels quickly and are used short-term. The polymers contain polyethylene glycol, which retains fluid in the stool and is used short-term.

Combinations use two or more types, such as stool softener with stimulant and should be used only short-term.

ENEMAS

The following are different types of enemas:

- **Medicated retention** enemas may contain antibiotics, nutritives, or anti-helminthics.
- **Oil retention** enemas use mineral oil to coat and soften stool in the rectum. Usually 3-8 ounces is used. Oil retention enemas come prepackaged in single use bulb-type devices. This enema is mild and often used for children who require enemas. It is also useful as the first step in removal of an impaction because it lubricates the stool.
- **Tap water** (hypotonic) enemas are used for mechanical flushing of the rectum, but tap water if used consistently can deplete electrolytes as well as causing acute water intoxication, especially in children and the elderly, if water is retained. However, the risk if very slight if small volumes of water, which do not overwhelm the system, are used. Volume is usually 500-1000 mL, and they are effective in 15-20 minutes.

SURGICAL TREATMENTS FOR FECAL INCONTINENCE

Surgical options for the treatment of fecal incontinence include:

- **Rectal sphincteroplasty** involves a curved incision around the anus, loosening the sphincter muscle and then cutting away weak or damaged muscle from the anal sphincter. The remaining muscle is overlapped and reattached in order to strengthen the sphincter. The bowel is cleansed preoperatively and diet restricted to prevent passage of stool to protect the incision from infection immediately postoperatively. Constipation and hard stools might damage the surgical repair, so tool softeners or laxatives may be used initially. Activities that could strain the surgical site, such as sports or sexual activity, need to be avoided for 2-3 months.

Continence Care: Intervention and Treatment

- **Gracilis muscle transplant** uses muscle usually removed from inner thigh and transplanted to circle the rectal sphincter and provide muscle tone to compensate for loss of nerve function. Postoperative repair is similar to that of sphincteroplasty.
- **Colostomy/ileostomy for fecal diversion** involves removing all or part of the colon and diverting stool to a stoma in the abdominal wall.

ARTIFICIAL ANAL SPHINCTER

The artificial anal sphincter consists of an inflatable cuff surgically implanted around the anal sphincter to prevent fecal leakage, a reservoir in the lower abdomen, and a pump with a button to push usually in the labia of females or scrotum of males. The artificial sphincter is used for intractable fecal incontinence. The procedure is usually done with a general or a spinal anesthesia after cleansing bowel preparation. There are different pressure settings available for the cuffs. Following surgery, the cuff is usually not inflated for about 6-8 weeks while the tissue is healing. The cuff is deflated when a person wants to have a bowel movement, and it automatically reinflates in about 10 minutes. Activities that apply pressure to the rectal area, such as bicycle riding, may cause trauma and irritation. Infection can occur because of fecal contamination of the tissues, and mechanical failure can necessitate removal or replacement of the device.

CONTINENT APPENDICOSTOMY (MALONE CONTINENCE ENEMA [MACE] PROCEDURE)

Continent appendicostomy (Malone continence enema [MACE] procedure) is frequently used with children who suffer neuromuscular impairment, resulting from congenital disorders (myelomeningocele), anorectal malformations, spinal injuries, and Hirschsprung's disease. It can also be used for adults with intractable constipation. In this procedure, the appendix or part of the cecum is brought to abdominal wall to form a stoma, usually at the umbilicus, to provide an open channel into the ascending colon for insertion of a catheter to provide antegrade irrigation. The Malone procedure may be done with and open procedure or a laparoscopy. A catheter is placed through the channel during surgery and left in place for about 3 weeks to allow healing. An antegrade enema is usually given about the 2nd day postoperatively and then every 2-3 days or as needed to control evacuation. Successful control of fecal incontinence is about 90% with this procedure.

MACE IRRIGATIONS

MACE irrigations are usually done with tap water, although normal saline may be used, about 900 mL average for an adult, but ranging from 500 mL to 2000 mL. For children 50 mL is used initially and then the amount is increased gradually with each irrigation, until optimum results are achieved. Sometimes, people are advised to add a small amount of mineral oil or Fleet's enema:

- Gather supplies and equipment
- Insert latex free straight or Foley catheter with 5 mL balloon (usually 12-14 Fr.) into stoma to prescribed distance. Inflate balloon if using Foley. Using a Foley catheter frees both hands as the balloon holds the catheter in place.
- Attach enema bag and tubing and slowly instill solution.
- Clamp tube.
- Deflate Foley/remove catheter.
- Cleanse equipment and wash catheter, which should be replaced every 2-3 weeks.

DIETARY MANAGEMENT OF BOWEL DYSFUNCTION

Dietary management requires identifying foods that increase bowel dysfunction by keeping a list of foods for a week to correlate with bowel activity. **Foods** to avoid include spicy, cured, or smoked meats and fatty and greasy foods that often cause diarrhea and fecal incontinence. Lactose intolerants should avoid dairy products. Caffeine, alcohol, and artificial sweeteners, such as aspartame, NutraSweet, and saccharine can act as laxatives so they and foods that contain them, like sugar-free gum and diet soda, should be avoided, although Splenda and stevia are usually acceptable.

- **Several small meals** instead of large meals may reduce bowel contractions.
- **Fiber** increased to 20-30 grams per day makes stool formed and easier to control although too much can cause bloating and gas, so it's important to add fiber slowly to the diet. Eating whole fruits, whole grains, and vegetables increases fiber.
- **Fluid intake** should be at least 8 glasses, especially water, daily to prevent constipation and impaction.

FIBER IN THE DIET

Most constipation is caused by insufficient fiber in the diet, especially if people eat a lot of processed foods. An adequate amount of fiber is 20-30 grams daily. There are both soluble and insoluble forms of fiber, and both add bulk to the stool and are not absorbed into the body. Some foods have both types:

- **Soluble fiber** dissolves in liquids to form a gel-like substance, one reason why liquids are so important in conjunction with fiber in the diet. Soluble fiber slows the movement of stool through the gastrointestinal system. Food sources include bananas, starches (potatoes, bread), cheese, dried beans, nuts apples, oranges, and oatmeal.
- **Insoluble fiber** changes little with the digestive process and increases the speed of stool through the colon, so too much can result in diarrhea. Food sources of insoluble fiber include oat bran, seeds, skins of fruits and vegetables and nuts.

INCREASING FIBER IN THE DIET AND PROMOTING OPTIMUM BOWEL HEALTH

Establishing a regular routine of eating certain types of foods easiest does increasing fiber. Foods that are high in fiber are often also rich sources of nutrients:

- Start the day with bran cereal, or add 1-2 Tablespoons bran to other foods.
- Substitute whole or dried fruit (including the skin when possible) for juice.
- Eat whole grain breads instead of white bread.
- Eat vegetables, such as broccoli, or dried beans.
- Eat a handful of nuts each day.
- Eat a big salad at least once a day.

Changing how a person eats can also help maintain good bowel function:

- Instead of 3 big meals, eat 5 or 6 small meals.
- Drink at least 8 glasses of liquid a day and drink before meals to help absorb soluble fiber.
- Avoid foods and drinks that trigger diarrhea or constipation

Continence Care: Intervention and Treatment

Continence Care: Education and Referral

Patient and Health Care Professional Education

PATIENT EDUCATION FOR WOUND MANAGEMENT

Patients should be educated on the following elements of wound management:

- **Infection control**: Topics include the importance of hand hygiene, methods for disposal of soiled materials, the risk of healthcare-associated infections (including asking healthcare providers to wash hands), appropriate use of antibiotics, and appropriate wound care.
- **Repositioning**: The need for repositioning, the manner, positions, and frequency vary depending on the patient's condition, but the patient should be apprised of the importance of repositioning to prevent skin breakdown and shown how to reposition, encouraging the patient to reposition at least every 2 hours.
- **Trauma avoidance**: Topics include fall prevention and safe driving as well as measures to improve home safety, such as removal of throw rugs and clutter, improved lighting, installation of handrails and safety bars, and use of shower chairs. Some patients may need information about avoiding choking, fire safety, and safe use of tools (such as knives and clippers)

TOBACCO CESSATION

Smoking releases carbon monoxide and hydrogen cyanide in the blood and interferes with the delivery of oxygen to the tissues, and nicotine is a vasoconstrictor, resulting in slowed healing. Smoking also increases platelet clumping, increasing risk of clotting. Patients should learn about the effects of smoking on healing and should be provided tobacco cessation aids. A number of medical treatments can assist patients through the withdrawal period, during which the person may experience anxiety, irritability, and nicotine craving. Many of the of the medications contain nicotine, but it is released in a slower manner to avoid the sudden increase in nicotine ("rush") associated with smoking: Nicotine patch, nicotine inhaler, nicotine gum, nicotine lozenge, and nicotine nasal spray. Prescription medications that are taken before quitting and then for up to 6 months include bupropion SR and varenicline. Smoking cessation programs include support groups, online forums (StopSmokingCenter.net) and informational websites (Smokefree.gov). The HHS recommends the 5A program: Ask, advise, assess, assist, and arrange followup.

BEHAVIORAL STRATEGIES
DIETARY MANAGEMENT TO CONTROL URINARY INCONTINENCE

Dietary management of urinary incontinence requires some modifications.

- **Foods** that are bladder irritants, such as spicy foods, citrus fruits, and tomatoes should be avoided altogether or rarely eaten. Most sugar substitutes should be avoided although Splenda and stevia may be used.
- **Fluid intake** may be limited to less than the optimal 60 ounces per day although too much restriction can result in dehydration and constipation, further aggravating the incontinence. A good plan is to spread intake out through the day and restrict fluids in the evening, especially if nocturia or enuresis is a problem. Alcohol, which has a diuretic effect, should be avoided or used only occasionally. Apple juice or grape juice can be substituted for orange juice or cranberry juice as they are less irritating to the bladder. De-caffeinated tea and coffee should be used or coffee limited to one cup per day. Carbonated drinks, most of which contain caffeine should be avoided.

BEHAVIORAL TECHNIQUES FOR TREATMENT OF URINARY INCONTINENCE

Behavioral techniques for treating urinary incontinence include:

- **Biofeedback**: Training to control bladder and sphincter muscles.
- **Bladder training**: Training to lengthen time between urination: may include double voiding to make sure bladder empties completely. Relaxation techniques are used to control urge to urinate. Timed urination, scheduled usually every 2-4 hours, helps to prevent incontinence.
- **Diet**: Avoid foods that irritate the bladder, such as acidic foods. Alcohol and caffeine intake may need to be limited. Monitoring fluid intake and reducing fluids in the evening are often helpful.
- **Electrical stimulation**: Pelvic floor muscles are stimulated by the temporary insertion of electrodes into the rectum or vagina. Because it can take months for treatment to be effective, and there are many side effects, it is often used only for those who haven't responded to other treatments and have severe incontinence.
- **Kegel (pelvic floor) exercises**: Strengthen the pelvic floor muscles and the urinary sphincter. They are usually done 3-4 times daily, for stress incontinence.

PELVIC MUSCLE EXERCISES AND METHODS TO ISOLATE PELVIC FLOOR MUSCLES

Pelvic muscle exercises, also known as Kegel exercises, are used to strengthen the periurethral and pelvic muscles in order to increase control of urination and fecal incontinence. Basic exercises involve tightening the muscles 3-4 times daily for about 3 seconds and then relaxing for the same period, repeating about 10 times and gradually increasing the time tightening the muscles to 5-10 seconds.

Isolating the right muscles to tighten is important. Tightening the stomach, leg, or other muscles will not help. People should not hold their breath during the exercises because this may tighten other muscles. There are three methods to check that the pelvic floor muscles are flexing:

1. Stop flow of urine in the midst of urination.
2. Pull in the anus as though trying to stop from passing flatus.
3. In supine position, place finger inside the vagina and squeeze as though trying to stop urine. Tightness should be felt.

POSITIONS FOR PELVIC FLOOR MUSCLE EXERCISES

Pelvic floor muscle exercises can be done anywhere, such as at work or while sitting in a restaurant, as they will not be obvious to others. It's important that people establish a schedule for exercises and try to maintain the schedule, even if not at home. These exercises can be done in different positions:

- **Sitting** exercises are done in a straight-back chair with a firm seat and with feet planted on the floor or legs stretched out and ankles crossed.
- **Reclining** exercises are done lying flat with head on a pillow and knees bent, with feet apart slightly. Knees may be supported with a pillow to prevent tightening of thigh muscles.
- **Standing** exercises are done while holding onto a surface, such as a chair or counter, for support. Knees should be bent slightly with feet about 1 foot apart. Alternately, one can lean against a counter with hips flexed.

PFES

Pelvic floor electrical stimulation (PFES) is the application of low-grade electrical stimulation to the pelvic floor muscles to provide a passive contraction, stimulating the pelvic muscles to contract. It is used to rehabilitate weakened muscles. PFES of the pudendal nerve causes a pudendal nerve reflex loop that results in muscle contraction. PFES is used to assist with isolating the pelvic floor muscles for those who have not been successful with Kegel exercises. It increases the strength of pelvic muscle contraction, it decreases ineffective and uninhibited contraction of the detrusor muscle, and it helps to normalize pelvic muscle relaxation. PFES is applied with skin electrodes around the anus or with vaginal or rectal sensor probes. PFES is often done in conjunction with biofeedback because PFES makes the person more aware of pelvic floor muscle activity and biofeedback helps the person to gain control of the bladder by using these muscles.

COMPONENTS

Key components of PFES units:

- **Waveform** is shape of the impulse on a graph. The waveform for muscle stimulation is rectangular, bi-phasic, and bipolar, a type not damaging to tissue.
- **Amplitude** is strength and intensity of current, which must be enough to create an "anal wink."
- **Ramping** is the speed with which the current reaches the muscles. The faster the current rises, the more discomfort is felt.
- **Frequency rate** is the number of pulses or hertz (Hz) per second. The frequency rate for stress incontinence is 50 Hz, which builds muscle and tightens urethral sphincters; for urge incontinence, 13 Hz, which calms the detrusor muscle and prevents bladder contractions.
- **On/off time** is the ratio of time the muscle is exposed to electrical current and time the muscle recovers. Time on must be less than time off. A typical ratio is 1:2, such as on 5 seconds and off 10.

PHARMACOLOGICAL TREATMENTS FOR URINARY INCONTINENCE

Pharmacological treatments are those oral and topical medications that have helped control urinary incontinence:

- **Adrenergic agents**, such as or Sudafed, increase pressure on urethra and prevent stress incontinence.
- **Antibiotics**, such as Bactrim, treat urinary infections that exacerbate incontinence.
- **Anticholinergics**, such as oxybutynin and tolterodine serve to relax detrusor and pelvic floor muscles and reduce frequency. They may also increase bladder capacity and are useful for overactive bladder because they block the chemicals that stimulate bladder nerves.
- **Estrogens**, such as Premarin (oral) and Estrace (topical) improve muscles tone and prevent atrophic changes of the mucosa.
- **Serotonin norepinephrine reuptake inhibitor** duloxetine (Cymbalta) increases urethral sphincter contraction during storage phase.
- **Smooth muscle relaxants** to relieve bladder spasms.
- **Tricyclic antidepressants**, such as imipramine, increase urinary sphincter tone and decrease bladder spasms.
- **Urinary analgesics**, such as phenazopyridine, alleviate spasms and discomfort caused by urinary infections.

VOIDING DIARIES

BLADDER DIARY

Bladder diary is a complete daily record of all urinations and episodes of urinary incontinence. The diary is usually kept for 3-5 days as part of the urological assessment and includes the following:

- **Time** must be recorded to document patterns of urination.
- **Amount** of urination should be estimated (small, medium, or large) or measured as directed.
- **Intake** should be recorded to determine if fluids are contributing to incontinence or urinary problems.

- **Incontinence** should be characterized by estimations of amount. A small volume of less than 30 mL is enough to wet underwear. A moderate volume of 30-60 mL is enough to soak underwear with overflow down legs. A large volume of more than 60 mL is usually enough to soak clothes and run onto floor or furniture.
- **Incontinence** should be characterized by activity and sensation of urge at time of incontinence to help determine the type of incontinence.

BOWEL DIARY

Bowel diary is a complete daily record of all defecations and episodes of fecal or flatal incontinence. The diary is usually kept for 3-5 days as part of the intestinal assessment and includes the following:

- **Time** of each event should be carefully documented.
- **Type** of bowel movement should be noted, using the Bristol Stool Form Scale or other guide: hard lumps, sausage-shaped, cracked sausage-shaped, smooth and snake-like, soft blobs, fluffy pieces, or liquid.
- **Amount** of stool should be estimated.
- **Abnormalities** such as blood or mucous and the need for finger splinting or straining should be noted.
- **Fecal incontinence** should be characterized by amount and type and activity at the time of incontinence.
- **Flatal incontinence** should be noted.
- **Intake** of both food and fluids should be recorded to see if intake relates to bowel activities.
- **Medications** should all be recorded, including laxatives, vitamins, and any over-the-counter preparations.

EMPTYING MANEUVER TO CONTROL URINARY INCONTINENCE

TRIGGER VOIDING

Trigger voiding is a technique that is useful for those with spinal cord injuries or neurogenic bladders. It involves finding the "trigger" that initiates contraction of the bladder. One method is **suprapubic tapping**, in which the person drums the fingers over the bladder area, above the pubic bone. Usually the suprapubic area is tapped 7 or 8 times, followed by a rest period of 3 seconds, and then the tapping is repeated. The rhythmic tapping is believed to produce an effect on the tension receptors in the bladder wall, activating the reflex arc that results in contraction of the bladder. Trigger mechanisms may vary from one individual to another, so some trial and error is involved. Other common triggers are pulling pubic hairs, stroking the inner thighs or abdomen, digital anal stimulation and dilation, listening to running water, placing hands in warm water, pouring warm water over perineum, or drinking warm fluids.

CREDÉ MANEUVER

Credé maneuver uses direct compression over the bladder area to prompt contraction of the detrusor muscle or to complete emptying of the bladder. The technique involves applying manual pressure above the pubic bone. Pressure should be firm and even, not abrupt, and begin with a slight upward pressure followed by downward pressure. Pressure should be maintained while the bladder empties but stopped immediately if pain occurs. The Credé maneuver should not be used if the bladder is grossly distended. The Credé maneuver is usually used in conjunction with a scheduled voiding program for chronic urinary incontinence.

DOUBLE VOIDING

Double voiding is a technique used with mild to moderate urinary retention. The person urinates, attempting to empty the bladder, and then stays on the toilet for 2-10 minutes and tries to urinate again. Alternately, after the initial urination, the person may stand for a brief period, sit back down, and then urinate for the second time.

SKIN CARE TO PREVENT IRRITATION FROM FECAL OR URINARY INCONTINENCE

Cleanse skin with water after each episode of incontinence. Soap tends to be drying and can cause irritation, but if soap is needed, people can use baby wash, which is quite mild, or disposable pre-moistened alcohol-free, perfume-free wipes. After cleansing, the area should be dried thoroughly, patting dry or using a hair dryer on low heat.

Apply cream or powder if there is any sign of skin irritation. Moisture-barrier creams, such as Desitin and A & D ointment can prevent urine or feces from directly contacting skin. Non-medicated, non-perfumed talcum powder or cornstarch may help to keep perineal area dry.

Wear loose clothing to allow for airflow as tight clothes can make skin irritation worse. Many synthetic fibers, such as polyester, constrict air and should be avoided. Underwear should be 100% cotton.

Incontinence pads should contain an absorbent wicking layer to keep moisture away from the skin and should be changed promptly when soiled.

EDUCATING HEALTH CARE PROVIDERS ON INCONTINENCE CARE PRINCIPLES

The continence care nurse's role in educating health care providers on **incontinence care** principles includes mentoring, role modeling, and providing information:

- Explaining the different types and causes of both fecal and urinary incontinence.
- Identifying signs of incontinence and asking pertinent questions about a history of incontinence and urinary tract infections.
- Assessing factors that may contribute to incontinence, including a discussion of dietary and fluid intake and review of medications.
- Developing a personalized plan of care and toileting program as appropriate for each patient with individualized goals based on multiple factors, including type of incontinence, cognition, barriers, mobility, dependence, medications, and resources.
- Assessing potential barriers to implementation of the plan (lighting, inaccessible bathroom, analgesics, cognitive impairments) and developing compensatory measures.
- Developing and education plan for both the patient and appropriate caregivers in preparation for discharge or transfer.
- Determining appropriate methods for evaluating the effectiveness of the care plan and carrying out ongoing monitoring of patient.

Multidisciplinary Collaboration

RESOURCES FOR PATIENTS

Resources available to the patient include:

- **Support and advocacy**: Support groups are available through many medical centers and hospitals as well as online. Many are sponsored by national organizations and are generally free of cost and available to patients and/or families. National organizations also often provide information about clinical trials and current research.
- **Access to supplies**: Many manufacturers provides assistance programs for those unable to afford supplies, such as dressings, and some national organizations may also provide assistance. Some patients may be eligible for Medicaid, which will cover the costs of necessary supplies and equipment.
- **Post-acute care**: This level of care is less intense than that provided by an acute hospital. Post-acute care may be provided after acute hospitalization or instead of acute hospitalization. Medical treatments can be continued with post-acute care but the focus is more commonly on rehabilitation.

COMMUNITY AND NATIONAL ORGANIZATIONS TO ASSIST THOSE MANAGING URINARY INCONTINENCE

There are a number of community and national organizations that can provide information and support to those who have urinary incontinence. Many of the sites listed below provide printable information sheets, lists of urologists, pictures and diagrams, information about clinical trials, newsletters, message boards, and print material, such as booklets. They are invaluable resources for persons and caregivers dealing with incontinence or other urinary conditions.

- National Institute on Aging Information Center
- National Association for Continence
- Simon Foundation for Continence
- National Institute of Diabetes and Digestive and Kidney Diseases
- American Urological Association/Urology Health.org

RESOURCES FOR PATIENTS SUFFERING FROM FUNCTIONAL INCONTINENCE

Functional incontinence is incontinence that is due to physical or mental disabilities that prevent a person from being able to get to the bathroom.

- **Physical Therapy**: This service can help to individualize an exercise program that can help patients to strengthen the muscles of their pelvic floor. If there are physical mobility issues limiting a person's ability to use the bathroom, they can help with strengthening and increasing the ROM of the muscles necessary.
- **Occupational Therapy**: This can help with improving the patient's ability to perform their activities of daily living. Training can be given in transferring to the toilet, evaluating for a raised toilet seat or grab bars that could help a person in transferring, improving trunk mobility and balance, and cognitive and sequencing skills.
- **Social Worker**: This can help to address some of the psychosocial issues associated with incontinence. The patients may have problems with depression and anxiety due to their incontinence. They may be limiting their social contacts because of the risk of embarrassment, thus resulting in a low self-esteem.

Continence Care: Education and Referral

MAKING APPROPRIATE CONSULTATIONS AND REFERRALS

REFERRALS TO SOCIAL SERVICES OR MENTAL HEALTH SERVICES

Patients often face many challenges and complex medical and emotional needs. The nurse plays an important role in identifying the appropriateness of **referrals** for specialized support:

- **Social services**: Costs of wound care products can be high, and patients may lack adequate income to pay for supplies or may have no or inadequate insurance. Some patients, especially older adults, may be unable to care for themselves without assistance or may lack transportation. Patients are often unaware of services for which they may be eligible. Social workers can assist patients to identify needs and government or community programs that can provide assistance.
- **Mental health professionals**: Depression, shame, and anxiety associated with wound care and body image issues may cause patients to refuse care, avoid assuming responsibility for care, or avoid social contacts. Patients may feel overwhelmed and hopeless and have difficulty expressing feelings. Those with cognitive decline may be confused. It's important to be alert to signs of distress, to utilize screening tools (such as PHQ-9 or GAD-7), and to refer patients to mental health professionals.

CONSULTS

Patients with symptoms or needs that exceed the nurse's scope of practice or suggest underlying pathology may require **consultation** with an appropriate specialist:

- **Gastroenterology**: GI specialist may help to manage underlying disease, adjust medications, and carry out diagnostic procedures, such as endoscopy. Indications include high output ostomies, persistent diarrhea, failure of fistulae to close, and stomal complications, and short bowel syndrome.
- **Genitourinary**: GU specialist may carry out diagnostic procedures, such as cystoscopy, provide interventions (Botox, artificial sphincter), or place long-term SP catheters. Indications include incontinence, urinary retention, hematuria, and recurrent UTIs.
- **Oncology**: Oncologist may provide guidance regarding disease, modify treatments to aid wound healing, and initiate palliative care when appropriate. Indications include malignant wounds, fungating tumors, issues of wound healing associated with chemotherapy or radiation, and need for pain control.
- **Gynecology**: Gynecologist may may hormones, fit pessaries, carry out surgical repairs, and coordinate pelvic floor rehabilitation. Indications include rectovaginal and vesicovaginal fistulae, prolapse, incontinence, and chronic vulvar skin breakdown associated with incontinence.

Handoff/Transition of Patients with Incontinence

Hand-off/transition procedures for patients with incontinence should be documented and adequate time allowed for communication, including questions from the receiving party. Important elements that must be covered include:

- Demographic information, such as name, diagnoses, address, telephone number.
- List of medications and treatments.
- Physical impairments that may impact ability to self-care, such as vision impairment and impaired mobility.
- Type of incontinence (urinary and/or fecal).
- History of incontinence and conditions under which incontinence occurs.
- Complications, such as moisture-associated skin damage, dermatitis, ulcerations, maceration, fungal infections.
- Interventions utilized in the past and in the present to manage incontinence, and patient response.
- Supplies and/or equipment that is needed by the patient (catheter supplies, bedside commode).
- Education of patient/caregiver regarding incontinence, treatments, skin care, and precautions (signs of infection, skin deterioration), preventive measures, and response.
- Psychosocial factors that may present a barrier to incontinence care, such as cognitive impairments, poverty, lack of support system.
- Nutritional guidelines/interventions, such as limiting fluids in the evening and increasing fiber in diet.

Continence Care: Education and Referral

CWOCN Practice Test

Want to take this practice test in an online interactive format?
Check out the online resources page, which includes interactive practice questions
and much more: **mometrix.com/resources719/cwocn**

Wound Care

1. Which of the following extends from a wound under normal tissue and connects two structures, such as the wound and an organ?

    a. undermining
    b. fistula
    c. tunneling
    d. abscess

2. A patient has a wound on the right hip with tunneling and fistulae. Which of the following is *MOST* indicative of an abscess formation?

    a. increased purulent discharge
    b. increased wound pain
    c. increased erythema and swelling at wound perimeter
    d. erythematous, painful, swollen area 3 cm from wound perimeter

3. Which of the following laboratory tests is the most effective to monitor acute changes in nutritional status?

    a. total protein
    b. albumin
    c. prealbumin
    d. transferrin

4. On the eighth day of wound care, granulation tissue is evident about the wound perimeter, and the wound is beginning to contract. The wound is in which of the following phases of healing?

    a. proliferation
    b. inflammation
    c. hemostasis
    d. maturation

5. Which of the following is the correct procedure for applying Eutectic Mixture of Local Anesthetics (EMLA Cream) to a wound prior to debridement?

    a. apply a thin layer (1/8 inch thick) to the wound for 15 minutes, leaving the wound open
    b. apply a thick layer (1/4 inch thick) to the wound, extending 1/2 inch past the wound onto surrounding tissue, and cover with plastic wrap for 20 to 60 minutes
    c. apply a thick layer (1/4 inch thick) to the wound surface only and cover with plastic wrap for 15 minutes
    d. apply a thin layer (1/8 inch thick) to the wound surface only and cover with a loose dry dressing for 20 to 60 minutes

6. When doing a routine dressing change for a healing decubitus ulcer on the right hip, which is the most appropriate cleaning solution?

   a. povidone-iodine solution
   b. hydrogen peroxide
   c. alcohol
   d. normal saline

7. Which of the following wound irrigation devices will provide approximately 8 psi in irrigant pressure to the wound surface?

   a. 35-mL syringe with 19-gauge Angiocath
   b. 250-mL squeeze bottle
   c. bulb syringe
   d. 6-mL syringe with 19-gauge Angiocath

8. Which of the following is the most important criterion when assessing a patient's level of wound pain?

   a. patient's behavior
   b. type of wound
   c. patient's report of pain
   d. patient's facial expression

9. Which of the following is likely to have the *MOST* negative effect on wound healing for a 65-year-old woman?

   a. hypoalbuminemia
   b. BMI of 20.2
   c. BMI of 28
   d. vegan diet

10. Which of the following is the most definitive method for obtaining a wound specimen for culture and sensitivities?

   a. tissue biopsy
   b. sterile swab of wound
   c. needle biopsy
   d. sterile swab of discharge

11. A patient with an infected abdominal wound is taking a number of drugs. Which of the following is most likely to impair healing?

   a. phenytoin
   b. corticosteroid
   c. prostaglandin
   d. estrogen

12. A burn extending into the dermis with obvious blistering would be classified as

   a. first degree.
   b. second degree.
   c. third degree.
   d. full thickness.

CWOCN Practice Test

13. Which of the following results from smoking cigarettes?

    a.   vasodilation

    b.   vasoconstriction

    c.   increased oxygen transport

    d.   increased oxygen tension

14. When calculating the ankle-brachial index (ABI), if the ankle systolic pressure is 90 mmHg and the brachial systolic pressure is 120 mmHg, what is the ABI?

    a.   1.33

    b.   13.3

    c.   7.5

    d.   0.75

15. Using transcutaneous oxygen pressure measurement (TCPO2), which of the following values indicates that oxygenation is adequate for healing?

    a.   18 mm Hg

    b.   20 mm Hg

    c.   30 mm Hg

    d.   42 mm Hg

16. The method of closure that involves leaving the wound open and allowing it to close naturally through granulation and epithelialization is healing by

    a.   primary or first intention.

    b.   secondary or second intention.

    c.   tertiary or third intention.

    d.   quaternary prevention.

17. A patient's laboratory results show a serum sodium of 155 mEq/L and a serum osmolality of 300 mOsm/kg. The most likely cause is

    a.   infection.

    b.   overhydration.

    c.   dehydration.

    d.   malnutrition.

18. Autolytic debridement is most effective for

    a.   chronic wounds.

    b.   large burns.

    c.   small wounds without infection.

    d.   necrotic wounds.

19. Enzymatic debridement requires application of enzymes

    a.   1 to 2 times daily.

    b.   3 to 4 times daily.

    c.   1 to 2 times weekly.

    d.   3 to 4 times weekly.

20. Which of the following indicates that sharp instrument debridement must be discontinued?

    a.   purulent discharge occurs

    b.   black eschar is removed

    c.   pain and bleeding occur

    d.   patient complains of fatigue

21. A patient has second and third degree burns on 30% of the body and is in severe pain. Which method of debridement is most indicated?

a. autolytic debridement
b. enzymatic debridement
c. sharp instrument debridement
d. surgical debridement

22. Which method of mechanical debridement may cause damage to granulation tissue and is generally contraindicated?

a. wet-to-dry dressings
b. whirlpool bath
c. irrigation under pressure
d. ultrasound treatment

23. Which of the following topical antimicrobials is most appropriate to treat nasal colonization of *Staphylococcus aureus* in a patient with an open wound?

a. cadexomer iodine
b. metronidazole
c. mupirocin (Bactroban®)
d. silver sulfadiazine

24. Which of the following is a contraindication to negative pressure wound therapy?

a. chronic Stage IV pressure ulcer
b. wound malignancy
c. unresponsive arterial ulcer
d. dehiscent surgical wound

25. Which of the following is the primary goal in referring a patient for multidisciplinary consultation?

a. prevention of complications
b. treatment of complications
c. education
d. identification of outcomes

26. Becaplermin (Regranex®) gel is indicated for which type of wound?

a. venous stasis ulcer
b. pressure ulcer
c. sutured/stapled wound
d. diabetic ulcer

27. Which of the following types of dressing is indicated for treatment of a full-thickness infected wound with large amount of exudate?

a. alginate
b. hydrocolloid
c. hydrogel
d. semipermeable film

CWOCN Practice Test

28. What hyperbaric oxygen therapy (HBOT) treatment regimen is usually recommended for chronic wounds and lower extremity diabetic ulcers?

a. compression at 2 ATA 3 times 60 minutes daily for 48 hours
b. compression at 2 to 2.4 ATA for 90 minutes daily for at least 30 treatments
c. compression at 3 ATA for 2 to 4 hour periods 3 to 4 times daily
d. compression at 3 to 2.5 ATA for 60 to 90 minutes 2 times daily for 2 to 3 days and then decreasing frequency over 4 to 6 days

29. Which NPIAP stage is a pressure ulcer characterized by deep full-thickness ulceration that exposes subcutaneous tissue with possible presence of slough, tunneling, and undermining but without visibility of underlying muscle, tendon, or bone?

a. stage I
b. stage II
c. stage III
d. stage IV

30. What is the most common cause of shear?

a. "sheet burn"
b. elevating the head of the bed >30°
c. lifting the patient with a pull sheet
d. turning the patient side to side

31. What is the minimal thickness of a support surface for a chair?

a. one inch
b. two inches
c. three inches
d. four inches

32. When turning and repositioning patients, what is the preferred position for the patient to reduce pressure?

a. prone
b. supine
c. 30° lateral
d. 90° side-lying

33. On the Braden scale for predicting risk of developing pressure sores, a patient scores 2 (1 to 4 or 1 to 3 scale) on each of 6 parameters (total score 12). What is the patient's risk of developing a pressure sore?

a. very minimal risk
b. breakpoint for risk
c. high risk
d. extremely high risk (worst score)

34. Which type of overlay support surface is best for moisture control?

a. rubber
b. plastic
c. gel
d. foam

35. Which of the following characteristics indicates venous insufficiency?

    a. pain ranges from intermittent to severe constant
    b. pulses are absent or weak
    c. brownish discoloration is evident about ankles and anterior tibial area
    d. rubor occurs on dependency and pallor on foot elevation

36. Which of the following is a typical example of a peripheral ulcer caused by arterial insufficiency?

    a. deep, circular, necrotic ulcer on toe tips
    b. irregular ulcer on medial malleolus
    c. round ulcer on anterior tibial area
    d. irregular ulcer on lateral malleolus

37. When assessing for capillary refill, arterial occlusion is indicated with a refill time of

    a. 15 seconds.
    b. <2 seconds.
    c. >20 seconds.
    d. >2 to 3 seconds.

38. A pulse graded as 1 on a 0 to 4 scale of intensity could be described as

    a. strong and bounding.
    b. weak, difficult to palpate.
    c. absent.
    d. normal, as expected.

39. Which of the following off-loading measures is usually the MOST effective for treatment of neuropathic ulcers?

    a. total contact cast
    b. removable cast walkers
    c. wheelchairs
    d. half-shoes

40. Which of the following is characteristic of Charcot arthropathy (Charcot foot)?

    a. severe pain and inflammation
    b. high arch and hypersensitivity
    c. muscle spasms, increased pain, and inflammation
    d. weak muscles, reduced sensation, inflammation, and collapsed arch

41. Which of the following is necessary to manage peripheral lymphedema of the legs?

    a. daily diuretics
    b. static compression bandaging
    c. off-loading
    d. bed rest

42. Which measurement must be used to evaluate the safety of static compression therapy to manage edema?

    a. capillary refill time
    b. venous refill time
    c. ankle-brachial index
    d. blood pressure

CWOCN Practice Test

43. Which of the following pharmacological measures is used to maximize perfusion with intermittent claudication?

    a. antiplatelet agents, such as Plavix®

    b. vasodilators, such as cilostazol (Pletal®)

    c. thrombolytics

    d. anticoagulants, such as warfarin (Coumadin®)

44. Which of the following may be a subtle indication of infection with arterial insufficiency?

    a. fever and chills

    b. decrease in necrotic area

    c. decreased pain or edema

    d. fluctuance of periwound tissue

45. A patient with venous insufficiency requires compression therapy and has Unna's boot applied but must be on bed rest for four weeks. Which action is correct?

    a. continue Unna's boot therapy during bed rest, but change 2 times weekly

    b. continue Unna's boot therapy, but keep leg elevated

    c. discontinue Unna's boot therapy during the bed rest period

    d. continue Unna's boot therapy, but change only every 2 weeks

46. When doing the nylon monofilament test, how many test sites should be used?

    a. 2

    b. 4

    c. 8

    d. 10

47. The *NEXT* step in wound care for a traumatic wound, such as a dog bite, after stabilizing the patient's condition and stopping bleeding is

    a. administer antibiotics

    b. administer tetanus toxoid/immune globulin as indicated

    c. flush wound with copious amounts of normal saline under pressure

    d. scrub wound with povidone-iodine

48. A patient with pemphigus vulgaris has generalized lesions with ulcerations and crusting, causing the patient's skin to adhere to the bed sheets. The patient is mobile and otherwise healthy and is seeking recommendations to self-manage this issue. What should the wound care nurse recommend?

    a. ensure bed sheets are always clean and dry

    b. set an alarm to turn frequently during the night

    c. place a piece of soft plastic over the sheets

    d. use an alternating pressure mattress

49. What is the most effective treatment for a fungating neoplastic wound of the breast that is oozing blood from eroded vasculature?

    a. charcoal dressing

    b. hemostatic dressing and cauterization with silver nitrate

    c. cleansing with ionic solution

    d. surgical debridement

50. One of the primary treatments for contact dermatitis with an itching, blistering rash is

   a. nonadherent dressings.

   b. topical corticosteroid.

   c. antibiotics.

   d. cleansing with povidone-iodine.

51. How many grams of protein per kilogram should the average person with a pressure sore receive each day?

   a. 1.25 to 1.5 g/kg

   b. 1.5 to 2 g/kg

   c. 2 to 2.5 g/kg

   d. 2.5 to 3 g/kg

52. If a patient is about to be discharged home from an acute care hospital unit but has poor insurance coverage and is concerned about the costs of dressing supplies, but best referral is likely

   a. community agency.

   b. social worker.

   c. national charity.

   d. faith-based organization.

53. If a patient with a chronic leg wound comes to an appointment and the wound has deteriorated because the patient has been changing the dressing one time weekly instead of every 3 days, the MOST appropriate response is,

   a. "Let's talk about how I can help you to adhere to the plan of care."

   b. "Your wound is deteriorating because you aren't adhering to the plan of care."

   c. "Why didn't you change your dressings according to the plan of care?"

   d. "If you don't take care of this wound, you might lose your leg."

54. A toe-brachial index should be assessed rather than the ankle-brachial index for patients with

   a. pain on walking.

   b. history of atherosclerosis.

   c. vascular calcification.

   d. hypertension.

55. A patient's transcutaneous oxygen pressure measurement (TCPO2) is 18 mm Hg, which indicates

   a. adequate oxygenation.

   b. slight impairment.

   c. equivocal finding.

   d. marked ischemia.

56. If a patient scheduled for hyperbaric oxygen therapy presents with a severe upper respiratory infection, the treatment should generally be

   a. withheld.

   b. given for a shorter period of time.

   c. given for a longer period of time.

   d. given as usual.

57. If using the PQRST method of pain assessment, an appropriate question to begin the assessment with is

    a. "Does the pain move or stay in one place?"
    b. "When did the pain start?"
    c. "What causes the pain?"
    d. "What does the pain feel like?"

58. Excessive collagen production at the site of a wound leads to

    a. inflammation.
    b. abnormal scarring.
    c. Dehydration of the wound
    d. rapid healing.

59. Hydrocolloid dressings with silver are appropriate for

    a. dry infected wounds.
    b. dry clean wounds.
    c. infected wounds without heavy exudate.
    d. infected wounds with mild to moderate exudate.

60. Which of the following drugs may impede wound healing?

    a. NSAIDs
    b. levothyroxine
    c. insulin
    d. ferrous sulfate

61. Which class of therapeutic compression stockings is appropriate for refractory venous ulcers and lymphedema?

    a. class 1: 20-30 mm Hg.
    b. class 2: 30-40 mm Hg.
    c. class 3: 40-50 mm Hg.
    d. class 4: 50-60 mm Hg.

62. A patient has been prescribed becaplermin gel (Regranex®) according to standard protocol for wound treatment. How many hours out of 24 should the gel be in place on the wound?

    a. 6
    b. 12
    c. 18
    d. 24

63. Which comment by the patient suggests that the patient may benefit from a referral to a nutritionist?

    a. "I try to eat my three meals within a 14-hour timespan so that I fast for 10 hours."
    b. "I've been eating a vegetarian diet for two years."
    c. "I limit my meat intake to 4 ounces daily and eat more fruits and vegetables."
    d. "I'm substituting honey for sugar in everything, so my carbohydrate intake is lower."

64. If teaching a caregiver to use pillow bridging to prevent pressure ulcers for an immobile patient, how many pillows should be employed?

    a. 2
    b. 4
    c. 5
    d. 7

65. When assessing a patient with diabetes, it's important to remember that diabetic patients tend to lose protective sensation after

    a.   10 to 15 years.
    b.   8 to 10 years.
    c.   5 to 8 years.
    d.   3 to 5 years.

66. Which of the following steroid dermatologic agents has the highest potency?

    a.   hydrocortisone acetate
    b.   desonide
    c.   triamcinolone
    d.   betamethasone dipropionate

67. If a patient with a slow-healing coccygeal wound is having negative pressure wound therapy (NPWT) and the nurse is assessing the wound with the DIME acronym, the M refers to

    a.   mobility.
    b.   maceration.
    c.   moisture balance.
    d.   malodor.

68. If a patient complains of severe pain during dressing changes and has an analgesic order, the analgesic should generally be administered

    a.   60 to 90 minutes before treatment.
    b.   30 to 60 minutes before treatment.
    c.   15 to 30 minutes before treatment.
    d.   5 to 15 minutes before treatment.

69. Which of the following types of debridement is MOST indicated for a wound with large amounts of unviable tissue and increasing cellulitis?

    a.   sharp debridement
    b.   enzymatic debridement
    c.   wet-to-dry debridement
    d.   autolytic debridement

70. The MOST accurate method of measuring the size and depth of a wound is a

    a.   ruler.
    b.   comparison with known object, such as a coin.
    c.   photograph.
    d.   stereophotogrammetry.

71. Undermining most often occurs as the result of

    a.   friction.
    b.   shear.
    c.   direct trauma.
    d.   direct pressure.

72. The odor of a wound should be assessed

    a.   before the dressing is removed.
    b.   before cleaning the wound.
    c.   after cleaning the wound.
    d.   at all stages of dressing change.

73. If exudate covers less than two-thirds, but more than one-third of a dressing after it is removed, the amount of exudate would be classified as

a. small.
b. moderate.
c. large.
d. excessive.

74. Moisture-associated skin damage (MASD) most often results in

a. maceration of periwound skin.
b. wound infection.
c. eschar development.
d. undermining.

75. Under CMS regulations, how long must a patient have an unsuccessful trial with static compression therapy before switching to intermittent pneumatic compression therapy?

a. 1 month
b. 2 months
c. 4 months
d. 6 months

76. If the edges of a wound are rolled inward, this may indicate any of the following etiologies EXCEPT

a. infection.
b. dehydration.
c. hypoxia.
d. basement membrane formation.

77. When developing the care plan for a patient, the MOST effective method of prioritizing a list of goals is to

a. review the history and physical.
b. ask the physician.
c. ask the patient.
d. refer to a care plan guide.

78. The initial sign of an infection in a chronic wound is often

a. delayed healing.
b. serosanguinous drainage.
c. purulent drainage.
d. pain.

79. When using the STONES mnemonic to help identify a deep infection, the "O" stands for

a. oxygenation.
b. obesity.
c. occlusion.
d. os (bone).

80. When applying a lidocaine 2% soak to a wound, how long should the saturated gauze be left in place prior to debridement of the wound?

a. 30 to 60 seconds
b. 1 to 2 minutes
c. 3 to 5 minutes
d. 6 to 8 minutes

81. Which of the following support surfaces has low moisture retention?

   a. air fluidized
   b. static flotation (air, water)
   c. alternating air
   d. foam

82. When assessing venous flow with duplex ultrasound, retrograde flow is classified as abnormal if it persists for

   a. more than 0.5 second.
   b. more than 1.0 second.
   c. more than 1.5 seconds.
   d. more than 2 seconds.

83. Hot tub folliculitis is most often caused by

   a. *Staphylococcus aureus.*
   b. *Escherichia coli.*
   c. *Enterobacter.*
   d. *Pseudomonas aeruginosa*

84. The use of topical silver-based creams, such as Silvadene®, should be limited to

   a. one week.
   b. two weeks.
   c. three weeks.
   d. four weeks.

85. Which of the following is a contraindication for the use of transparent film dressings?

   a. the wound has a small amount of exudate
   b. the dressing is applied to protect a pressure spot
   c. the wound is covered with dry eschar
   d. the wound has a suspected bacterial infection

86. Which of the following are the two primary factors that determine how damaging pressure will be to the tissue?

   a. duration and magnitude
   b. oxygenation and nutrition
   c. duration and oxygenation
   d. magnitude and nutrition

87. When evaluating support surfaces, what does *immersion* refer to?

   a. the thickness of the support surface
   b. the duration that a patient can be left in one position on the support surface
   c. the depth the patient's body penetrates the support surface
   d. the amount of pressure that the support surface can actually support

88. If a patient's wound has developed epibole and a closed edge, what intervention is needed to increase healing?

   a. a moist healing environment
   b. debridement of the epibole
   c. application of topical antibiotics
   d. compression therapy

89. Foam mattresses tend to "bottom out" and should be replaced after about

    a.   3 months.

    b.   12 months.

    c.   2 years.

    d.   3 years.

90. Which of the following is a contraindication for use of electrical stimulation to promote healing?

    a.   pacemaker

    b.   diabetic neuropathy

    c.   renal disease

    d.   edema

91. Which of the following is a recommended position for a patient on a horizontal surface?

    a.   prone position with rotation of 40 degrees to the right or left

    b.   supine position with rotation of 40 degrees to the right or left

    c.   supine position with head of bed elevated ≤30 degrees and knees flexed

    d.   supine position with head of bed elevated ≤35 degree and feet blocked

92. A patient on a continuous or intermittent lateral rotation support surface is at risk for

    a.   friction injury.

    b.   shear injury.

    c.   pressure injury.

    d.   moisture injury.

93. Lower extremity girth measurement to assess edema should be done at the metatarsal head, both malleoli, and

    a.   2, 8, 14, and 18 cm above the lateral malleolus and lower edge of patella.

    b.   2, 4, and 8 cm above the lateral malleolus and lower edge of patella.

    c.   8 and 16 cm above the lateral malleolus and lower edge of patella.

    d.   3, 12, and 18 cm above the lateral malleolus and lower edge of patella.

94. If a diabetic patient has a stage IV sacral ulcer with undermining from 4 to 8 o'clock to 1 cm, a heavy volume of exudate, and a bioburden, which of the following dressings is MOST indicated?

    a.   packing wound with calcium alginate and covering with bordered foam dressing

    b.   packing wound with silver alginate and covering with bordered foam dressing

    c.   packing the wound with normal-saline saturated gauze and covered with absorptive dressing

    d.   packing wound with a wound filler (starch copolymers) and covering with absorptive dressing

95. If an overweight patient's weight is at the upper limit for a specialty mattress, the correct intervention is to

    a.   consider the patient's weight distribution.

    b.   utilize the specialty mattress for the patient's weight.

    c.   utilize a bariatric mattress.

    d.   utilize the specialty mattress for the patient's weight with additional support surface.

96. When educating a patient with mild cognitive impairment (MCI) about wound care, one way to deal with the communication barrier is to

    a.   also instruct a caregiver.

    b.   write everything down.

    c.   break instructions into small steps.

    d.   repeat the instructions numerous times.

97. Biologic therapy with maggots is contraindicated with

  a. a wound that has not responded to other treatments.
  b. infected wound.
  c. painful wound.
  d. exposed blood vessels.

98. When carrying out limb volume measurements by the circumferential method, measurements are taken on the hand and arm every

  a. 4 cm.
  b. 6 cm.
  c. 10 cm.
  d. 14 cm.

99. The Braden scale for risk of developing pressure sores assesses 6 different areas: sensory perception, moisture, activity, mobility, usual nutrition pattern, and

  a. friction and shear.
  b. mental status.
  c. pain level.
  d. risk of fall.

100. If a patient has a total contact cast applied for offloading for a plantar neuropathic foot ulcer, how frequently should the TCC be changed?

  a. every 4 to 5 days
  b. every 1 to 2 weeks
  c. every 2 to 4 weeks
  d. every 4 to 5 weeks

101. When using Doppler ultrasound to evaluate blood flow, at what angle to the skin should the transducer be held?

  a. 20 degrees
  b. 45 degrees
  c. 75 degrees
  d. 90 degrees

102. An essential role of fat in the diet is to

  a. provide the most available source of energy.
  b. serve as a component of antibodies and the immune system.
  c. maintain the normal function of the cell membrane.
  d. increase the activation of white blood cells at the wound site.

103. When educating a patient with peripheral arterial disease about self-care, which of the following should the patient be advised poses the greatest risk for decreasing circulation?

  a. drinking one glass of wine daily
  b. smoking cigarettes
  c. using cannabidiol (CBD) cream to reduce pain
  d. drinking 2 cups of coffee daily

104. The Braden Q scale was designed specifically for which population?

  a. pediatric
  b. geriatric
  c. obstetric
  d. disabled

CWOCN Practice Test

105. If the nurse is teaching a hearing-impaired patient to do dressing changes, and the patient nods the head and appears to understand, which of the following is the MOST effective method of ensuring the patient understands the information?

    a. provide information in writing/visual form as well
    b. provide instructions to a family member
    c. ask the patient if the instructions are clear
    d. ask the patient to do a return demonstration

106. If collagenase is being applied to a wound for debridement, the wound's pH must stay within the range of

    a. 2 to 4.
    b. 4 to 6.
    c. 6 to 8.
    d. 8 to 10.

107. If a patient who is malnourished has the following nursing diagnosis on the plan of care, "Imbalanced nutrition, less than body requirements," which of the following is an appropriate desired outcome?

    a. provide supplements if diet remains insufficient
    b. patient will improve activity level and show increased energy
    c. ensure well-balanced healthy diet
    d. patient will maintain adequate nutrition evidenced by weight within normal range

108. Which of the following is a contraindication to surgical/sharp debridement of a wound?

    a. diabetic neuropathy
    b. ischemic tissue
    c. underlying infection
    d. deep extensive wound

109. The best method of attaching dressings to vascular leg ulcers is

    a. paper tape.
    b. ACE bandage.
    c. liquid adhesive.
    d. tube gauze/netting.

110. If a patient has a diabetic ulcer with minimal to moderate exudate and a small amount of eschar that requires debridement, which of the following dressing choices is MOST appropriate for autolytic debridement?

    a. gauze
    b. hydrogel
    c. alginate
    d. hydrocolloid

111. Compression of tissue impairs circulation and can result in ischemia and pressure injury when the skin perfusion pressure falls to below

    a. 5 to 10 mmHg
    b. 10 to 20 mm Hg.
    c. 30 to 40 mm Hg.
    d. 50 to 60 mm Hg.

112. If a patient score 13 total points in the 5 categories of the Norton Plus Pressure Ulcer Scale and checks positive for diabetes, hypertension, and hemoglobin, what is the patient's risk for pressure ulcers?

a. high risk
b. moderate risk
c. low risk
d. no risk

113. The 5 basic elements of a skin assessment include (1) temperature, (2) color, (3) moisture, (4) integrity, and (5)

a. pain.
b. turgor.
c. sensation.
d. edema.

114. If the healthcare provider is using the NERDS mnemonic to identify a superficial infection, the "D" stands for

a. Degeneration.
b. Data.
c. Dusky.
d. Debris.

115. If a wound is characterized by a defective matrix and cell debris that are impairing healing, which of the following is the correct intervention?

a. negative pressure wound therapy
b. moisture-balancing dressings
c. antimicrobials
d. debridement

116. Calluses on the bottom of the foot most often occur because of

a. improperly fitted shoes.
b. shoes that are too soft.
c. dampness, such as from excessive perspiration.
d. going barefoot.

117. With the TIME wound bed preparation approach, the "M" stands for

a. mechanical debridement.
b. measure of wound.
c. moisture balance.
d. maintenance of circulation.

118. In a chronic wound, which phase of wound healing is generally prolonged?

a. hemostasis
b. inflammatory
c. proliferative
d. maturation

CWOCN Practice Test

119. If an older adult was admitted to the hospital with severe malnutrition and pressure sores and was started on a high protein diet, which of the following laboratory tests is the BEST measure of short-term change in nutritional status?

    a.   prealbumin
    b.   albumin
    c.   transferrin
    d.   total protein

120. In a wound, a biofilm may take on the appearance of

    a.   necrosis.
    b.   slough.
    c.   serosanguinous discharge.
    d.   purulent discharge.

Ostomy Care

1. A 57-year-old male is diagnosed with stage III cancer of the bladder with invasion of the muscle tissue. Which primary treatment is *MOST* common?

- a. partial or segmental cystectomy
- b. interstitial radiation only
- c. radical cystectomy with urinary diversion and chemotherapy
- d. chemotherapy only

2. Which of the following stomal complications indicates a need for surgical intervention?

- a. slight bleeding when changing stomal appliance
- b. slow oozing at one area of the mucocutaneous juncture
- c. slow bleeding at mucocutaneous juncture and caput medusa
- d. frank bleeding from the mucocutaneous juncture

3. Within what period of time postoperatively should an ileostomy begin to excrete stool?

- a. immediately
- b. 24 to 48 hours
- c. 2 to 3 days
- d. 4 to 5 days

4. A male patient develops painful red pustular lesions about the peristomal area. The most likely diagnosis is

- a. candidiasis.
- b. folliculitis.
- c. contact dermatitis.
- d. trauma.

5. A patient with a colostomy develops herpes zoster with lesions in the peristomal area. The draining lesions are interfering with pouch adhesion. The *BEST* solution is to

- a. apply hydrocolloid dressing to lesions.
- b. apply barrier paste to lesions.
- c. leave appliance off until the lesions heal.
- d. mechanically debride lesions by washing and drying.

6. Which is the most effective type of pouching system for a retracted stoma?

- a. concave pouching system
- b. large pouching system without rigid rings
- c. transparent pouching system
- d. convex pouching system with a belt

7. In the PLISSIT model for communicating about sexuality, at which level should the nurse discuss topics such as the use of lubricants and pouch covers?

- a. level one
- b. level two
- c. level three
- d. level four

8. Peristomal abscess is most commonly associated with

   a. Crohn's disease.
   b. systemic bacterial infection.
   c. paralytic ileus.
   d. ulcerative colitis.

9. Which is the *MOST* common method to ensure correct placement of the stoma during surgery?

   a. careful written instructions
   b. marking site with permanent marker or tattoo
   c. marking site by making circular scratches with a small-gauge needle
   d. photograph of abdomen with site indicated

10. Which type of colostomy creates one or two stomas, usually in the upper abdomen in the middle or on the right side?

   a. descending
   b. transverse
   c. ascending
   d. end

11. A loop colostomy is usually performed for

   a. simplicity of procedure.
   b. inflammatory bowel disease.
   c. permanent fecal diversion.
   d. short-term fecal diversion.

12. When a patient is doing a colostomy irrigation, what is the correct level for the bottom of the irrigation bag?

   a. above the head
   b. shoulder level
   c. level with the stoma
   d. level with the umbilicus

13. Which of the following groups of symptoms indicates obstruction of an ileostomy?

   a. dry mouth and tongue, poor skin turgor, weight loss, diarrhea, and lethargy
   b. high fever, abdominal cramping, dry mouth, poor skin turgor, and bloody diarrhea
   c. palpitations, lethargy, fatigue, tinnitus, dyspnea, and headache
   d. edematous stoma, high-pitched bowel sounds, obvious peristaltic waves, distension, dry mouth, abdominal pain, nausea, and vomiting

14. Which of the following is most important to avoid fluid and electrolyte imbalance with an ileostomy?

   a. increase intake of high fiber foods to slow absorption
   b. increase intake of water with diarrhea
   c. take routine antidiarrheal medication
   d. monitor intake and output

15. What is the correct volume and type of fluid to use for an ileostomy lavage?

   a. 500 to 1500 mL warm tap water
   b. 500 mL normal saline
   c. 100 mL warm tap water
   d. 30 to 50 mL normal saline

16. After ileostomy takedown, the BEST functional result is

a. 8 to10 stools per day with no incontinence.
b. 6 to 8 stools per day with nighttime incontinence.
c. 4 to 5 stools per day with no or little incontinence.
d. 6 to 8 stools per day with occasional day and night incontinence.

17. A patient with a loop ileostomy and a retained distal segment of bowel has copious anal discharge of mucus. The most likely cause is

a. normal mucus production.
b. diversion colitis.
c. anastomotic leak.
d. fluid and electrolyte imbalance.

18. In which instance is the surgical intervention of a strictureplasty appropriate for treating Crohn's disease?

a. when the stricture created by the disease is excessively long or several diseased portions of the bowel connect to one another
b. when a diseased portion of the bowel connects to a healthy portion of the bowel
c. when both the colon and the rectum are infected by the disease
d. surgical interventions are contraindicated in the case of Crohn's disease

19. Which of the following complies with the AMA guidelines for informed consent for a patient facing surgery for severe inflammatory bowel disease?

a. the patient is advised to have the ileostomy with Kock pouch because the surgeon has more experience with that procedure
b. the patient is provided a brief summary of possible complications
c. the patient is provided with a number of surgical options
d. the patient is advised to relax and focus on thinking positively

20. Megacolon is associated with which of the following disorders?

a. necrotizing enterocolitis
b. Hirschsprung's disease
c. ulcerative colitis
d. Crohn's disease

21. An imperforate anus with no external opening but rectum in normal position with normal function and no connection to the GU tract is classified as

a. atypical anomalies.
b. low anomalies.
c. intermediate anomalies.
d. high anomalies.

22. Which of the following symptoms are typical of an overactive neurogenic bladder?

a. dribbling
b. straining to urinate
c. urgency
d. retention

23. If the peristomal skin about an ileostomy becomes irritated, which medication(s) may be indicated?

    a. oral antibiotics
    b. topical corticosteroid spray
    c. topical corticosteroid spray and nystatin powder
    d. topical antibiotic ointment

24. What change in ileostomy care is common during pregnancy?

    a. no changes
    b. change in size of appliances
    c. diet modifications
    d. decrease in ileostomy activity

25. The most common colorectal cancers are

    a. adenocarcinomas.
    b. lymphomas.
    c. melanomas.
    d. sarcomas.

26. The nurse is teaching a 45-year-old woman with a colostomy to do irrigations. The nurse has prepared written directions and a video, but the patient ignores them and picks up the equipment and looks at each part, trying to figure it out. The patient's learning style is probably

    a. auditory.
    b. visual.
    c. kinesthetic.
    d. mixed.

27. A 30-year-old woman is hospitalized with severe depression and is incontinent of urine, although the urinary system is normal. The most appropriate nursing diagnosis is

    a. functional urinary incontinence.
    b. stress urinary incontinence.
    c. overflow urinary incontinence.
    d. urge urinary incontinence.

28. Which foods should be included in the diet of those with an ileostomy to reduce odor?

    a. spinach and parsley
    b. milk products
    c. fish
    d. broccoli and asparagus

29. Which agents can be used by those with ileostomies to treat constipation?

    a. osmotic agents, such as Milk of Magnesia®
    b. stimulant agents (such as Dulcolax®)
    c. mineral oil
    d. stool softeners, such as Colace®

30. A 72-year-old female is being discharged from the acute hospital with a colostomy. She is intelligent and cooperative, but is very nervous about caring for her colostomy at home, despite demonstrations and practice. Which is the MOST effective solution?

    a.   a home health agency referral
    b.   printed materials about colostomy care
    c.   a video showing colostomy care
    d.   instruction of family member to assist

31. Ureteral stents are placed postoperatively with a urostomy. On day three, the urine becomes cloudy with purulent discharge. Which action is indicated?

    a.   stent removal
    b.   gentle irrigation with 5 to 10 mL of normal saline
    c.   irrigation under pressure with 5 to 10 mL of normal saline
    d.   surgical revision

32. One of the *FIRST* indications of urostomy infection is

    a.   change in character and/or amount of urine.
    b.   fever and chills.
    c.   backache.
    d.   nausea and vomiting.

33. The *BEST* method to obtain a urine specimen for a culture and sensitivity from a patient with a urostomy is to

    a.   drain urine from the urostomy bag into a sterile container.
    b.   remove bag, cleanse peristomal skin, and hold sterile container below stoma.
    c.   remove bag, apply a new bag, and drain urine from the new bag into a sterile container.
    d.   remove bag, cleanse peristomal skin, and catheterize stoma with #14 straight catheter to obtain specimen.

34. Which is the *BEST* method to manage mucus in the urine after a urostomy?

    a.   increase fluid intake
    b.   acidify urine
    c.   irrigate urostomy
    d.   limit dairy products

35. Which of the following medications may not be absorbed completely or at all with continent cutaneous fecal diversions?

    a.   liquid medications
    b.   enteric-coated medications
    c.   uncoated medications
    d.   parenteral medications

36. Which of the following sets of symptoms would most likely indicate pouchitis for an individual with fecal diversion?

    a.   decrease in frequency of stools, abdominal pain, itching, and fever
    b.   increase in frequency of stools, dehydration, abdominal pain, and fever
    c.   itching, dehydration, bloody stools, and fever.
    d.   decrease in frequency of stools, dehydration, and fever

CWOCN Practice Test

37. Which is the *MOST* appropriate method of cleansing the perianal area after ileal pouch anal anastomosis (IPAA)?

    a.   scrub the area with soap and water
    b.   rinse with warm water using a squirt bottle or spray
    c.   wash the area gently with povidone-iodine solution
    d.   wash gently with chlorhexidine gluconate 4% (Hibiclens®) solution

38. Which of the following breakfast choices is best to maintain acidic urine after continent cutaneous urinary diversions?

    a.   fruit plate, yogurt, and tea
    b.   orange juice, sliced bananas with yogurt, milk
    c.   cheese, sliced oranges and apples, and milk
    d.   cranberry juice, scrambled eggs, whole grain toast, and prunes

39. What is the target intubation schedule for one month after surgery for continent cutaneous urinary diversion?

    a.   every 2 hours during the day and every 3 hours at night
    b.   every 3 hours during the day and every 4 hours at night
    c.   every 4 hours during the day and every 5 hours at night
    d.   every 5 hours during the day and every 6 hours at night

40. Which of the following is utilized to promote bladder control after removal of the postoperative Foley catheter for orthotopic neobladder?

    a.   pelvic floor/Kegel exercises
    b.   scheduled straight catheterizations
    c.   scheduled urination every 2 to 4 hours indefinitely
    d.   fluid restriction in the evening

41. Where do most anorectal fistulae originate?

    a.   perineal skin
    b.   rectum
    c.   anal glands
    d.   anal sphincter

42. What type of nutritional support is indicated with enterocutaneous fistulae affecting both the small intestine and the colon?

    a.   enteral nutrition
    b.   total parenteral nutrition (TPN)
    c.   oral liquid diet
    d.   oral soft diet

43. A fistula that drains 300 mL in 24 hours would be classified by volume as

    a.   low output.
    b.   small to medium output.
    c.   high output.
    d.   extreme output.

44. Using the Parks classification system for anorectal fistulae, how would a fistula that extends from the internal sphincter, down to the perineum, and up to a blind tract or into the rectum be classified?

   a. intersphincteric
   b. transsphincteric
   c. suprasphincteric
   d. extrasphincteric

45. Which treatment option should be used *FIRST* for peristomal hyperplasia about an enteral feeding tube?

   a. cauterization with silver nitrate
   b. application of topical corticosteroid (such as triamcinolone or Kenalog)
   c. debridement
   d. resiting of tube

46. The *FIRST* step in cauterization of peristomal hyperplasia with silver nitrate sticks is to

   a. moisten the silver nitrate sticks with sterile water.
   b. reapply 2 to 3 times weekly until resolved.
   c. run the tip of the silver nitrate stick over the hyperplastic tissue using a rolling motion.
   d. apply a skin barrier around the hyperplastic tissue.

47. How much space should be left between the external bumper and the skin to prevent excessive traction and buried bumper syndrome?

   a. 0.5 cm
   b. 1.0 cm
   c. 1.5 cm
   d. 2 cm

48. Which of the following is indicated to prevent occlusion of enteral feeding tubes used for intermittent or continuous feeding?

   a. flush with 30 mL water every 8 hours or after feedings and medication administration
   b. flush with 30 mL water every 8 hours and before feedings and medication administration
   c. flush with 30 mL of water every 4 hours
   d. flush with 30 mL of water every 4 hours and before and after feedings and medication administration

49. The patient has a percutaneous endoscopic gastrostomy (PEG) and has developed leakage about the tube. What INITIAL intervention is indicated?

   a. check the balloon to ensure adequate inflation
   b. stabilize the tube with the bumper and external stabilizer
   c. replace the tube
   d. apply barrier ointment

50. Which is the BEST method for nighttime management of a urostomy?

   a. empty the bag right before bed
   b. attach a leg bag to the appliance to hold overflow
   c. limit fluid intake in the evening to decrease urinary output
   d. attach a long tube and an overnight urinary drainage bag

51. A patient with an ileostomy has developed hyponatremia when the sodium value drops to

   a. <145 mEq.
   b. <135 mEq.
   c. <130 mEq.
   d. <125 mEq.

52. A low profile percutaneous feeding tube is recommended for pediatric patients because

    a. it is less uncomfortable.

    b. it is easier to insert.

    c. it is less likely to become dislodged.

    d. it has fewer complications.

53. Which of the following is a critical element of active listening?

    a. providing feedback

    b. remaining passive

    c. focusing only the speaker's words

    d. making constant eye contact

54. Which of the following is a measure to prevent buried bumper syndrome with a percutaneous endoscopic gastrostomy (PEG) tube?

    a. rotate the tube daily

    b. place a dressing under the external fixation device

    c. flush the tube before feedings

    d. mark the tube where it exits the skin

55. When using a closed suction system to manage a high-output fistula, the suction catheter is positioned

    a. 4 to 5 cm inside the fistula orifice.

    b. 1 to 2 cm inside the fistula orifice.

    c. 4 cm away from the fistula orifice.

    d. next to the fistula orifice.

56. How long after a percutaneous endoscopic gastrostomy (PEG) is performed is the tract usually mature and well-healed enough for placement of a balloon gastrostomy tube (G-tube)?

    a. 4 to 7 days

    b. 2 to 4 weeks

    c. 1 to 2 months

    d. 3 to 4 months

57. If a patient complains of difficulty keeping a seal of an ostomy appliance because of a bulge on one side of the stoma, the most likely cause is

    a. parastomal hernia.

    b. tumor.

    c. abscess.

    d. constipation.

58. Management of severe stomal stenosis usually requires

    a. intermittent use of a dilator.

    b. surgical repair.

    c. regular use of a dilator.

    d. dietary modifications.

59. If a patient with a colostomy has a new onset of loose stools, the nurse should initially review the patient's

    a. medication history.

    b. activity level.

    c. fluid intake.

    d. food history.

60. **If an ostomy pouch has a drainable spout, it is usually positioned at**

    a. 12 o'clock.
    b. 9 o'clock.
    c. 6 o'clock.
    d. 3 o'clock.

61. **An ostomy pouch with a deodorizing gas filter works best with**

    a. any type of output.
    b. formed stool.
    c. semi-liquid stool.
    d. liquid stool.

62. **When preparing a cut-to-fit ostomy pouch, the patient should be taught to**

    a. trace the stoma on a piece of plastic wrap.
    b. measure the stoma diameter with a ruler.
    c. start with a small opening and gradually enlarge.
    d. make a template out of a piece of paper and use as a pattern.

63. **Stomal retraction is most common in patients who are**

    a. young adults.
    b. older adults.
    c. very thin.
    d. obese.

64. **A clear pouch should be used over the stoma in the immediate postoperative period in order to**

    a. monitor output.
    b. begin patient acceptance of stoma.
    c. allow stomal assessment.
    d. prevent mechanical trauma.

65. **If the patient is markedly obese with a very large abdomen, the stoma**

    a. should be sited as usual.
    b. may need to be sited higher than usual.
    c. may need to be sited lower than usual.
    d. should be on the usual beltline.

66. **If, following an emergent traumatic injury, a 25-year old patient required a colectomy and permanent end colostomy, but the patient has become increasingly withdrawn and shows evidence of suicidal ideation, the most appropriate response is to**

    a. refer the patient for psychological counseling.
    b. ask a volunteer ostomate to visit the patient.
    c. suggest the patient join a support group.
    d. encourage the patient to participate in care.

67. **If a patient develops granulomas at the peristomal skin/stoma juncture, the treatment of choice is usually**

    a. surgical debridement.
    b. mechanical debridement.
    c. electrical cauterization.
    d. silver nitrate cauterization.

68. Sodium phosphate bowel prep is usually more acceptable to patients than polyethylene glycol preparations because sodium phosphate

 a. works faster.
 b. spares electrolytes.
 c. has a pleasant taste.
 d. has low volume.

69. The two primary concerns of ostomy patients are

 a. inconvenience and discomfort.
 b. embarrassment and shame.
 c. odor control and leakage.
 d. pain and physical limitations.

70. When assessing the postoperative condition of a fecal stoma, the nurse expects the stoma to be

 a. flush with the skin.
 b. deep red in color.
 c. light pink in color.
 d. grossly edematous.

71. Ideally a stoma, such as for an end ileostomy, should protrude from the skin by approximately

 a. 1 to 2 cm.
 b. 2 to 3 cm.
 c. 3 to 4 cm.
 d. 4 to 5 cm.

72. The ideal site for a stoma is in which muscle?

 a. internal oblique
 b. external oblique
 c. rectus abdominus
 d. latissimus dorsi

73. Following construction of an Indiana pouch, irrigation is usually carried out with

 a. 20 to 30 mL NS two times daily.
 b. 20 to 30 mL NS four times daily.
 c. 30 to 60 mL NS two times daily.
 d. 30 to 60 mL NS four times daily.

74. The continent ileostomy (Kock pouch) is currently

 a. the procedure of choice for ulcerative colitis.
 b. used primarily as a backup for IPAA failure.
 c. no longer advised because of complications.
 d. used only for patients with Crohn's disease.

75. The ileal pouch anal anastomosis (IPAA) is not routinely recommended for patients with Crohn's disease because of

 a. increased risk of pouch failure/pouch-associated fistulae.
 b. increased risk of postoperative hemorrhage.
 c. patient resistance to the procedure.
 d. prolonged period of healing and limited mobility required.

76. **Patients with a perineal wound should be reminded to avoid using a donut cushion because**

    a. it provides no relief from discomfort.
    b. it causes increased blood flow and risk of bleeding.
    c. it causes pulling of the incision and decreased blood flow.
    d. it increases the risk of skin irritation.

77. **If a patient with inflammatory bowel disease presents with hair loss, weight loss, balance problems, decreased energy and fatigue, the nurse should suspect**

    a. electrolyte imbalance.
    b. systemic infection.
    c. depression/anxiety.
    d. malnutrition.

78. **The most common surgical procedure for Crohn's disease is removal of the**

    a. terminal jejunum and proximal ileum.
    b. terminal ileum and cecum.
    c. cecum and proximal ascending colon.
    d. ileum only.

79. **With extensive ulcerative colitis, the distance (measured from the anal verge) of involved tissue is**

    a. 20 cm.
    b. 35 to 40 cm.
    c. >60 cm.
    d. entire colon.

80. **If a patient with an ileal pouch anal anastomosis (IPAA) experiences anal burning and loose stools after eating certain foods, the treatment may include**

    a. bile salt binding agents.
    b. simethicone.
    c. loperamide.
    d. corticosteroid.

81. **If a patient has developed skin irritation about a biliary tube, the best solution is to apply**

    a. barrier paste.
    b. barrier cream.
    c. barrier wafer cut to fit around tube.
    d. alcohol-free liquid skin barrier.

82. **The most common cause of bladder cancer is**

    a. genetic predisposition.
    b. smoking (tobacco).
    c. alcohol abuse.
    d. environmental toxins.

83. **If siting both a fecal and a urinary stoma, the urinary stoma should be**

    a. the same height as the fecal stoma.
    b. at least one inch lower than the fecal stoma.
    c. at least one inch higher than the fecal stoma.
    d. on the opposite side of the abdomen from the fecal stoma.

84. A patient with an ileostomy should be advised that the best way to take fluids is

a. by themselves without food.
b. together with food.
c. before eating.
d. after eating.

85. What percentage of patients with an ileal pouch anal anastomosis (IPAA) develop chronic pouchitis?

a. 5%
b. 10%
c. 30%
d. 40%

86. If a patient has familial adenomatous polyposis (FAP), the chance of developing colon cancer by age 40 is

a. 100%.
b. 75%.
c. 50%.
d. 25%.

87. A moderate output enterocutaneous fistula is one with an output of

a. 100 to 200 mL/24 hours.
b. 500 to 700 mL/24 hours.
c. 200 to 500 mL/24 hours.
d. 50 to 100 mL/24 hours.

88. Modifiable risk factors for the development of colorectal cancer include

a. age.
b. high fat/low fiber diet.
c. disease.
d. genetic predisposition.

89. If the physician has ordered that a nephrostomy tube be flushed because of mucus and sediment in the urine, the irrigation should be done with

a. 30 to 40 mL NS.
b. 20 to 30 mL NS.
c. 10 to 20 mL NS.
d. 5 to 10 mL NS.

90. Which of the following is characteristic of ulcerative colitis?

a. superficial mucosal penetration
b. patchy areas of inflammation
c. presence of fistulae
d. presence of granulomas

91. The first step in managing stomal trauma is to

a. change the type/size of pouch.
b. apply topical antibiotic to prevent infection.
c. identify the cause.
d. apply skin barrier cream to the stoma.

92. If a patient has a proximal enterocutaneous fistula, the primary concern is

a. odor.
b. cutaneous periwound condition.
c. pain.
d. nutrition.

93. Most cases of metastatic melanoma to the gastrointestinal system occur in the

a. rectum.
b. stomach.
c. small intestine.
d. colon.

94. A patient with a high output ileostomy should avoid drinking excessive hypotonic fluids, such as water, fruit juice, and soda, because they

a. increase risk of hypernatremia.
b. increase risk of hyponatremia.
c. can lead to increased thirst.
d. increase risk of leakage.

95. If a patient has an ileal pouch anal anastomosis (IPAA) and has become pregnant, the patient should be advised that she may experience

a. increased frequency of stools and fecal incontinence.
b. increased incidence of pouchitis.
c. decreased frequency of stools.
d. increased risk of stillbirth.

96. If a patient is undergoing video capsule endoscopy for Crohn's disease, a primary concern is

a. infection.
b. capsule retention.
c. intestinal perforation.
d. allergic response.

97. If an 80-year-old male patient lives with his 72-year-old wife and is about to be discharged with a new colostomy that will require irrigations, but the patient is too frail to carry out the irrigations independently and his wife is still confused about the procedure, which of the following is likely the BEST plan?

a. transfer the patient to a convalescent hospital
b. keep the patient in the hospital until the wife is more capable
c. advise the patient to hire someone to assist with the irrigations
d. refer the patient to a home health agency for assistance

98. If, when the urostomy appliance is removed after 4 days, the skin is clear but there is erosion in the peristomal area of the barrier of the appliance, this means that

a. the appliance should be changed less frequently.
b. the appliance could be changed more frequently.
c. the appliance performed as expected.
d. the appliance was the wrong size.

99. If a 64-year-old female client has recently had surgery for colon cancer and has a colostomy, but the client has been resistive to educational efforts and refuses to look at the colostomy, the MOST appropriate intervention is

    a. remain supportive and encourage client to express feelings.
    b. remind the client that she will have to soon assume self-care.
    c. insist that the client assist in care of the colostomy.
    d. ask a family member to assume responsibility for colostomy care.

100. If a Vietnamese immigrant patient had surgery for a bowel resection and colostomy but has not requested pain medicine in the 6 hours after returning from the recovery room to his room on the surgical unit, the nurse should assume the patient

    a. has no pain.
    b. is insensitive to pain.
    c. is reluctant to complain of pain.
    d. has not recovered from anesthesia.

101. When teaching a patient to irrigate a colostomy, how much fluid should the patient be advised to use for the irrigation?

    a. 200 to 500 mL
    b. 500 to 700 mL
    c. 500 to 1000 mL
    d. 1000 to 1500 mL

102. Which of the following is the best choice to protect the skin from drainage from a high-output fistula?

    a. moisture barrier powder
    b. skin barrier spray
    c. absorbant dressings
    d. moisture barrier cream

103. When siting the stoma for a woman who is 6 months pregnant, the stoma site should be

    a. in the same position as for non-pregnant patients.
    b. in the same horizontal plane as the umbilicus.
    c. more medial than the usual site.
    d. more lateral than the usual site.

104. Most bacteria that is ingested orally is eliminated by

    a. gastric alkalinity.
    b. gastric acidity.
    c. intestinal bile.
    d. intestinal villi.

105. Absorption of nutrients, electrolytes, vitamins, and minerals takes place primarily in the

    a. stomach.
    b. small intestine.
    c. ascending colon.
    d. descending colon.

106. Penrose drains are usually kept in a wound postoperatively for

a. 1 to 2 days.
b. 2 to 3 days.
c. 3 to 5 days.
d. 6 to 7 days.

107. Most colorectal lymphomas are located in the

a. cecum/ascending colon.
b. transverse colon.
c. descending colon
d. sigmoid colon/rectum.

108. If a patient is diagnosed with rectal cancer, which of the following TNM classifications generally indicate the need for transanal excision only?

a. T4
b. T3N2
c. T2N0
d. T1N0

109. Most electrolyte loss occurs through

a. urine.
b. respirations.
c. feces.
d. perspiration.

110. If a colonoscopy shows a fragmented polyp with invasive cancer, the likely treatment will be

a. remove the polyp and observe the patient.
b. adjuvant therapy only.
c. colectomy, removal of lymph nodes, and possible diversion.
d. colectomy, removal of lymph nodes, diversion, and adjuvant therapy.

111. Carcinoid tumors are most common in which of the following ethnic groups?

a. Asians
b. African Americans
c. Hispanics
d. Caucasians

112. Which of the following makes patients with Crohn's disease more refractory to treatment?

a. older age
b. obesity
c. alcohol use
d. smoking

113. A patient with Crohn's disease is especially at risk for which of the following vitamin deficiencies?

a. B12
b. B6
c. C
d. D

114. With ulcerative colitis, which of the following is an indication for urgent surgery?

    a.   chronic steroid dependency
    b.   refractory disease
    c.   adenocarcinoma
    d.   toxic megacolon

115. If a patient has a subtotal colectomy with ileostomy and a Hartman's pouch for Crohn's disease, the patient should be told to expect

    a.   no issues with the Hartman's pouch.
    b.   to feel the urge to defecate and pass mucus periodically.
    c.   to feel no urge to defecate but leak mucus.
    d.   periodic cramping pain in the Hartman's pouch.

116. If a male patient who is 6 weeks postoperative with an ileal pouch anal anastomosis (IPAA) complains of difficulty achieving an erection and engaging in sexual activity and seems quite distressed, the MOST appropriate referral is to a

    a.   urologist.
    b.   gastroenterologist.
    c.   sex therapist.
    d.   psychologist.

117. If a patient with Crohn's disease is considering surgery to create an ileostomy, the most important role of the nurse is to

    a.   provide encouragement and reassurance.
    b.   stress the positive aspects of an ileostomy.
    c.   stress the negative aspects of an ileostomy.
    d.   provide information about the procedure.

118. When a patient undergoing a 3-stage proctocolectomy and ileal pouch anal anastomosis (IPAA) procedure has the end ileostomy changed to a temporary loop ileostomy, the patient is especially at increased risk of

    a.   infection.
    b.   dehydration.
    c.   dehiscence.
    d.   hemorrhage.

119. If a patient has an ileostomy, which type of foods is most indicated to thicken the stool?

    a.   fats
    b.   dairy foods
    c.   starchy foods
    d.   high protein foods

120. Which of the following is a contraindication to negative pressure wound therapy (NPWT) for an enterocutaneous fistula?

    a.   exposed bowel at wound base
    b.   lack of pseudostoma
    c.   no potential for spontaneous closure
    d.   indications of infection in the wound

Continence Care

1. Which is the *BEST* solution for chemical trauma in the perianal and genital area from incontinence of urine and feces in an 87-year-old patient?

    a. apply moisture barrier paste
    b. apply solid moisture barrier
    c. apply skin barrier powder
    d. leave skin open to the air

2. What percentage of the fluid does the colon absorb from the stool as the stool traverses the bowel?

    a. 30%
    b. 40%
    c. 60%
    d. 90%

3. Which of the following occurs during phase I (filling/storing) of the urination process?

    a. spinal nerves contract the detrusor muscles
    b. spinal nerves relax internal sphincter muscles
    c. neurotransmitters signal the detrusor muscles to relax
    d. external sphincter muscles relax

4. With the Bristol Stool Form, which of the following stool types is described as sausage-shaped and lumpy with cracks on the surface?

    a. type 1
    b. type 2
    c. type 3
    d. type 4

5. Postinfectious irritable bowel syndrome (PI-IBS) is characterized most commonly by

    a. fever.
    b. altered bowel habits with chronic diarrhea.
    c. constipation.
    d. flu-like symptoms.

6. Which of the following is a typical a symptom associated with rectoceles?

    a. chronic constipation
    b. chronic diarrhea
    c. pulling sensation in pelvic area
    d. vaginal discharge

7. The PRIMARY cause of fecal incontinence with anorectal fistulae is

    a. pain.
    b. inflammation and tissue damage.
    c. loss of sensation.
    d. leakage of stool from fistula.

8. Which of the following disorders can result in chronic constipation and incontinence because of damage to the myelin sheath and underlying nerve fibers in the brain, eyes, and spinal cord?

    a. Amyotrophic lateral sclerosis (ALS)
    b. Parkinson's disease (PD)
    c. Muscular dystrophy (MD)
    d. Multiple sclerosis (MS)

CWOCN Practice Test

9. The Q-tip test measures

    a. strength of the pelvic floor muscles.

    b. duration of bladder contractions.

    c. length of urethra.

    d. mobility and axis position of the urethra.

10. During the provocative stress test (urinary cough test), what position should the patient be placed in for the first part of the test?

    a. supine position

    b. standing with one leg on stool

    c. prone

    d. sitting

11. Which of the following is included on the mini-mental status exam?

    a. reading text and then summarizing

    b. timed reading test

    c. counting backward by 7s or spelling "world" backward

    d. drawing the face of a clock with 12 numbers and hands indicating a specific time

12. Which test measures the pressure of the anal sphincter muscles, degree of rectal sensation, and neural reflexes?

    a. anal wink

    b. bulbocavernosus reflex

    c. endoanal ultrasound

    d. anal manometry

13. Which of the following groups of foods should be avoided to prevent gas with a colostomy?

    a. cabbage, broccoli, kale, onions, turnips, brussel sprouts, asparagus, dried beans, fish, eggs, and strong cheeses

    b. applesauce, bananas, cheese, creamy peanut butter, potatoes, rice, pasta, marshmallows

    c. apple juice, prune juice fresh fruit, raw vegetables, spicy foods, fried foods

    d. dried fruits, fruits with skin, tree nuts, popcorn, whole corn, bean sprouts, celery, and large servings of raw fruits or vegetables

14. When patients keep a bladder diary, which description is estimated as equaling 30 to 60 mL volume of urinary incontinence?

    a. slight spot of dampness in underwear

    b. underwear wet

    c. underwear soaked with overflow down legs

    d. clothes soaked and overflow on floor or furniture

15. The patient is scheduled for anal sphincter electromyography. Which of the patient's medications should be stopped prior to the EMG?

    a. stool softener

    b. anticholinergic

    c. antibiotic

    d. warfarin

16. The normal specific gravity of urine is

a. 1.000 to 1.010.
b. 1.010 to 1.015.
c. 1.015 to 1.025.
d. 1.025 to 1.035.

17. When a person is doing a 24-hour pad test at home, which of the following is necessary?

a. sealing wet pads in plastic bags and storing
b. counting the number of pads used in a day
c. leaving the same pad in place for 24 hours
d. changing pads every 8 hours

18. Which of the following tests assess bladder capacity and pressure, including how full the bladder is when the urge to urinate is felt?

a. electromyography
b. uroflowmetry
c. pressure flow study
d. cystometry

19. A reduced Valsalva leak point pressure indicates

a. stress incontinence.
b. urge incontinence.
c. functional incontinence.
d. overflow incontinence.

20. When fitting a patient with a pessary for second-degree cystocele, which is correct?

a. the smallest possible pessary should be used
b. a finger should pass easily between the vaginal wall and the pessary
c. a finger should not be able to pass between the vaginal wall and the pessary.
d. should always begin with ring pessaries

21. Chronic pelvic pain syndrome results from

a. unknown etiology.
b. bacterial infection.
c. trauma.
d. viral infection.

22. Which of the following medical treatments is used to reduce urinary frequency and incontinence in patients with multiple sclerosis?

a. prophylactic low dose antibiotics
b. diuretics (such as furosemide)
c. anticholinergics (such as oxybutynin or tolterodine)
d. muscle relaxers (such as baclofen)

23. The average age for menopause is

a. 50.
b. 49.
c. 53.
d. 51.

CWOCN Practice Test

371

24. Which of the following is the *MOST* significant factor in developing urinary incontinence?

    a. obesity
    b. diuretic use
    c. history of human papillomavirus
    d. history of oral contraceptive use

25. In a functional assessment, support from family or friends is evaluated as

    a. nonfunction related.
    b. psychological function.
    c. sensory function.
    d. social function.

26. Which environmental factor may *MOST* likely contribute to incontinence in a patient with severe rheumatoid arthritis affecting the hips, knees, and ankles?

    a. bathroom is on the second floor from kitchen and living room
    b. throw rugs are in place in the hall leading to bathroom
    c. hallway to bathroom is not lit
    d. toilet is too low

27. Which of the following is a bladder irritant?

    a. watermelon
    b. milk
    c. artificial sweetener (aspartame, saccharine)
    d. beef

28. The "knack" is

    a. a method to prevent fecal incontinence.
    b. a method to strengthen pelvic floor muscles.
    c. a method to prevent urge incontinence.
    d. a method to prevent stress incontinence.

29. The "quick flicks" method treats urinary incontinence by

    a. improving contractility.
    b. improving endurance.
    c. improving sensory awareness.
    d. reducing muscle spasms.

30. Which of the following is *MOST* important in controlling constipation?

    a. taking daily stool softener
    b. increasing exercise
    c. increasing dietary fiber and fluids
    d. taking laxatives

31. Incontinence of liquid stool and engorged hemorrhoids are *MOST* indicative of

    a. constipation.
    b. diarrhea.
    c. fecal impaction.
    d. rectal cancer.

32. Which of the following is a good source of soluble fiber?

    a. oat bran
    b. seeds
    c. skins of fruits
    d. bananas

33. When is the best time for scheduled defecation?

    a. 20 to 30 minutes before a meal
    b. 20 to 30 minutes after a meal
    c. first thing in the morning
    d. last thing at night

34. A woman with a coccygeal ulcer has occasional urinary incontinence but has no urinary infection. Which should be the *INITIAL* step in controlling her incontinence?

    a. limited fluid intake
    b. insertion of Foley catheter
    c. anticholinergic medication (such as oxybutynin)
    d. scheduled urination

35. Black tarry stools may be caused by

    a. Rifadin®.
    b. Pepto-Bismol®.
    c. Kaopectate.
    d. Beta-carotene.

36. With nocturnal enuresis, which medication can be taken at bedtime by a female patient to reduce urinary production?

    a. oxybutynin
    b. imipramine
    c. desmopressin
    d. tamsulosin

37. With vaginal weights, correct size is determined by

    a. vaginal measurements.
    b. the heaviest weight that fits comfortably.
    c. the ability to hold the weight for one minute.
    d. the smallest weight that doesn't fall out.

38. The treatment of choice for urge incontinence is

    a. anticholinergics.
    b. reducing bladder irritants.
    c. surgical repair.
    d. bladder training.

39. Which is the *INITIAL* treatment of choice for a male who develops bladder outlet obstruction from benign prostatic hypertrophy?

    a. intermittent catheterization to empty bladder
    b. transurethral prostatectomy
    c. medications, such as alpha-blocker and 5-alpha reductase inhibitor
    d. transurethral needle ablation

40. **The treatment of choice for a male with detrusor sphincter dyssynergia is**
   a. insertion of urethral stent.
   b. external sphincterectomy.
   c. long-term catheterization.
   d. urinary diversion.

41. **Which of the following is recommended to manage detrusor hyperactivity with impaired contractile function (DHIC)?**
   a. anticholinergics
   b. indwelling catheter
   c. double voiding and Credé maneuver
   d. urinary diversion

42. **The most appropriate fecal containment product for an elderly bedridden patient with diminished level of consciousness, intact skin, and incontinence of approximately 400 mL of semi-liquid stool daily is**
   a. fecal pouch with skin barrier.
   b. fecal containment system.
   c. disposable underwear with skin barrier.
   d. refastenable briefs with skin barrier.

43. **A patient with mild dementia lives alone and has increasing urge incontinence, because she forgets to comply with scheduled urination. The best solution is**
   a. disposable underwear.
   b. long-term catheterization.
   c. an alarm.
   d. telephone reminders.

44. **A male using a penile clamp to control moderate urinary incontinence after prostatectomy should release the clamp and urinate**
   a. when the bladder feels full.
   b. every 4 to 6 hours.
   c. after each meal.
   d. every 2 hours.

45. **Which of the following is the *MOST* effective for a physically active woman to use during periods of strenuous exercise to prevent stress incontinence?**
   a. absorbent pads
   b. tampon
   c. urethral plug
   d. valved catheter

46. **The *PRIMARY* purpose of sensory motor reeducation using biofeedback for fecal incontinence is to**
   a. assist in contraction of anal sphincters.
   b. increase sensory perception and control of the muscles of defecation.
   c. assist in relaxation of external anal sphincters.
   d. prevent fecal impaction.

47. Overuse of phosphate enemas to control constipation puts a person at risk for

a. hypermagnesemia and hypocalcemia.
b. hypomagnesemia and hypercalcemia.
c. hypophosphatemia and hypercalcemia.
d. hyperphosphatemia and hypocalcemia.

48. Which of the following procedures is done to expand bladder capacity?

a. augmentation cystoplasty
b. sling procedure
c. tension-free vaginal tape procedure (TVT)
d. retropubic suspension

49. For clean intermittent catheterization at home, which methods of sterilization are MOST effective after first cleaning and drying catheters?

a. boil for 5 minutes or microwave for 3 minutes on high
b. boil for 10 minutes OR microwave on high for 6 minutes with a glass of water in the microwave
c. boil for 5 to 8 minutes
d. microwave for 4 minutes on high with a glass of water in the microwave

50. During pelvic floor electrical stimulation, which serves as a guide that adequate amplitude has been set?

a. anal wink occurs
b. the patient reports muscle contractions
c. standardized setting guidelines have been used
d. the patient feels pain

51. For female patients undergoing anal sphincteroplasty, the most common problem in the postoperative period is

a. infection.
b. difficulty urinating.
c. severe pain.
d. separation of sutures.

52. The first indication that a patient may develop fecal incontinence is

a. flatus incontinence.
b. chronic constipation.
c. mucus incontinence.
d. chronic diarrhea.

53. If a patient is diagnosed with detrusor external sphincter dyssynergia (DESD), the nurse expects the treatment plan to include

a. indwelling catheter.
b. urinary diversion.
c. augmentation cystoplasty.
d. clean intermittent catheterization.

54. If a patient has quit smoking and has been chewing sugar free gum and snacking on carrots, nuts, and celery all day to control cravings, but has developed bloating and recurrent diarrhea, the most likely cause of the diarrhea is

    a. sugar free chewing gum.
    b. carrots.
    c. nuts.
    d. celery.

55. If using ultrasound scanning to decrease obsessive toileting for a patient with overactive bladder, the patient should be urged to delay urination if the bladder volume is less than

    a. 50 to 75 mL.
    b. 100 to 150 mL.
    c. 175 to 200 mL.
    d. 200 to 225 mL.

56. Patients with fecal incontinence often try to self-manage for years before discussing the problem with healthcare providers primarily because they

    a. don't believe help is available.
    b. don't want to bother the healthcare provider.
    c. feel shame and embarrassment about the incontinence.
    d. aren't concerned about the fecal incontinence.

57. The most common cause of fecal incontinence in females is

    a. neurological disease.
    b. obstetric trauma.
    c. constipation and straining.
    d. irritable bowel syndrome.

58. When treating urge urinary incontinence with pelvic floor electrical stimulation, the frequency rate, pps/Hz, should be set at

    a. 13 pps.
    b. 20 pps.
    c. 50 pps.
    d. 100 pps.

59. If a patient is undergoing bladder training and is trying to resist the urge to urinate for one-hour periods but feels a strong urge to urinate after 40 minutes, the patient should be advised to

    a. urinate.
    b. avoid urinating for 20 minutes.
    c. avoid urinating for 1 to 3 minutes.
    d. practice distraction techniques.

60. If the urinalysis is positive for leukocyte esterase, this usually indicates

    a. normal finding.
    b. pregnancy.
    c. pyuria.
    d. fungal infection.

61. Which of the following types of pessaries is MOST appropriate for treatment for cystocele and stress urinary incontinence?

    a. Gehring with knob.
    b. donut.
    c. ring.
    d. Gelhorn soft silicone with standard stem.

62. Smoking increases the risk of urinary incontinence, especially

    a. urge incontinence.
    b. stress incontinence.
    c. overflow incontinence.
    d. functional incontinence.

63. Reservoir fecal incontinence is associated with

    a. anal sphincter damage.
    b. constipation/fecal impaction.
    c. neurological impairment.
    d. decreased colonic or rectal capacity.

64. Which of the following tests is used to determine the amount of fecal material the rectum can accommodate and how effectively the stool is expelled?

    a. anorectal ultrasonography
    b. balloon expulsion test
    c. proctography
    d. anal manometry

65. For patients with fecal incontinence, the most troubling physical effect is generally

    a. sensation of incomplete emptying of bowels.
    b. rectal irritation.
    c. cramping.
    d. urgency.

66. Which of the following medications may relieve flatus incontinence?

    a. psyllium fiber
    b. simethicone
    c. docusate sodium
    d. loperamide

67. During an interview, older patients often fail to mention urinary incontinence because they

    a. forget about it.
    b. don't feel it is burdensome.
    c. believe it is a natural part of aging.
    d. successfully manage it.

68. If a patient with no previous fecal incontinence has developed a sudden onset of slow leakage of stool and a feeling of rectal discomfort, the patient should first be assessed for

    a. rectal cancer.
    b. fecal impaction.
    c. medication-associated incontinence.
    d. internal hemorrhoids.

69. The most common cause of urinary obstruction in older males is

    a.   benign prostatic hyperplasia.
    b.   tumor.
    c.   infection.
    d.   prostatitis.

70. If, following a urethral bulking injection of silicone polymers (Macroplastique®), the patient develops urinary retention, the recommended intervention is

    a.   oxybutynin.
    b.   aspiration of bulking material.
    c.   indwelling catheter.
    d.   intermittent catheterization.

71. Which type of imaging is generally the test of choice for identification of the specific type of fecal incontinence that a patient has?

    a.   X-ray
    b.   CT scan
    c.   anal endoscopic sonography
    d.   MRI

72. If a patient with stress incontinence has been doing Kegel exercises but still finds she experiences occasional slight incontinence when she coughs or sneezes, the nurse should recommend the use of

    a.   the "knack."
    b.   anticholinergics/antimuscarinics.
    c.   adult briefs.
    d.   urethral plug.

73. If a female patient complains of new onset of urinary incontinence, which of the following medications may be implicated?

    a.   stool softener (Colace®)
    b.   thyroid hormone, levothyroxine
    c.   antidiabetic medication, metformin
    d.   alpha blocker, doxazosin (Cardura®)

74. Which of the following is the most common complication after midurethral sling surgery to correct stress incontinence?

    a.   infection
    b.   urinary retention
    c.   cystocele
    d.   erosion of mesh into the urethra

75. If a patient is taking mirabegron (Myrbetriq®) for treatment of overactive bladder, which of the following should be routinely assessed?

    a.   platelet count
    b.   glucose
    c.   blood pressure
    d.   WBC count

76. Which of the following is a contraindication to the use of an internal bowel management system?

    a. diabetes
    b. clotting disorder
    c. neurological disease
    d. heart disease

77. If urinary incontinence is associated with atrophic vaginitis, treatment may include

    a. anticholinergic/antimuscarinic drugs.
    b. muscle relaxant.
    c. topical estrogen cream or vaginal ring.
    d. oral estrogen.

78. What dietary modification is most indicated to help patients control fecal incontinence?

    a. increased fiber
    b. decreased fiber
    c. limited fruit and vegetables
    d. fluid restriction

79. If, when adjusting the amplitude for pelvic floor electrical stimulation, the anal wink is absent, this indicates

    a. a normal response.
    b. nontherapeutic stimulation.
    c. the need for increased ramping.
    d. the need to increase the on/off to a 2:1 ratio.

80. If a patient has been wearing a pessary but has developed chronic constipation associated with the pessary, the BEST solution is to

    a. stop using the pessary.
    b. take stool softeners.
    c. change to a different size or type of pessary.
    d. modify the diet to add more fluids and fiber.

81. The internal fecal management system should be used consecutively for no more than

    a. 29 consecutive days.
    b. 20 consecutive days.
    c. 15 consecutive days.
    d. 7 consecutive days.

82. If a post-menopausal patient has a vaginal balloon (Eclipse® system) inserted to control fecal incontinence, the patient should be advised to remove the device for cleaning

    a. monthly.
    b. every 3 weeks.
    c. every 2 weeks.
    d. every week.

83. When reviewing a patient's management of clean intermittent catheterization, which of the following may indicate increased risk of complications?

    a. carrying out intermittent catheterization 3 times daily
    b. having a urinary output of 1300 mL per day
    c. draining a volume of 200 to 350 mL per catheterization
    d. emptying the bladder completely with each catheterization

84. The saline infusion test is given to assess capacity to retain stool by

    a. triggering peristalsis.

    b. flushing the rectum.

    c. softening the stool.

    d. simulating diarrhea.

85. If a patient with Parkinson's disease has increasing urinary incontinence, has fallen 3 times in recent months, suffers from depression, and exhibits functional decline, these problems would be best categorized as

    a. co-morbidities.

    b. geriatric syndromes.

    c. disabilities.

    d. incidental disorders.

86. What is the normal functional capacity of the bladder?

    a. 200 to 300 mL

    b. 300 to 400 mL

    c. 400 to 600 mL

    d. 600 to 800 mL

87. If a family member complains that an 80-year-old patient with multiple health problems (including arthritis) repeatedly urinates on the floor during the night on the way to the bathroom, which is down the hall, the best solution is likely

    a. bedside commode.

    b. catheterization.

    c. fluid restriction in the evening.

    d. adult briefs.

88. If, as part of a bowel-training program, the patient has daily scheduled defecation, what is the BEST time to schedule a bowel movement?

    a. first thing in the morning after arising

    b. at bedtime

    c. 2 hours after a meal

    d. 20 to 30 minutes after a meal

89. If a patient has developed urinary incontinence and has been researching all different treatment options and comes with a list of questions for the physician, the type of coping strategy this exemplifies is

    a. cognitive adaptation.

    b. behavioral adaptation.

    c. emotion-focused adaptation.

    d. avoidance/denial.

90. If a patient is undergoing the balloon (50 mL) expulsion test to assess defecatory disorders, and the patient requires 4 minutes to expel the balloon, this indicates

    a. normal defecation.

    b. hyperactive bowel.

    c. dyssynergic defecatory muscle action.

    d. decreased rectal capacity.

91. If an outbreak of *Clostridioides difficile* has resulted in 20 patients in a medical-surgical unit becoming infected and developing severe diarrhea, the breakdown in process that likely caused the outbreak is related to

a. ventilation.
b. handwashing.
c. housekeeping.
d. food handling.

92. Which of the following is likely to have the greatest impact on a patient's access to quality healthcare?

a. socioeconomic status
b. age and gender
c. race/ethnicity
d. place of residence

93. The most important factor in ensuring compliance with the treatment regimen is

a. education.
b. follow-up.
c. therapeutic relationship.
d. cost.

94. Which of the following is an example of functional incontinence?

a. the patient must strain to initiate urine flow and often leaks urine
b. the patient has impaired mobility and often cannot get to the toilet in time
c. the patient tends to leak urine when engaging in strenuous exercise
d. the patient experiences sudden intense urge to urinate and leakage of urine

95. If a 76-year-old female patient complains of nocturnal enuresis but denies having any problem during the daytime, the likely contributing cause is

a. urinary tract infection.
b. nocturnal confusion.
c. medication-associated sphincter impairment.
d. nocturnal polyuria.

96. Overactive bladder in males is most often associated with

a. cancer.
b. dementia.
c. bladder outlet obstruction.
d. smoking.

97. If a patient with urinary incontinence shows the nurse a small notebook that lists all the available toilets in the shopping area of the town, this is an example of

a. toilet mapping.
b. obsessive behavior.
c. risk mitigation.
d. self-care.

98. Strategies for defensive urination include

a. restricting fluid intake prior to activities to decrease urination.
b. urinating on a scheduled basis and before activities.
c. urinating and then waiting for a moment and urinating again.
d. wearing absorbant pads to contain urinary leakage.

99. When assessing a patient's manual dexterity and ability to handle self-care, which of the following activities may be used to assess fine motor skills?

  a. lifting the arm from the lap and placing on a table
  b. flexing and extending the elbow
  c. picking up pencils from a table top and placing in a cup
  d. raising the arms over the head while holding weights

100. If a 4-year-old male patient has developed retentive encopresis with leakage of stool, the primary interventions are

  a. psychological counseling.
  b. reward system.
  c. stool softeners and laxatives.
  d. scheduled toileting and dietary changes.

101. When assessing a patient for reversible causes of urinary incontinence using the PRAISED mnemonic, the D stands for

  a. diuretic use.
  b. dehydration/delirium.
  c. briefs.
  d. dementia.

102. If a patient with severe urge incontinence is learning to manage urgency and feels a strong urge to urinate, the patient should

  a. walk slowly to the bathroom.
  b. rush to the bathroom.
  c. sit and wait until the urge passes.
  d. sit on the toilet but try to withhold urination briefly.

103. As part of the bowel diary, the patient is provided a Bristol stool form in order to

  a. help to quantify the amount of stool.
  b. keep tract of the time and date of defecation.
  c. help to identify the type of stool passed.
  d. correlate diet with defecation times.

104. The most common type of urinary incontinence in long-term care facilities is

  a. stress.
  b. overflow.
  c. functional.
  d. urge.

105. Reflex incontinence is urinary leakage that

  a. occurs without a warning sensation.
  b. is accompanied by pain.
  c. is preceded by feeling of urgency.
  d. occurs in response to abdominal pressure.

106. Normal micturition is controlled by the

  a. spinal cord.
  b. bladder.
  c. central nervous system.
  d. urinary sphincters.

107. If a patient is learning pelvic floor exercises to increase muscle strength, for the first week or two, the patient should aim to be able to tighten and hold for

a. 1 second.
b. 5 seconds.
c. 10 seconds.
d. 15 seconds.

108. For a patient with dementia who forgets where the bathroom is and doesn't recognize the bathroom if the door is shut, resulting in periodic urinary incontinence, the best solution is likely

a. adult briefs.
b. prompted voiding.
c. bladder training
d. habit training.

109. In a healthy person, the normal frequency of urination during waking hours is every

a. 1 to 2 hours.
b. 2 to 3 hours.
c. 1 to 4 hours.
d. 2 to 6 hours.

110. If a patient complains that it takes at least 60 seconds to initiate urinary flow, as part of assessment the nurse considers that the normal duration is

a. 15 seconds.
b. 30 seconds.
c. 45 seconds.
d. 60 seconds.

111. A patient is considered to have chronic constipation if the patient has bowel movements fewer than

a. 5 times per week.
b. 4 times per week.
c. 3 times per week.
d. 2 times per week.

112. If a patient needs to increase fiber in the diet, which of the following provides the most concentrated form of dietary fiber?

a. whole grain bread
b. fresh fruits
c. fresh vegetables
d. unprocessed wheat bran

113. Prompted voiding is appropriate for a patient having

a. <2 episodes of urinary incontinence in 12 hours.
b. <4 episodes of urinary incontinence in 12 hours.
c. <6 episode of urinary incontinence in 12 hours.
d. <8 episodes of urinary incontinence in 12 hours.

114. Bisacodyl laxative tablets are classified as

a. stimulants.
b. prokinetic agents.
c. osmotic agents.
d. lubricants.

CWOCN Practice Test

115. Which of the following may increase intestinal fluid secretion and liquid stools?

a. dairy products
b. starchy foods
c. caffeine
d. spicy foods

116. Upon the digital rectal exam for a male patient, a hard lump is felt in the prostate, likely indicating

a. normal prostate.
b. a tumor.
c. hyperplasia.
d. prostatitis.

117. If a bedbound patient is incontinent of frequent loose stools and wears adult briefs but has developed incontinence-associated skin damage, the best solution is likely

a. fecal containment device.
b. more frequent cleansing of skin with soap and water.
c. using underpads only to allow air to reach skin.
d. changing adult briefs every 2 hours.

118. When utilizing habit training for a patient with urinary incontinence and toileting is scheduled every 3 hours, what is the best response to a patient who has the urge to urinate in 2.5 hours?

a. ask the patient to try to wait 5 minutes before urinating
b. ask the patient to try to wait 15 minutes before urinating
c. ask the patient to try to wait 30 minutes before urinating
d. advise the patient to go ahead and urinate

119. If the nurse notes an itchy red oozing rash in the labial folds, under abdominal rolls, in the underarms, and under the breasts of a very obese patient, this most likely indicates

a. intertriginous dermatitis.
b. contact dermatitis.
c. cellulitis.
d. mechanical irritant dermatitis.

120. The most common psychiatric comorbidity with urinary incontinence is

a. generalized anxiety disorder.
b. depression.
c. bipolar disease.
d. obsessive-compulsive disorder.

Answer Key and Explanations

Wound Care

1. B: A fistula extends under normal tissue away from the wound and connects two structures, such as the wound and an organ or the wound and the skin. Undermining occurs when damaged tissue lies underneath intact skin about the wound perimeter. Tunneling is damaged tissue extending from the wound under normal tissue but not opening to the skin or other structures. An abscess is a collection of purulent material in a localized area, often occurring with a fistula.

2. D: Abscesses often form in conjunction with fistulae. Typical indications include erythema, pain, and swelling above the localized area of the abscess. If the abscess is deep within the tissue or within an internal organ, however, obvious signs of abscess formation may not be evident, and symptoms may be less specific, including general malaise, abdominal pain, chills, fever, lethargy, diarrhea, and anorexia. Additional symptoms may be specific to the site of the abscess; for example, a perirenal abscess may cause flank pain.

3. C: Prealbumin is most commonly monitored for acute changes in nutritional status because it has a half-life of only 2 to 3 days. Prealbumin decreases quickly when nutrition is inadequate and rises quickly in response to increased protein intake. Protein intake must be adequate to maintain normal levels of prealbumin.

- Normal value: 16 to 40 mg/dL
- Mild deficiency: 10 to 15mg/dL
- Moderate deficiency: 5 to 9 mg/dL
- Severe deficiency: <5 mg/dL

Total protein levels and transferrin levels may be influenced by many factors, so they are not reliable measures of nutritional status. Albumin has a half-life of 18 to 20 days, so it is more sensitive to long-term protein deficiencies than to short-term deficiencies.

4. A: Proliferation (days 5 to 20) is characterized by granulation tissue starting to form at wound perimeter, contracting the wound, and epithelialization, resulting in scar formation. Hemostasis (within minutes) occurs as platelets seal off the vessels and the clotting mechanism begins. Inflammation (days 1 to days 4 to 6) is characterized by erythema and edema as phagocytosis removes debris. During maturation or remodeling (days 21 plus), scar tissue continues to form until the scar has about 80% of its original tissue strength and the wound closes; the underlying tissue continues to remodel for up to 18 months.

5. B: Eutectic Mixture of Local Anesthetics (EMLA Cream) is applied thickly (1/4 inch) to both the surface of the wound and surrounding tissue, extending about 1/2 inch past the wound. After application, the wound must be covered with plastic wrap for 20 to 60 minutes to numb the tissue. EMLA cream is effective for about an hour after the wrapping is removed. EMLA can interact with a number of different medications, such as antiarrhythmics, anticonvulsants, and acetaminophen, so medications should be carefully reviewed prior to administration.

6. D: Normal saline is the most appropriate wound-cleansing solution. Antiseptic solutions should be avoided as they may damage granulation tissue and retard healing because they interfere with fibroblast cells necessary for healing of the wound, cause increased pain, and do not significantly reduce overall bacterial load. In heavily-contaminated or necrotic wounds, topical antiseptic solutions, such as dilute povidone-iodine or hydrogen peroxide, may be used for a short period of time to reduce surface bacteria and foul odor.

7. A: A 35-mL syringe with 19-gauge needle provides irrigation pressure at about 8 psi. A squeeze bottle (250 mL) provides about 4.5 psi, but a bulb syringe usually only provides ≤2 psi. Both syringe/catheter and needle

385

size affect irrigant pressure. Pressures <4 psi do not provide adequate wound cleansing, but pressures >15 psi can result in wound trauma.

- 6 mL/19 gauge = 30 psi
- 12 mL/19 gauge = 20 psi
- 12 mL/22 gauge = 13 psi
- 35mL/21 gauge = 6 psi
- 35mL/25 gauge = 4 psi

8. C: Perceptions and expressions of pain vary widely from one individual to another, so the most important criterion for evaluating pain is the patient's own report of pain. Cultural differences have a role in how people express pain, with some cultures typically appearing more stoic than others. Using a 1 to 10 pain scale is an effective tool for people who are cognitively alert. If people are not able to report their pain level, then observation of behavior and facial expressions may give clues to their need for pain medication.

9. A: Hypoalbuminemia is likely to have the most negative effect on wound healing. Hypoalbuminemia is an indication of protein malnutrition (kwashiorkor) and may cause delayed wound healing because of inadequate nutrition. A BMI of 20.2 is within normal range (18.5 to 24.9) and indicates normal weight. A person with a BMI of 29 is overweight, but not obese. Both being underweight (BMI <18.5) and obese (BMI ☐30) can interfere with the body's ability to heal. BMI alone is not adequate to assess nutritional status or healing ability, and vegan diets can provide adequate nutrition.

10. A: The most definitive method of obtaining a wound specimen for culture and sensitivities is a tissue biopsy. A needle biopsy can also provide an adequate sample in many cases. Swabbing a wound with a sterile applicator often does not provide an adequate sample, because this method obtains material only from the wound surface, which may include both pathogenic agents from the wound and contamination from skin bacteria. The tissue itself must be cultured, not just the discharge.

11. B: Corticosteroids may impair wound healing by interfering with vascular proliferation and epithelialization. The anti-inflammatory effect may interfere with the inflammatory phase of healing by decreasing migration of macrophages and polymorphonuclear leukocytes to the wound, interfering with angiogenesis, and increasing susceptibility to wound infection. Other drugs that may impair healing include vasoconstrictors, NSAIDs, aspirin, colchicine, immunosuppressant's, DMARDS (anti-rheumatoid-arthritis drugs), and anticoagulants. Some drugs appear to promote wound healing, including phenytoin, prostaglandin, and estrogen.

12. B: A burn extending into the dermis with obvious blistering would be classified as a second-degree burn. A first-degree burn is superficial and involves only the epidermis. First and second-degree burns, like other wounds, may also be classified as partial-thickness injuries, because the vessels and glands necessary for healing remain intact. A third-degree burn, also classified as a full-thickness injury, extends through the dermis and into the underlying subcutaneous tissue and may extend through vessels, nerves, muscle and even to the bone.

13. B: The nicotine in cigarettes is a powerful vasoconstrictor and interferes with oxygen transport. The carbon monoxide from smoking displaces oxygen on hemoglobin, decreasing the level of oxygen in the blood. Vasoconstriction reduces delivery of nutrients needed for healing. Peripheral blood flow can be reduced by 50% for up to 60 minutes after smoking a cigarette, and oxygen tension may be reduced for 120 minutes. Additionally, nicotine increases the heart rate and blood pressure, so the heart requires more oxygen to function adequately while receiving less.

14. D: The ankle-brachial index (ABI) examination evaluates peripheral arterial disease of the lower extremities. The ankle and brachial systolic pressures are obtained, and then the ankle systolic pressure is divided by the brachial systolic pressure to obtain the ABI. If the ankle systolic pressure is 90 and the brachial systolic pressure is 120: 90 divided by 120 = 0.75. Normal value is 1 to 1.1 with lower values indicating decreasing perfusion. A value of 0.75 indicates severe disease and ischemia.

15. D: Transcutaneous oxygen pressure measurement (TCPO2) is a noninvasive test that measures dermal oxygen to show the effectiveness of oxygen in the skin and tissues. A value of >40 mm Hg indicates adequate oxygenation for healing. Values of 20 to 40 mm Hg are equivocal findings, and values < 20 mm Hg indicate marked ischemia, affecting healing. Two or three different sites on the lower extremities should be tested to give a more accurate demonstration of oxygenation. TCPO2 is often used to determine if oxygen transport is sufficient for hyperbaric therapy.

16. B: Secondary healing (healing by second intention) involves leaving the wound open and allowing it to close through granulation and epithelialization. Primary healing (healing by first intention) involves surgically closing a wound by suturing, flaps, or split or full-thickness grafts to completely cover the wound. Tertiary healing (healing by third intention) is also sometimes called delayed primary closure because it involves first debriding the wound and allowing it to begin healing while open and then later closing the wound through suturing or grafts. Quaternary prevention includes activities to prevent iatrogenic disorders/effects.

17. C: Increased serum sodium and serum osmolality indicate dehydration. Serum sodium measures the sodium level in the blood.

- Normal values: 135 to 150 mEq/L
- Dehydration: >150 mEq/L

Serum osmolality measures the concentration of ions, such as sodium, chloride, potassium, glucose, and urea, in the blood. Levels increase with dehydration, which stimulates the antidiuretic hormone, resulting in increased water reabsorption and more concentrated urine in an effort to compensate.

- Normal levels: 285 to 295 mill-osmoles per kilogram/ H_2O
- Dehydration: >295 mOsm/kg/ H_2O

18. C: Autolytic debridement is effective for small wounds without infection, but it is slower than other types of debridement. Autolytic debridement requires an occlusive or semi-occlusive dressing to create a warm moist wound environment. Any moisture-retentive dressing, such as hydrocolloids, alginate, and hydrogels, and transparent film, can promote some degree of autolytic debridement, but because of drainage and odor, surrounding tissue must be protected with some type of skin barrier to prevent tissue maceration.

19. A: Enzymatic (chemical) debridement requires application of enzymes 1 to 2 times daily and is most effective for a wound with necrosis and eschar, which must be crosshatched if it is dry. Enzymes include the following:

- Collagenase, applied 1 time daily. Wound pH must remain at 6 to 8 or the enzyme deactivates. Deactivated by Burrows solutions, hexachlorophene, and heavy metals.
- Papain/urea combinations, applied 1 to 2 times daily. Wound pH must remain at 3 to 12. Deactivated by hydrogen peroxide and heavy metals.

20. C: Pain and bleeding indicate that viable tissue is being debrided, so debridement must be discontinued. Only necrotic tissue/eschar should be removed by sharp debridement, removing small layers at a time to prevent injury to viable tissue. Purulent discharge often occurs with an infected wound. While patient fatigue is a concern, positioning the patient for comfort, explaining the procedure, and reassuring the patient may help the patient tolerate continuing the procedure until the wound is adequately debrided.

21. D: Surgical debridement is most commonly used when very large amounts of tissue must be debrided, such as with extensive burns, or when immediate debridement is needed in order to effectively treat a serious wound infection. General anesthesia allows extensive debridement to be done without the patient suffering associated pain and trauma, although postoperative pain is common. One advantage is that most debridement can be done in one procedure. Lasers may also be used for surgical debridement, with pulsed lasers posing less risk to adjacent tissue than continuous lasers.

22. A: In the past, wet-to-dry gauze dressings were frequently used for wound care; however, wet-to-dry dressings have little use in current wound care unless the wound is very small because the gauze adheres to the wound and can disrupt granulation or epithelization. While a whirlpool bath may effectively cleanse debris from a wound, concerns about cross infection have resulted in less frequent use of the whirlpool. Ultrasound may effectively débride wounds. Irrigating a wound with pressurized solution can be effective if the pressure remains in the optimal range, usually 8 to 12 psi.

23. C: Mupirocin is effective against Gram-positive organisms, such as *Staphylococcus aureus* and MRSA, and is used for treating nasal colonization to decrease risk of wound infection. Cadexomer iodine is effective against a wide range of bacteria, viruses, and fungi and is placed in the wound where beads of iodine swell in contact with exudate, releasing the iodine into the wound. Metronidazole is effective against bacterial infections, such as MRSA. Silver sulfadiazine is often used to treat burns and is effective against Gram-positive organisms, including *Staph*, MRSA, and Strep.

24. B: Contraindications to negative pressure wound therapy include wound malignancy, untreated osteomyelitis, exposed blood vessels or organs, and nonenteric, unexplored fistulas. Negative pressure therapy uses subatmospheric (negative) pressure with a suction unit and a semi occlusion vapor-permeable dressing. The suction reduces periwound and interstitial edema, decompressing vessels, improving circulation, stimulating production of new cells, increasing the rate of granulation and reepithelialization, and decreasing colonization of bacteria. NPWT is used for a variety of difficult-to-heal wounds, especially those that show less than 30% healing in 4 weeks of postdebridement treatment or those with excessive exudate.

25. A: The primary goal in referring a patient for multidisciplinary consultation is to prevent complications. A multidisciplinary team is composed of experts in a number of different fields, collaborating to address the complex problems associated with wound care and underlying pathology. Instead of the serial approach to problem-solving involved in the traditional model of care, where referrals are made in response to problems that arise with little communication among specialists, the multidisciplinary approach attempts to identify potential problems and institute preventive measures at the onset, with all members communicating and sharing information.

26. D: Becaplermin (Regranex®) gel is indicated for treatment of peripheral diabetic ulcers extending into subcutaneous tissue or deeper with adequate perfusion. Application follows debridement and usually about 3 weeks offloading if healing is not adequate. Becaplermin is a growth factor derived from human platelets. It is not approved for use with pressure ulcers and stasis ulcers and should not be used with closed (sutured/stapled) wounds. Becaplermin is associated with increased risk of developing malignancy and increased risk of death from existing malignancy.

27. A: Alginates are effective for infected full-thickness wounds with undermining, tunneling, and large amounts of exudate. They are made from brown seaweed and absorb exudate, forming a hydrophilic gel that conforms to the shape of the wound. Hydrocolloids are effective for clean wounds with granulation and minimal to moderate exudate, but they increase the risk of anaerobic infection and hypergranulation. Hydrogels are effective for partial- or full-thickness wounds that are dry or have a small amount of exudate. Hydrogels can be used with necrotic and infected wounds. Semipermeable film is effective over intravenous sites or dry, shallow, partial-thickness wounds.

28. B: The usual hyperbaric oxygen therapy (HBOT) for chronic wounds and lower extremity diabetic ulcers is compression at 2 to 2.4 ATA for 90 minutes daily, with at least 30 treatments. Oxygen toxicity may occur with treatment over 90 minutes. Hyperbaric oxygen therapy (HBOT) is treatment in a high-pressure chamber while breathing 100% oxygen, which increases available oxygen to tissues by 10 to 20 times, improving perfusion. HBOT results in:

- Hyperoxygenation of blood and tissue.
- Vasoconstriction, reducing capillary leakage.
- Angiogenesis, because of increased fibroblasts and collagen.
- Increased effectiveness of antibiotics needing active transport across cell walls (fluoroquinolone, amphotericin B, aminoglycosides).

29. C: This is a stage III ulcer. NPIAP stages include:

- Suspected deep tissue injury: purple/reddish discoloration and boggy, mushy, or firm tissue
- Stage I: skin intact with localized non-blanching reddened area, often over bony prominences
- Stage II: abrasion, blister, or slightly depressed area with red/pink wound bed, partial-thickness skin loss, but no slough
- Stage III: deep, full-thickness ulceration that exposes subcutaneous tissue with possible presence of slough, tunneling and undermining without visibility of underlying muscle, tendon, or bone
- Stage IV: deep, full-thickness ulceration with extensive damage, necrosis of tissue extending to muscle, bone, tendons, or joints
- Unstageable: cannot be staged before debridement because of the extent of slough/eschar

30. B: The most common cause of shear is elevation of the bed >30°. Shear occurs when the skin stays in place and the underlying tissue in the deep fascia over the bony prominences stretches and slides, damaging tissue and vessels, which become thrombosed, often resulting in undermining and deep ulceration. Friction against the sheets holds the skin in place while the body slides down the bed, causing pressure and damage in the sacrococcygeal area. The head of the bed should be maintained <30° except for the brief periods when the patient is lifted with a pull sheet or lifting device and turned, at least every 2 hours.

31. A: Support surface material should provide at least one inch of support under areas to be protected when in use to prevent "bottoming out." (Check by placing a hand palm up under the overlay, below the pressure point.) Static support surfaces are appropriate for patients who can change position without increasing pressure to an ulcer. Those needing assistance to move require dynamic support surfaces. Dynamic support surfaces are also needed when static pressure devices provide less than an inch of support.

32. C: The 30° lateral position is better than the 90° side-lying or supine positions because it prevents pressure over bony prominences. Prone (face down) is not comfortable for most patients and requires careful positioning. Devices such as pillows or foam should be used to correctly position patients so that bony prominences are protected and not in direct contact with each other. Patients should not be positioned on ulcers. Goals for repositioning and a turning schedule of at least every 2 hours should be established for each individual and documented.

33. C: A Braden score of 12 indicates high risk. The Braden scale rates 5 areas (sensory perception, moisture, activity, mobility, and usual nutrition pattern) with a 1 to 4 scale and one area (friction and shear) with a 1 to 3 scale. Lower scores correlate with increased risk. The scores for all six items are totaled, and a risk is assigned according to the number.

- 23 (best score): excellent prognosis with very minimal risk
- ≤16: breakpoint for risk of pressure ulcer (will vary somewhat for different populations)
- 12 to 14: high risk
- 6 (worst score): very poor prognosis with strong likelihood of developing pressure ulcer

34. D: Foam overlays provide the best moisture control for preventing moisture damage to skin. Some materials, such as rubber, plastic, or gel, may increase perspiration and moisture, while some porous materials, including some types of foam, may reduce perspiration. Foam varies considerably in density and indentation load definition (ILD). ILD is the number of pounds of pressure needed to make an indentation in a 4-inch foam of 25% of its thickness, using an indentation of 50 square inches. Foam can be closed-cell (resistant) or open-cell (viscoelastic). Open-cell foam is temperature-sensitive, helping it to mold to the body as it reaches the patient's body temperature.

35. C: Venous insufficiency is characterized by hemosiderin staining (brownish discoloration) about the ankles and anterior tibial area. Pain is usually aching and cramping, and peripheral pulses are present. Lipodermatosclerosis occurs in the lower leg area as the tissue becomes fibrotic from fibrin and protein (collagen) deposits, causing the skin to feel waxy and the tissue to harden, with narrowing of the tissue around the ankle compared to proximal tissue above. Venous (stasis) dermatitis is inflammation of the epidermis and dermis, resulting in scaly, erythematous, crusty, weepy, itchy skin, usually in the lower leg (ankle and tibia).

36. A: Arterial ulcers are characterized by painful, deep, circular, often necrotic ulcers on toe tips, toe webs, heels or other pressure areas, with little edema of extremity. Because circulation is impaired, peripheral pulses are weak or absent, and skin is pale, shiny, and cool, with loss of hair on toes and feet and little edema. Nails are thick with ridges. Rubor occurs on dependency, and pallor occurs on foot elevation. Venous ulcers, by contrast, are typically superficial, irregular ulcers on the medial or lateral malleolus and sometimes on the anterior tibial area, with varying pain and moderate to severe edema of extremity.

37. D: Capillary refill time >2 to 3 seconds indicates arterial occlusion. To assess capillary refill, grasp the toenail bed between the thumb and index finger and apply pressure for several seconds to cause blanching. Release the nail and count the seconds until the nail regains normal color. Check both feet and more than one nail bed. Assess venous refill time with the patient lying supine for a few moments and then have the patient sit with the feet dependent. Observe the veins on the dorsum of the foot and count the seconds before normal filling. Venous occlusion is indicated with times >20 seconds.

38. B: A pulse graded 1 would be weak and difficult to palpate. Pulses should first be evaluated with the patient in a supine position and then again with the legs dependent, checking bilaterally and proximally to distally to determine if the intensity of pulse decreases distally. Pedal pulses should be examined at both the posterior tibialis and the dorsalis pedis. The pulse should be evaluated for rate, rhythm, and intensity, which is usually graded on a 0–4 scale.

- 0 – pulse absent
- 1 – weak, difficult to palpate
- 2 – normal, as expected
- 3 – full
- 4 – strong and bounding

39. A: Total contact casts (TCCs) encase the lower extremity in a walking cast that equalizes pressure of the plantar surface. The casts may have windows over pressure ulcers to allow observation and treatment. TCC is more successful than other off-loading measures, possibly because people restrict activity more. Removable cast walkers allow patients to remove the casts, but studies show that people only use them 28% of the time, decreasing effectiveness. Wheelchairs allow dependency of using a limb but prevents pressure. Half-shoes may have a high walking heel with the front of the foot elevated off of the ground.

40. D: Charcot arthropathy results from neuropathy that weakens the muscles of the foot and reduces sensation. As muscles supporting the bones weaken, the bones become weak and fracture easily. Because of the lack of sensation, the patient may be unaware of the fracture and continue to walk, causing further deformity. It causes inflammation, swelling, and increased temperature in the foot, but usually no pain. In time, the joint dislocation causes the arch to collapse. Treatment includes:

- Compression bandages for 2 to 3 weeks.
- Total contact or non–weight-bearing cast for up to 9 months.
- Gradual weight-bearing after skin has resumed its normal temperature.

41. B: Lymphedema is managed with static compression bandaging during the day, providing 40 to 60 mmHg pressure. Bandaging may be removed at night if the limb is elevated. Dynamic compression may be used, but it can displace fluid or further damage lymphatics if not monitored carefully. Diuretics do not help. Lymphedema is a dysfunction of the lymphatic system, resulting in a debilitating, progressive disease. Proteins, lipids, and fluids accumulate in interstitial spaces, causing pronounced induration, edema, and fibrosis of tissues, resulting in distention and thick fibrotic skin with orange discoloration (peau d'orange). Scaly keratotic debris collects, and the skin develops cracks and leaks of lymphatic fluid.

42. C: Static compression is contraindicated if the ankle brachial index (ABI) is <0.5. Compression therapy serves as a preventive and therapeutic treatment to eliminate edema. It is contraindicated in those with heart failure or peripheral arterial disease, because it may further impair compromised arterial circulation.

- High-level compression provides therapeutic compression at 30 to 40 mmHg at the ankle. Some may provide pressure at 40 to 50 mmHg. ABI should be >0.8.
- Low-level compression provides modified pressure up to 23mmHg at the ankle. ABI must be >0.5 and <0.8. While this level is less than therapeutic, even low levels of pressure may provide some therapeutic benefit.

43. B: While vasodilators may divert blood from ischemic areas, some, such as cilostazol (Pletal®) or pentoxifylline (Trental®), may be indicated. Vasodilators dilate arteries and decrease clotting and are used for control of intermittent claudication. If medications do not relieve symptoms, surgical intervention, such as bypass grafts, angioplasty, and even amputation (if ischemia is irreversible), may be necessary. Surgery is indicated with ABI <0.5 or >0.5 if the patient fails to respond to medication and lifestyle changes or with intolerable, incapacitating pain.

44. D: Subtle indications of infection with arterial insufficiency include fluctuance (soft, wavelike texture) of periwound tissue on palpation, increased pain in the ischemic limb, or ulcer and/or increased edema, increased area of necrosis, and slight erythema about wound perimeter. Because of the lack of circulation, the normal signs of inflammation and infection may not be evident with arterial insufficiency, so observing for subtle signs of infection is critically important. Prompt identification and treatment is necessary to prevent cellulitis and/or osteomyelitis, which might necessitate amputation.

45. C: Unna's boot (ViscoPaste®) is a gauze wrap impregnated with zinc oxide, glycerin, or gelatin to provide a supporting compression "boot" to support the calf muscle pump during ambulation, so it is not suitable for non-ambulatory patients and should be discontinued during the bed rest period. The bandage must be applied carefully, without tension. It may either be left open to dry or covered with an elastic or self-adherent wrap. The dressings are changed according to individual needs, determined by a decrease in edema, the amount of exudate, and hygiene, with dressing changes ranging from twice weekly to once every other week.

46. D: The nylon monofilament test is evaluated according to how many of 10 test sites the patient is able to detect, with <4 indicative of decreased sensation. To test, use this procedure:

- Ask the patient to indicate when the monofilament pressure is felt.
- Grasp a length of #10 monofilament in the instrument provided.
- Touch the monofilament against the bottom of the foot, and then press the monofilament into the foot until the line buckles.

- Test the great, 3rd, and 5th toes.
- Test the left, medial, and right areas of the ball of the foot.
- Test the right and left of the arch.
- Test the middle of the heel.
- Test the dorsal aspect of the foot.

47. C: Traumatic injuries are usually contaminated, and once the patient is stable and the bleeding is controlled, the wound should be flushed with copious amounts of isotonic normal saline under pressure (8 to12 psi), usually 100 to 200 mL of irrigant per inch of wound. Prophylactic antibiotics may be given for 3 to 7 days for superficial wounds and up to 14 days with evidence of infection. Tetanus toxoid or tetanus immune globulin may be necessary if vaccination is not current. Animal bites may also require rabies postexposure prophylaxis (PEP).

48. A: Pemphigus vulgaris (PV), an autoimmune disorder causing blistering of both the skin and the mucus membranes (presenting symptom in 50 to 70% of patients), creates burn-like wounds, which may heal slowly or not at all, often starting in the mouth and genital areas. Untreated, the disorder can lead to death. Blisters on skin rupture, causing ulcerations, and those in folds may develop hypergranulation and crusting. Treatment includes corticosteroids, immunosuppressive drugs, and plasmapheresis to remove antibodies. Ensuring that bed sheets are always clean and dry will help keep the patient's skin from sticking to them and prevent the introduction of infection.

49. B: The ulcers of fungating neoplastic wounds bleed as the vasculature erodes, so hemostatic dressings (gel foam, alginates) and cauterization with silver nitrate may be necessary. Using nonadherent dressings or long-term dressing reduces trauma. Charcoal dressings control odor, and ionic cleansers or antiseptics may be used to cleanse the wound. A foam, alginate, or hydrofiber dressing or wound pouch is used to manage exudate. Skin sealants, barrier ointments, and hydrocolloid wafers to anchor tape protect periwound tissue.

50. B: With contact dermatitis, topical corticosteroid is used to control inflammation and itching. Skin should be gently cleansed with water or oatmeal bath and left open without dressings. Antibiotics are needed only if a secondary infection occurs. Caladryl® lotion may relieve itching, and antihistamines may reduce allergic response. Contact dermatitis is a localized response to contact with an allergen, resulting in a rash that may blister and itch. Common allergens include poison oak, poison ivy, latex, benzocaine, nickel, and preservatives, but people may react to a wide range of items, preparations, and products.

51. A: The average person with a pressure sore should receive 1.25 to 1.5 g/kg per day, but the patient's kidney function should be assessed to determine if the person can tolerate high levels of protein. Protein has important roles in healing, increasing synthesis of collagen and proliferation of epidermal cells. Protein also has immune properties, is a component of antibodies, and takes part in chemical reactions throughout the body. Each gram of protein provides 4 kilocalories.

52. B: If a patient is about to be discharged home from an acute care hospital unit but has poor insurance coverage and is concerned about the costs of dressing supplies, the best referral is likely a social worker. A social worker can help the patient find resources, including community resources, and determine if the patient may be eligible for Medicaid or for manufacturer's patient assistance programs and assist the patient with applying for appropriate programs.

53. A: If a patient with a chronic leg wound comes to an appointment and the wound has deteriorated because the patient has been changing the dressing one time weekly instead of every 3 days, the most appropriate response is, "Let's talk about how I can help you to adhere to the plan of care." This is a non-judgmental response that may encourage the patient to share rather than being defensive. There can be many reasons why a patient doesn't adhere to the plan of care, including inability to pay for supplies.

54. C: A toe-brachial index should be assessed rather than the ankle-brachial index for patients with vascular calcification. If vessels are calcified, then correct measurements are impossible because the vessels cannot be compressed. The vessels in the toe are much smaller so the calcification that is present rarely encircles the entire vessel, so the vessel can be compressed for testing. A pressure of at least 50 mm Hg is required for healing; 20 to 30 mm Hg indicates vascular compromise, which can impair healing of lesions.

55. D: Marked ischemia. Transcutaneous oxygen pressure measurement (TCPO2) assesses dermal oxygen and is used to determine if oxygenation is sufficient for hyperbaric oxygen treatment, to determine the optimum site for amputation, and to determine the degree of hypoxia in tissues. Contact gel and electrodes are applied to the lower extremities to determine variations in oxygen tension. Test results:

- >40 mm Hg adequate oxygenation for healing.
- 20-40 mm Hg equivocal finding.
- <20 mmHg marked ischemia, affecting healing.

56. A: If a patient scheduled for hyperbaric oxygen therapy presents with a severe upper respiratory infection, the treatment should generally be withheld because an upper respiratory infection increases the risk of developing barotrauma. URIs are considered a relative contraindication. Other relative contraindications include lung disorders (such as COPD and asthma), high fever, pregnancy, seizure disorders (the threshold for seizures may be lowered), medical devices (may malfunction unless approved for hyperbaric oxygen therapy), abnormalities of the eustachian tube, and claustrophobia.

57. C: "What causes the pain?"

PQRST Method of pain assessment

P	Perception/Provoking factors	What causes the pain? What relieves the pain or makes it worse?
Q	Quality of pain	What does the pain feel like? Would you describe the pain as sharp, dull, stabbing, shock-like, aching, burning?
R	Radiation	Does the pain move or stay in one place?
S	Severity	Can you rank the pain on a scale of 1 to 10?
T	Time (onset and duration)	When did the pain start? How long did it last?

58. B: Excessive collagen production at the site of a wound leads to abnormal scarring. This often results from dehydration of the tissue, which stimulates keratinocytes to produce cytokines. These in turn cause fibroblasts to release collagen. Hydrating agents, such as silicone sheets/gels (dimethicone) should be applied to the scar to maintain hydration and prevent transepidermal water loss (TEWL). TEWL increases when the barrier function of the skin is impaired. TEWL can be affected by both intrinsic factors (inadequate intake of fluids, fever) and environmental factors (temperature, humidity).

59. D: Hydrocolloid dressings with silver are appropriate for infected wounds with mild to moderate exudate. The silver requires exudate in order to be released, but hydrocolloid dressings are inappropriate with heavy exudate. The silver has antimicrobial action. The hydrocolloid dressing can be left in place for up to a week before changing the dressing, but this may depend on the amount of exudate. Hydrocolloid dressings with silver deactivate enzymatic agents used for debridement.

60. A: Medications that may impede wound healing include NSAIDs and steroids. Steroids, especially, have a negative effect on healing and may increase the risk of skin breakdown. Patients' medication lists should be reviewed if wound healing is slow. Other drugs that may impede healing include anticoagulants, antibiotics (some classes), anti-angiogenesis agents, methotrexate, colchicine, and vasoconstrictive agents. Some drugs, such as levothyroxine, phenytoin, insulin, estrogen, and ferrous sulfate may improve wound healing.

61. C: Class 3 (40-50 mm Hg) therapeutic compression stockings are appropriate for refractory venous ulcers and lymphedema. Compression stockings may be used to prevent ulcers after edema is controlled or with existing ulcers when edema recedes. The stockings come in many sizes and colors and may extend from the foot to the knee or the groin. The stockings must be fitted properly and have the correct level of compression:

- Class I: 20-30 mm Hg (varicose veins).
- Class 2: 30-40 mm Hg (venous ulcers and prevention).
- Class 3: 40-50 mm Hg (refractory venous ulcers & lymphedema).
- Class 4: 50-60 mm Hg (lymphedema).

62. B: If a patient has been prescribed becaplermin gel (Regranex®), a growth factor derived from platelets, according to standard protocol for wound treatment, the gel should be left in place for 12 out of 24 hours. The wound is cleansed with saline or water, becaplermin gel is applied, and the wound is covered with a saline-moistened gauze dressing. After 12 hours, the dressing and gel is removed, and the wound is covered with saline-moistened gauze only for the remaining 12 hours.

63. D: The comment by the patient that suggests that the patient may benefit from a referral to a nutritionist is, "I'm substituting honey for sugar in everything, so my carbohydrate intake is lower." In fact, a teaspoon of honey has 7 g of carbohydrate compared to about 5 g per teaspoon of sugar. Sugar, honey, and maple syrup all metabolize in a similar manner in the body and should be limited in a healthy diet.

64. C: teaching a caregiver to use pillow bridging to prevent pressure ulcers for an immobile patient, five pillows should be employed:

- First under legs to elevate the heels.
- Second between the ankles.
- Third between the knees.
- Fourth behind the back.
- Fifth under the head.

In some cases, a small pillow may also be placed under the upper arm for comfort when the patient is positioned on the side.

65. A: When assessing a patient with diabetes, it's important to remember that diabetic patients tend to lose protective sensation after 10 to 15 years; therefore, patients may not feel a lesion and need to be educated about the importance of examining the feet daily, avoiding going barefoot, wearing well-fitting shoes, and seeing a physician if any abnormality is noted. Patients may also begin to develop neuropathic pain or numbness, which can interfere with recognition of skin lesions.

66. D: Betamethasone dipropionate (Diprolene®) has ultra-high potency as a steroid dermatologic agent. Hydrocortisone acetate and Desonide have low potency while triamcinolone has medium potency. Betamethasone, which comes in ointment, cream, and lotion forms, is used for lesions that are non-responsive to lower-level corticosteroids, as well as for lichen planus and insect bites. Betamethasone is typically applied twice daily.

67. C: If a patient with a slow-healing coccygeal wound is having negative pressure wound therapy (NPWT) and the nurse is assessing the wound with the DIME acronym, the D refers to debridement, I to infection/inflammation control, M to moisture balance and E to wound Edge preparation. Eschar must be removed from the wound prior to NPWT, and infection must be cleared. The moisture balance should be evaluated with each dressing change. If too dry, the wound healing will slow and eschar may form, so the negative pressure should be reduced or type of packing changed. If the wound is too moist, maceration may occur, and the pressure may need to be increased.

68. B: If a patient complains of severe pain during dressing changes and has an analgesic order, the analgesic should generally be administered 30 to 60 minutes before treatment to ensure that the medication has peaked. Soaking a dressing with water or NS may help to loosen it if it is adhering to the wound surface. The nurse should note any signs of infection, which generally increases wound pain, and clean the wound of exudate and any debris to reduce the bioburden.

69. A: The type of debridement most indicated for a wound with large amounts of unviable tissue and increasing cellulitis is sharp debridement because this is the fastest method of converting a necrotic wound to a clean wound and allows for better assessment and treatment of the cellulitis. Sharp debridement may be done as a one-time surgical procedure or as a series of sequential debridements. In some cases, laser debridement (considered a form of surgical debridement) may be done if the patient is not a candidate for operative debridement.

70. D: The most accurate method of measuring the size and depth of a wound is stereophotogrammetry (SPG), which creates images and measurements through the use of a digital camera and computer software. The software calculates the size. If measuring manually, a ruler should be used that measures in mm and cm, and the wound size should not be assessed by comparison with known objects, such as a coin.

71. B: Undermining most often occurs as the result of shear or when the surface opening of the wound is smaller than the damage under the surface. Undermining is often documented according to a clock face: "Undermining from 1 to 3 o'clock, extending 0.75 cm." A thorough description of the undermining should include how far it extends under the tissue and which areas have the most extensive undermining.

72. C: The odor of a wound should be assessed after the dressing is removed and the wound is cleaned because some wound treatments and dressings develop a malodor that may be mistaken for infection. Some infections have a distinctive odor. *Proteus*, for example, has an ammonia-like smell; *Pseudomonas aeruginosa*, a grape-like or sweet odor; and *Escherichia coli*, a floral odor.

73. B: If exudate covers less than two-thirds of a dressing after it is removed, the amount of exudate would be classified as moderate. If the drainage covers less than a third of the dressing, it is classified as a small amount. A large amount is drainage that covers more than two-thirds of the dressing. The amount of exudate provides important information about the condition of the wound and the patient's general condition.

74. A: Moisture-associated skin damage (MASD) most often results in maceration of periwound skin. MASD usually results from wound changes that cause excessive exudate or inadequate dressings to absorb the amount of exudate. With maceration, the skin becomes soft and irritated and often takes on a white, water-logged appearance. Skin barriers and more absorptive dressings, such as alginates, are indicated to better manage exudate.

75. D: Under CMS regulations, a patient must have an unsuccessful trial with static compression therapy for 6 months before switching to intermittent pneumatic compression (IPC) therapy. IPC may also be used if a patient is immobile. IPC devices are used on the lower leg or plantar area of the foot. IPC devices have a garment and a pneumatic pump that inflates the garment. Intermittent inflations occur segmentally up the leg, increasing venous return.

76. D: If the edges of a wound are rolled inward (also known as epibole), this may be caused by a variety of factors including infection, trauma, extreme dehydration, hypoxia, dysfunction of the wound bed, or insufficient basement membrane formation. In this case, the wound edge must be debrided so that the healing process can start again.

77. C: When developing the care plan for a patient, the most effective method of prioritizing a list of goals is to ask the patient what the patient feels is the most important. This patient-focused approach encourages the patient to take an active role in healthcare decisions and shows respect for the patient's autonomy. If the patient is unable to participate, then a parent or caregiver may provide useful insight into what is most important to the patient.

78. A: The initial sign of an infection in a chronic wound is often delayed healing. Typically, an uninfected healing ulcer should show improvement in 2 to 4 weeks, so if there is no sign of improvement, a wound culture is indicated. The classic signs of infection—erythema, increased temperature, purulent discharge, and edema—may or may not be present, and it can be difficult to distinguish among a deep infection, contamination, and colonization because the response to infection may be altered.

79. D: When using the STONES mnemonic to help identify a deep infection, the "O" stands for os (bone):

- S: Size is bigger.
- T: Temperature has increased.
- O: Bone is exposed or prone to exposure.
- N: New or satellite areas of tissue breakdown are evident.
- E: Exudate, erythema, and or edema are evident.
- S: Smell is present.

80. C: When applying a lidocaine 2% soak to a wound, the saturated gauze should be left in place prior to debridement of the wound for 3 to 5 minutes. The wound should be thoroughly cleansed with water, saline, or a wound cleaning solution before the gauze, saturated with 5 to 10 mL of lidocaine, is applied to cover the wound and periwound tissue. Before beginning debridement, the wound should be checked to ensure that it is thoroughly anesthetized.

81. A: Air fluidized and low air loss support surfaces have low moisture retention. Air-fluidized (high air loss) beds are special bed systems in which silicone beads are contained in a bathtub-like frame. There is a high flow of air through the beads. As the air flows through the beads, it "fluidizes" them so that they move, and provide support and redistribution of pressure in much the way water does. The air-fluidized bed is most commonly used for patients with multiple pressure ulcers, making positioning to avoid pressure on sores very difficult.

82. A: When assessing venous flow with duplex ultrasound, retrograde flow is classified as abnormal if it persists for more than 0.5 second. Various factors, such as trauma or thrombosis, may result in retrograde flow (reflux), which increases hydrostatic pressure and may cause veins to dilate and capillaries to burst. Retrograde flow occurs when the valves are impaired and the flow of blood is reversed when the patient is sitting or standing. Treatment generally includes the use of compression stockings to increase blood flow.

83. D: Hot tub folliculitis is most often caused by *Pseudomonas aeruginosa*. Pruritic pustular lesions usually occur within 1 to 4 days of exposure to contaminated water in a hot tub. Some patients may have flu-like symptoms in addition to the rash. Generally, the rash is self-limiting within about a week, but persistent or severe infections may require topical or oral antibiotics (such as ciprofloxacin for 5 days), especially in patients who are neutropenic.

84. B: The use of topical silver-based creams, such as Silvadene® (which contains silver sulfadiazine), should be limited to two weeks. Silver sulfadiazine is used to treat second- and third-degree burns and has been found to be effective in reducing bacterial levels. Use should be of limited duration because extended use may increase the risk of resistant bacteria. Additionally, studies have shown that bacterial levels usually decrease markedly within one week.

85. D: A contraindication to the use of transparent film dressings is when the wound has a suspected bacterial or fungal infection. Transparent film dressings should also be avoided with third-degree burns, moderate to heavy exudate, fragile skin, and skin at risk for periwound maceration. Transparent film can be used when a wound has no or minimal exudate or dry eschar that will be debrided and to help secure other dressings in place over the wound.

86. A: The two primary factors that determine how damaging pressure will be to the tissue are duration (the length of time the pressure occurs) and magnitude (the amount of pressure exerted). As the magnitude increases, the duration must decrease in order to protect the tissue. Pressure points of greatest concern include the sacrum, greater trochanters, ischial tuberosities, heels, and scapula. However, other areas may also be at risk, such as ears, depending on the position of the patient.

87. C: When evaluating support surfaces, *immersion* refers to the depth the patient's body penetrates the support surface and is a factor is the dispersal of pressure. For example, on a hard surface, the pressure is more localized to pressure points, but on a softer surface that allows greater immersion, the pressure is more dispersed. However, immersion is different from compression. If a support surface is too compressed, then the pressure localizes, regardless of the type of support surface.

88. B: If a patient's wound has developed epibole and a closed edge the intervention that is needed to increase healing is debridement of the epibole, which may be done surgically or conservatively, such as with silver nitrate. In some cases, vigorous scrubbing of the epibole with gauze or monofilament fiber dressings may be sufficient to open the tissue. Epibole occurs when upper epidermal cells proliferate over lower epidermal cells rather than across the open wound, causing a rolled edge to occur.

89. D: Foam mattresses tend to "bottom out" and should be replaced after about 3 years of use because foam begins to degrade over time. Two types of foam support surfaces are available: elastic and viscoelastic. Some are permeable (open-cell) to fluid and gas, and others are impermeable (closed cell). Support surfaces are often comprised of layers of different densities of foam and different configurations. Foam seat cushions, for example, may be flat, contoured to fit the shape of the person's buttocks, segmented, or cut out.

90. A: Electrical stimulation should be avoided with electronic implants, such as pacemakers, which may be negatively affected. Electrical stimulation is also contraindicated with malignancy, osteomyelitis, and presence of topical substances containing metal ions. A commonly used device provides high voltage pulsed current (HVPC) with pulse rate of 50 to 120 pps, peaks of 5 to 20 microsecond phase duration, voltage between 100 and 500 V, and amplitude between 80 and 200 V for wound healing. Pulse rate varies according to the targeted phase of healing: 30 pps during inflammatory stage and 100 to 150 pps during other phases. HPVC effectively increases blood flow and reduces edema and bacterial load.

91. C: A recommended position for a patient on a horizontal surface is supine with the head of the bed elevated ≤30 degrees and the knees flexed or the feet blocked. Patients may also be positioned prone or supine with rotation of 40 degrees to the right or left. Regardless of the position, the heels should be supported by pillows to reduce pressure on the heels and pillows may be placed between the knees if rotated to the side.

92. B: A patient on a continuous or intermittent lateral rotation support surface, which moves the patient about a longitudinal axis from side to side, is at risk for shear injuries every time their position is changed. Therefore, the patient must be carefully positioned and supported to prevent the development of ulcers or the worsening of existing ulcers. Lateral rotation support surfaces are often used for obese patients that are difficult to turn, but the support surfaces typically have a weight capacity, which may vary from 350 to 1000 pounds.

93. D: Lower extremity girth measurement to assess edema should be done at the metatarsal head, both malleoli, 3, 12, and 18 cm above the lateral malleolus and the lower edge of the patella. Measurement should be done distal to proximal and on both the left and right sides. Lower extremity girth measurement can provide accurate evaluation of changes in edema. The other method of assessment is volumetric measurement, which utilizes a tank and water displacement to determine the amount of edema.

94. B: If a diabetic patient has a large (7 x 3 x 1.5 cm) chronic stage IV sacral ulcer with undermining from 4 to 8 o'clock to 1 cm, a heavy volume of exudate, and a bioburden, the dressing that is most indicated is packing the wound with silver alginate and covering with bordered foam dressing. The silver alginate is indicated because of the volume of exudate and the bioburden, as silver has antimicrobial properties. The dressing will need to be changed on a daily basis.

95. A: If an overweight patient's weight is at the upper limit for a specialty mattress, the correct intervention is to consider the patient's weight distribution. If the patient's weight is evenly distributed, then the specialty mattress for the patient's weight is appropriate, but if the distribution is uneven—for example if the patient has very large hips—then a better choice is a bariatric mattress because the patient may bottom out on the weight-appropriate mattress.

96. C: When educating a patient with mild cognitive impairment (MCI) about wound care, one way to deal with the communication barrier is to break instructions into small steps because carrying out actions that require a number of sequential steps can be very confusing to patients with MCI. The healthcare provider should ask the patient what helps them to learn. Some patients may want to take notes while others may need illustrations or written guides.

97. D: Biologic therapy with maggots is contraindicated with exposed blood vessels because the maggots may cause the vessels to bleed. Maggots debride the wound because they secrete proteolytic enzymes as well as cytokines and growth factors. Maggot therapy is typically reserved for wounds that have not responded well to other therapies because patients often object to the use of maggots, which are usually left in the wound for about 48 hours. The maggots must be secured to the wound with a special "maggot cage" and gauze that allows air to circulate because lack of air will kill the maggots.

98. A: When carrying out limb volume measurements by the circumferential method, measurements are taken on the foot and leg every 10 cm with the foot in dorsiflexion position and on the hand and arm every 4 cm with the hand flat. The two other methods of limb volume measurements include water displacement (inserting a limb into a container with a measured volume of water and then measuring the overflow) and Perometer® (using an infrared laser system and software to calculate limb volume).

99. A: Friction and shear. Braden scale:

Sensory perception	(1) Completely limited, (2) very limited, (3) slightly limited, (4) no impairment
Moisture	(1) Constantly moist, (2) very moist, (3) occasionally moist, (4) rarely moist
Activity	(1) Bed, (2) chair, (3) occasional walk, (4) frequent walk
Mobility	(1) Immobile, (2) limited, (3) slightly limited, (4) no limitations
Usual nutrition pattern	(1) Very poor, (2) inadequate, (3) adequate, (4) excellent
Friction & shear	(1) Problem (skin frequently slides down sheets and needs help to move), (2) potential problem (skin slides somewhat during moves, needs assistance, (3) no apparent problem

100. B: If a patient has a total contact cast (TCC) applied for offloading for a plantar neuropathic foot ulcer, the TCC should be changed every 1 to 2 weeks. With the TCC, healing usually occurs within 6 to 8 weeks, primarily because it forces the patient to carry out offloading since it rests and immobilizes the area of the lesion. However, the cast may be uncomfortable and makes bathing difficult, so removable cast walkers are often utilized instead.

101. B: When using Doppler ultrasound to evaluate blood flow, conductive gel is placed on the end of the transducer or on the skin and the transducer is then held at approximately a 45-degree angle to the skin (pointing towards the patient's head, which can be anywhere from 30 to 60 degrees). The pulse is counted, noting the intensity, and a marking pen is used to mark the site where the pulse is heard. The echo is at a higher frequency when blood flow is in the direction of the transducer and lower frequency when it is in the opposite direction (representing the Doppler effect/frequency shift).

Answer Key and Explanations

102. C: An essential role of fat in the diet is to maintain the normal function of the cell membrane, permitting fat-soluble substances (such as vitamins A, D, E, and K) to move in and out of the cell. Fats can also serve as a source of energy when carbohydrates are deficient. Stored fat in the tissues provides insulation and protection against heat and cold. Fat provides 9 kcal/g compared to 4 kcal/g for proteins and carbohydrates.

103. B: When educating a patient with peripheral arterial disease about self-care, the patient should be advised that smoking cigarettes poses the greatest risk for decreasing circulation because the nicotine serves as a vasoconstrictor. With each cigarette, the smoker absorbs about 1 mg of nicotine, although this can vary among patients because of genetic differences and racial differences. Vaping and other smokeless tobacco products (such as chewing tobacco) also pose a risk to patients.

104. A: The Braden Q scale was designed specifically for the pediatric population. The scale is similar to the Braden scale although every category is scored from 1 (worst) to 4 (normal) and the descriptions are age appropriate. The categories include mobility, activity, sensory perception, moisture, friction/shear, and nutrition. The last category does not appear in the adult Braden scale and is tissue perfusion and oxygenation. This category is scored based on MAP, hemoglobin, and oxygen saturation.

105. D: If the nurse is teaching a hearing-impaired patient to do dressing changes, and the patient nods the head and appears to understand, the most effective method of ensuring the patient understands the information is to ask the patient to do a return demonstration. While presenting the information in more than one form (spoken and visual) is also helpful, some patients are unable to read or to follow written directions well, and patients may state that they understand even when they do not.

106. C: If collagenase is being applied to a wound for debridement, the wound's pH must stay within the range of 6 to 8 because otherwise inactivation will occur. Other substances that may inactivate the enzyme include Burrows solution, heavy metal ions, and hexachlorophene. If papain/urea compounds are utilized for enzymatic debridement, the pH must remain between 3 and 12, and heavy metal salts and hydrogen peroxide may inactivate the enzymes.

107. D: A desired outcome for a patient should clearly reflect the nursing diagnosis. Therefore, if the nursing diagnosis is, "Imbalanced nutrition—less than body requirements," the appropriate desired outcome is "Patient will maintain adequate nutrition evidenced by weight within normal range." A number of different outcomes may be listed under "evidenced by." Nursing interventions, such as "provide supplements..." are part of the plan of care and distinct from desired outcomes.

108. B: Ischemic tissue is a contraindication to surgical/sharp debridement because this indicates that the blood supply is inadequate for healing. Other contraindications include malignant lesions (because debridement may spread cancer cells), clotting disorders (anticoagulation is a relative contraindication), immunocompromise, and unstable medical condition. Surgical debridement is primarily used for wounds with an underlying infection, such as cellulitis or sepsis, when the need for debridement is urgent.

109. D: The best method of attaching dressings to vascular leg ulcers is tube gauze/netting, which holds the dressings in place but does not apply excessive pressure on the wound, because it's important to avoid any type of adhesive since the skin is likely to be friable. Adhesives may cause stripping of the skin and further ulceration. If adhesives must be used, silicone adhesives are likely to cause the least skin irritation.

110. D: If a client has a diabetic ulcer with minimal to moderate exudate and a small amount of eschar that requires debridement, the most appropriate dressing choice is a hydrocolloid (such as DuoDERM®, Exuderm®, and Replicare®). Hydrocolloids form a gelatinous mass that keeps the wound hydrated and provides an environment in which autolytic debridement can occur. Hydrocolloids can be used with wounds that have minimal to moderate exudate.

111. C: Compression of tissue impairs circulation and can result in ischemia and pressure injury when the skin perfusion pressure falls to below 30 to 40 mm Hg. Normal skin perfusion pressure may range from 50 mm Hg to 100 mm Hg. Skin perfusion pressure, which measures blood flow to a wound, may be assessed by applying sensors that detect oxygen about the wound in a normal room environment. The test may also be conducted in a hyperbaric chamber with the patient breathing 100% oxygen to determine if the oxygen content increases with hyperbaric oxygen treatment.

112. B: Score of ≤10 is high risk and 11 to 15 moderate risk on the Norton Plus Pressure Ulcer scale. Each category (physical condition, mental state, activity, mobility, and incontinence) is score from 1 (worst) to 4 (normal). A one-point deduction is made for each of the following categories for which the patient is positive: diabetes, hypertension, hematocrit (<41% for males and <36% for females), hemoglobin (<`4 g/dL for males and <12 g/dL for females), albumin level (<3.3 g/dL, fever (>99.6⬚F/37.6⬚C), polypharmacy (5 or more), and change in mental status to confused/lethargic within 24 hours. Thus, the patient's initial score was 13, minus 3 points for positive findings of diabetes, hypertension, and hemoglobin for a total score of 10.

113. B: The 5 basic elements of a skin assessment include:

1. <u>Temperature</u>: Normally warm to the touch. Cool may indicate impaired circulation, and hot may indicate inflammation or infection.
2. <u>Color</u>: Varies according to ethnicity, but pallor may indicate impaired circulation, while hyperpigmentation/hypopigmentation may indicate impaired circulation, disease or skin condition (altered melanin deposition).
3. <u>Moisture</u>: May vary from dry to moist, depending on general condition and skin disorders.
4. <u>Integrity</u>: Should be intact and free from open areas.
5. <u>Turgor</u>: Pinched skin should return to normal shape rapidly. Turgor may slow with dehydration and aging skin.

114. D: Debris. NERDS mnemonic to identify a superficial infection:

- N: Non-healing wound is present.
- E: Exudate is present from the wound.
- R: Red and bleeding surface granulation tissue is evident.
- D: Debris includes yellow or black necrotic tissue on the surface of the wound.
- S: Smell or malodor is present from the wound.

115. D: If a wound is characterized by a defective matrix and cell debris that are impairing healing, the correct intervention is debridement, which may be carried out episodically or continually, depending on the condition of the wound. Various methods of debridement may be utilized: autolytic, biological, sharp, mechanical, or surgical. The goal is to restore the wound base so that there is viable tissue that can begin the healing process.

116. A: Calluses on the bottom of the foot most often occur because of improperly fitted shoes, which cause the patient's weight to be unevenly distributed. As calluses thicken, they may begin to crack and fissure, causing pain and discomfort. Treatment includes soaking, filing or with pumice stone, and applying moisturizer. In some cases, inserts may be necessary to better distribute weight.

117. C: TIME wound bed preparation approach:

- **T:** Tissue nonviable or deficient: Carry out debridement.
- **I:** Infection/Inflammation: Administer topical/systemic antimicrobials, anti-inflammatories, and/or protease inhibitors.
- **M:** Moisture balance: Apply moisture-balancing dressings/therapy.
- **E.** Edge margin non-advancing or undermined: Utilize adjunctive therapies, bioengineered skin, debridement, and/or skin grafts.

118. B: In a chronic wound, the inflammatory phase is generally prolonged because of the presence in the wound of neutrophils, which produce proinflammatory cytokines. As new tissue forms, it tends to become degraded through the action of proteinases. Most chronic wounds have full-thickness loss of tissue, resulting in the absence of the basement membrane to which epithelial cells generally attach, making epithelialization a more complex and lengthy process. Chronic wounds are also susceptible to the growth of biofilms, which retard healing.

119. A: Prealbumin is the laboratory test that is the best measure of short-term change in nutritional status because it has a half-life of just 2 to 3 days. Prealbumin is a good measurement because it quickly decreases when nutrition is inadequate and rises quickly in response to increased protein intake. Protein intake must be adequate to maintain levels of prealbumin. Prealbumin is necessary for transportation of both thyroxine and vitamin A throughout the body. Values: Normal—16-40 mg/dL, mild deficiency—10-15mg/dL, moderate deficiency—5-9 mg/dL, and severe deficiency—<5 mg/dL.

120. B: In a wound, a biofilm may take on the appearance of slough, so it may be a challenge to differentiate the two, although a biofilm tends to have a shinier and more gel-like appearance from the extracellular polymeric matrix that encloses the biofilm. In fact, the biofilm causes a chronic inflammation that results in increased permeability of vessels and increased exudate, leading to the production of slough, so the presence of slough may be an indication that a biofilm is present. Treatment includes debridement and dressings and topical antibiotics to prevent reformation of the biofilm.

Ostomy Care

1. C: The most standard treatment for cancer that has invaded the muscle is radical cystectomy with urinary diversion. Chemotherapy may be done prior to or after surgery to improve survival rates, because recurrence rates are about 50%. In males, the bladder, prostate, seminal vesicles, and perivesical tissues are removed; in females, the bladder, uterus, ovaries, fallopian tubes, urethra, and anterior vaginal wall are removed. Urinary diversions may include an ileal conduit or an internal pouch, such as the Indiana pouch or neobladder (formed from part of the intestine).

2. D: Frank bleeding from the mucocutaneous juncture may indicate bleeding from a mesenteric artery, requiring surgery to open the incision and ligate the artery. A slight bleeding when changing of stomal appliance relates to mechanical trauma to the mucosa and is normal, unless it continues. Slow oozing usually stops, but may require cauterization. Oozing of blood may be caused by antiplatelet drugs, such as salicylates. Slow bleeding along with caput medusa (distention of veins about the umbilicus) is a complication related to portal hypertension.

3. B: An ileostomy should begin to function and excrete stool by 24 to 48 hours postoperatively, because digested food passes quickly into the small intestine in liquid form. A colostomy, however, may not pass stool for 4 to 5 days, varying somewhat with the position of the colostomy, which affects reabsorption of liquids. Because kidneys constantly produce urine, an ureterostomy should immediately produce urine. Stomas should be observed carefully to ensure that they are functioning properly. Delayed function may indicate obstruction or other complications.

4. B: Folliculitis is inflammation of the hair follicles by staphylococcus aureus. The lesions are often pustular, red, and painful. Folliculitis usually results from slight nicks in the skin from shaving with a razor, from friction, or from occlusion. Candidiasis is a fungal infection that causes inflammation with burning and itching and red patches, related to prolonged moisture on skin, usually from secretions or leakage under the pouch. Contact dermatitis may result from a hypersensitivity reaction to a particular chemical or product in the pouching system. Skin may be red, draining, and painful. Chemical trauma from secretions may look similar: red, draining, and painful.

5. A: Hydrocolloid dressing may be used to prevent fluid from herpetic lesions from interfering with the pouching system. Herpes zoster and herpes simplex, both viral illnesses, remain dormant, but can be triggered by illness or stress and can erupt in the peristomal area. Antiviral treatments may be used to speed healing. Herpetic lesions in the peristomal area may be irritated by pouch adhesive. While cool moist compresses may provide some relief from discomfort, the lesions should be allowed to open and dry on their own (usually within 2 to 3 weeks).

6. D: A convex pouching system with a belt is used for a retracted stoma because it fits snugly about the stoma to prevent leakage. Retraction occurs when the stoma pulls below the skin level. This is caused by tension below the stoma, which can be from a variety of factors, including excessive scar formation, obesity, inadequate stoma length, recurrence of active Crohn's disease, and improper excision of skin. In severe cases, achieving a seal about the stoma may be very difficult, and may require surgical revision.

7. C: Specific suggestions are given at Level 3 in the PLISSIT model:

- Level 1—Permission: giving the person permission to have feelings or attitudes and to do or not do something.
- Level 2—Limited Information: providing factual information, specifically related to needs and concerns of patient, that helps dispel misconceptions and fears.
- Level 3—Specific Suggestions: making recommendations when a person needs to take action or seek treatment with medical guidance.
- Level 4—Intensive Therapy: referring the patient to an appropriate specialist, for example if reconstructive surgery or psychotherapy is needed.

8. A: Peristomal abscess is common with active Crohn's disease distal to the stoma. Crohn's disease is a form of inflammatory bowel disease in which ulcerations occur in the small and sometimes in the large intestines. Peristomal abscess is characterized by open (from fistulae) and closed lesions that are painful, swollen, and erythematous. Peristomal abscess may also occur after stomal revision, because of contamination from skin bacteria. Colostomy irrigation may result in perforation that causes abscess formation. A peristomal abscess rarely heals spontaneously but requires surgical incision and drainage.

9. B: The most common method to ensure correct placement of the stoma during surgery is to mark the site with a permanent marker. The site is marked with an X or circle, and is usually covered with a transparent dressing to protect the markings. Markings will usually last for 1 to 3 weeks, but patients should be provided a marking pen and additional dressings in case markings fade. Tattooing is the most permanent method of marking, but is painful for the patient. Making circular scratches in the epidermis with a small-gauge needle is not recommended, because the break in the skin can lead to infection.

10. B: A transverse colostomy creates one or two stomas in the transverse colon, usually in the upper abdomen, in the middle or on the right side. A descending (sigmoid) colostomy (most common) creates a stoma from the end of the sigmoid colon, usually in the lower left abdomen. An ascending colostomy creates a stoma from the ascending portion of the colon on the right side of the abdomen. An end colostomy is a temporary procedure or a permanent procedure where a stoma is created proximal to an inoperable carcinoma to allow for fecal diversion and to prolong life.

11. D: A loop colostomy is usually performed for short-term fecal diversion. A loop colostomy creates one stoma with two openings, one for stool and the other for mucus, usually in the transverse colon. A supporting rod may be in place to maintain the stoma's position. This procedure is relatively easy and can be reversed in a simple operation. Indications include trauma, conditions requiring the bowel to heal and rest, such as cancer, and (in children) major pelvic surgery.

12. B: The bag should be at shoulder level. Follow this procedure:

1. Hang the bag with 500 to 1500 mL lukewarm water, with the bottom at shoulder level, and release air bubbles from the tubing.
2. Sit on or near toilet. Apply a long irrigation sleeve, placing the end into the toilet.
3. Lubricate the cone nozzle and insert it about 3 inches into stoma in the direction of the colon.
4. Holding the cone firmly in place to retain the fluid, open the clamp and let the fluid flow into colon slowly, over about 5 to 10 minutes. Hold the cone in place for a few seconds and then remove it.
5. Drain fecal output into the toilet for 10 to 15 minutes. The initial flow of fluids is usually followed by fecal material within 15 minutes.
6. Dry and clamp the end of the irrigation sleeve. Keep the bag in place for up to an hour if stool continues to drain. Remove the irrigation sleeve, cleanse peristomal area, and apply the pouch.

13. D: Indications of ileostomy obstruction include edematous stoma, high-pitched bowel sounds, obvious peristaltic waves, distension, dry mouth, abdominal pain, nausea, and vomiting. Obstruction is usually related to high-fiber foods. Other complications include

- Fluid and electrolyte imbalance: mouth and tongue dry, skin turgor poor, weight loss, diarrhea, and lethargy.
- Vitamin B12 deficiency: palpitations, lethargy, fatigue, tinnitus, dyspnea, and headache.
- Pouchitis: high fever, abdominal cramping, dry mouth, poor skin turgor, and bloody diarrhea.

14. D: Monitoring intake and output is most important in preventing fluid and electrolyte imbalance, along with ensuring adequate nutrition. During episodes of diarrhea, the patient should substitute water with Gatorade® or a similar sports drink designed to replenish electrolytes and supply nutrition. With electrolyte imbalance, increasing the oral intake of fluids is not sufficient, because these fluids will be excreted through the kidneys and may not correct the electrolyte imbalance. If stools are too liquid, the patient can increase fiber and, if stools are too dry, increase sodium. Antidiarrheal agents should be taken only as necessary when dietary changes are not sufficient, never routinely.

15. D: Lavage is NOT the same as an irrigation, which uses large volumes of fluid. About 30 to 50 mL of normal saline (NS) is used to prevent further dehydration, instilled with a catheter-tipped piston or bulb syringe with a 14 to 16 Fr catheter attached. Lavage is usually done after an abdominal x-ray has determined that food is the cause of a blockage.

1. Apply irrigation sleeve with the end in the toilet.
2. Do a digital exam to determine the direction of intestine.
3. Lubricate the catheter and gently insert it approximately 12 to 15 cms.
4. Slowly inject normal saline into the intestine and then slowly aspirate the entire amount with light to moderate pressure.
5. Repeat the procedure until the blockage is relieved.

16. C: After ileostomy takedown, the best functional result is 4 to 5 stools per day with no incontinence, but most procedures result in (at best) 95% continence during the daytime and 90% continence during the night. The ileoanal reservoir is usually quite small after surgery, so 8 to 10 stools per day is not unusual in the immediate postoperative period, putting the person at risk for fluid and electrolyte imbalances; the reservoir capacity will expand and stool frequency should decrease over a 6 to 12-month period.

17. B: While some anal mucus discharge is normal, copious discharge is often associated with diversion colitis, in which the distal segment becomes inflamed. Treatment includes rectal irrigation and topical steroids, as well as oral antibiotics. The perianal area should be cleansed and protective cream or ointment applied to prevent irritation of the skin. The mucus fistula should be checked each time the appliance is changed and discharged mucus gently wiped from the opening. The stoma should remain pink. Changes in color or swelling may indicate compromised circulation or infection.

18. B: A strictureplasty is a surgical procedure that widens the narrowed bowel in cases of chronic inflammation or scar tissue, such as that occurring with Crohn's disease. In this procedure, no aspect of the intestine is removed, preserving the bowel length. A strictureplasty is indicated when a diseased portion of the bowel connects to a healthy portion. The procedure widens the narrowed or scarred portion, and maintains the intestinal flow. If the strictures are extensive, part of the intestine will require removal (resection). If both the colon and the rectum are infected by the disease, the entire colon may need to be removed (colectomy). Approximately 70-90% of patients affected by Crohn's disease will require surgical intervention during their lifetime.

19. C: Providing the patient with a list of surgical options complies with the AMA guidelines for informed consent. Options should not be limited by a specific surgeon's area of expertise or experience, as a patient can be referred to other surgeons. The patient must be provided a complete list and explanation of possible complications, not a brief summary. While relaxing and focusing on thinking positively may have benefits, this advice is not part of informed consent.

20. B: Megacolon is associated with Hirschsprung's disease, a congenital disorder in which infants are born without intestinal ganglion nerve cells in part of or the entire colon, causing mechanical obstruction. Normally, nerves signal the colon to contract, pushing the stool through the colon, but the absence of propulsion in the segments without ganglions causes the fecal material to accumulate. Affected areas almost always include the rectum and distal colon, but in rare instances can "skip" segments and involve the entire colon and the small intestine. As fecal material collects, the segment of the bowel proximal to the defect distends, creating megacolon.

21. B: Imperforate anus with low anomalies: no external opening, but the rectum is otherwise in normal position through the puborectalis muscle, with normal function and no connection to the genitourinary tract.

22. C: An overactive neurogenic bladder is characterized by urgency, frequency, dysuria, urinary tract infection, and fever, while an underactive neurogenic bladder results in incontinence, dribbling, straining, inability to urinate, and retention. Neurogenic bladder is bladder dysfunction from lesions of the peripheral or central nervous system with traumatic or congenital etiologies or resulting from cerebrovascular accident or diabetic neuropathy. Nerve damage can cause an underactive bladder, which is unable to contract effectively to empty the bladder, or an overactive bladder, which contracts frequently and ineffectually.

23. C: Peristomal irritation, usually caused by chemical trauma from secretions, may be treated with corticosteroid (Kenalog®) spray, to reduce inflammation, and nystatin (Mycostatin®) powder, for fungal infections, which are common under appliances. Oral antibiotics are not indicated unless there are signs of folliculitis (pustules, erythema, and warmth). Topical antibiotics are not indicated for irritation, and ointments should not be used under appliances, as they will prevent the appliance from adhering. Alternative methods include applying a Stomahesive® wafer directly over irritated skin or applying karaya powder and then a karaya gum washer.

24. B: As the abdomen enlarges, the stoma often also enlarges and changes shape, becoming more oval. The stoma should be measured from time to time, and appliance size changed as necessary. The stoma usually returns to normal shortly after delivery. An ileostomy may be more active during pregnancy because of increased pressure. While adequate fluid intake and nutrition are important, no special diet modifications are indicated. There is a slight chance of blockage as the fetus grows and applies pressure, causing distention and pain. Treatment includes liquid diet and rest or intravenous fluids to rest the intestines.

25. A: Adenocarcinomas develop from epithelial tissue in adenomatous polyps and account for 90 to 95% of all colorectal cancers. Lymphomas are rare primary tumors that occur primarily in the rectum, while secondary metastatic tumors occur primarily in the colon. Melanomas are rare tumors that usually metastasize from other parts of body, accounting for <2% of colorectal cancers. Sarcomas (leiomyosarcoma) develop from smooth muscle and account for <2% of colorectal cancers, but >50% metastasize. Carcinoids are slow-growing tumors that rarely spread, most commonly found in the rectum and accounting for <1% of colorectal cancers.

26. C: Kinesthetic learners learn best by handling, doing, and practicing and should be allowed to handle supplies and equipment with minimal instruction. They benefit from demonstrating their understanding by doing the procedure. Visual learners learn best by seeing and reading, and they benefit from written directions, videos, diagrams, pictures, and demonstrations. Auditory learners learn best by listening and talking, so procedures should be explained during demonstrations. Auditory learners benefit from audiotapes and extra time for questions. While learning styles do vary some from person to person, all people do need learn from visual information, auditory information, and by hands-on learning. Different materials lend themselves to a different format, but where possible, the best practice when presenting information to others is to use a mixture of formats, including hands-on materials, visual, and auditory information to keep the materials engaging to all learners.

27. A: Functional urinary incontinence can occur when physical (impaired mobility) or mental (confusion, depression) disabilities prevent the person from controlling urination. Stress incontinence is characterized by small amounts of involuntary urinary leakage, often during physical activity. Overflow incontinence is characterized by small leakage of urine resulting from pressure on an over-distended bladder. Urge incontinence is caused by moderate to large amounts of involuntary urinary leakage caused by sudden urge to urinate and inability to hold urine.

28. A: Spinach and parsley have properties that help to eliminate odor in the intestinal tract. Most appliances are now odor proof, but leaking or improper cleaning of the appliance may lead to odor. If odor persists, bismuth subcarbonate tablets taken 3 to 4 times daily may effectively reduce odor. Additionally, a number of different deodorant tablets and drops are available to place inside of a pouch to reduce odor. Milk products, fish, broccoli, and asparagus may increase odor.

29. D: Stool softeners (DSS, Colace®) increase retention of fluid in the stool, helping to prevent constipation and impaction. Fiber and bulking agents may also be used. These include preparations made with methylcellulose (Citrucel®), psyllium (Metamucil®), and bran, which dissolve or swell in the intestines, promoting peristalsis. Osmotic (Milk of Magnesia®) and stimulant laxatives (Dulcolax®) should be avoided by those with ileostomies, as they can lead to increased diarrhea and electrolyte imbalance. They should be rarely used with any type of fecal diversion. Overuse can lead to bowel dysfunction. Mineral oil should not be used as a laxative.

30. A: The most effective solution is a home health agency referral, so a nurse can visit the patient in her home and provide further education and supervision. Printed materials and video are also helpful, but many people need hands-on experience and one-on-one instruction to feel secure about ostomy care. Patients are often overwhelmed with new information while in the hospital and are not able to fully comprehend what they need to do, even if they are alert and intelligent. Many people are reluctant to be assisted by family members, and they may be less motivated to be independent in care if they can depend on someone else.

31. A: In the case of suspected or confirmed infection indicated by pain, purulent discharge, or fever, the stent must be removed. Likely, antibiotics will also be prescribed. While stents are the primary management of urinary tract disease and postoperatively with a urostomy, risk of urinary tract infection is increased when any foreign body is introduced into the urinary tract. For this reason, the goal is to utilize ureteral stents as short as possible and to enforce infection prevention efforts to avoid this complication. Prior to stent insertion, a urine culture should be collected to determine (and treat) any pre-existing infection. Irrigation will not effectively treat an infection, nor would surgical revision.

32. A: While symptoms may vary, one of the first indications of a urostomy infection is usually a change in the character and/or amount of urine. The urine may become cloudy from mucus or purulent material. Hematuria may be present. Also, urine usually becomes concentrated and may be dark yellow, orange, or brownish in color and have a very strong or foul odor. Urinary output may decrease markedly. Other symptoms, such as fever, chills, back or flank pain (generally indicating infection has spread to the kidneys), and nausea and vomiting may also occur.

33. D: The best method to obtain a urine specimen from a urostomy is to remove the appliance, cleanse peristomal skin, and catheterize the stoma with a #14 straight catheter. A urine specimen should never be obtained from a bag that has been in use, because it is considered contaminated. If the stoma cannot be catheterized, an alternative method is to remove the appliance, cleanse the peristomal tissue, apply a new clean appliance, and obtain the specimen from the new bag. Do not hold a sterile cup below a stoma and attempt to obtain a specimen.

34. A: The best method to manage mucus in the urine after a urostomy is to increase fluid intake to 2 to 3 L daily to flush the mucus. Mucus production is normal. In the period immediately following, a marked increase in mucus in the urine may occur, but this will usually abate. Gentle irrigations will be done postsurgically to maintain patency of ureteral catheters. Acidifying the urine may help reduce crystal formation. Irrigating the urostomy is not recommended and may cause infection. Dairy products do not cause increased mucus.

35. B: Because of the loss of the colon, enteric-coated medications or time-release capsules spend less time in the intestine and may not be absorbed completely or at all. Uncoated tablets or liquid medications usually are absorbed; however, if food is passing through the ileostomy undigested, there may be decreased absorption of uncoated and liquid medications.

- Antidiabetics: Glucophage may not be absorbed properly.
- Birth control pills: These may not be completely absorbed, making them unreliable.
- Corticosteroids: Corticosteroids can cause sodium retention and fungal infection under the faceplate of the pouch because they suppress the immune system.
- Diuretics: May cause electrolyte imbalance.

36. B: One common indication of pouchitis is a steady increase in the frequency of stools. The patient may also develop fecal incontinence, watery, or bloody stools, and a feeling of urgency. Some may develop cramping abdominal pain. Dehydration and fever may occur with excessive loss of fluids. Pouchitis is a nonspecific inflammation of the mucosal lining of the internal (ileoanal, Kock, J, W, S) pouch created from part of the small intestine after colectomy. It usually occurs during the first 2 years after surgery and is most common among those with ulcerative colitis. Itching and a decrease in the frequency of stools do not indicate pouchitis.

37. B: With IPAA, seepage of fecal material and mucus from the anus may occur, especially at night. The combination of moisture and friction from walking or wiping the area with tissue can cause severe irritation, so the patient should rinse the perineal area with warm water using a squirt bottle or bulb syringe or gently wipe with cotton balls, Tucks®, or baby wipes. Patients should avoid washcloths, which are too rough, and soap, which may irritate because of alkalinity, and should pat dry, fan, or use a cool hair dryer. Preventive measures include skin barrier cream or ointment and positioning a soft dressing between buttocks.

38. D: Foods that produce acidic urine include grains and cereals, meats, cheese, corn, crackers, cranberries, eggs, pasta, nuts, rice, prunes, plums, fish, and poultry. The pH of the urine ranges normally from 4.6 to 8, in the acidic range, and patients should maintain acidity. Alkaline urine is more likely to become infected and develop crystals. Most meats and cereals produce acidic urine, but most fruits and vegetables produce alkaline urine. Drinking cranberry juice instead of orange juice can help to keep the urine acidic. Patients may also take daily vitamin C, with permission of physician.

39. D: The target intubation schedule for one month after surgery for continent cutaneous urinary diversion is usually every 5 hours during the day and every 6 hours during the night. Immediately after surgery, intubation is done every 2 hours, but as healing takes place, the time is extended until the pouch can hold increased amounts of urine. Patients must be cautioned to maintain a regular schedule to avoid infection and overdistention or rupture of the pouch.

40. A: Pelvic floor/Kegel exercises must be done both preoperatively and postoperatively. Because the neobladder does not expel urine, the abdominal muscles must tighten and the sphincter muscles relax. Scheduled urinations usually begin with every 2 hours during the day and 3 hours at night, extending time until reaching the target of every 4 hours during the day and once at night. Patients must sit to urinate and strain, often taking several minutes. Those who cannot completely empty the bladder may need to catheterize one or more times daily. Fluids should not be restricted.

41. C: Most anorectal fistulas originate in the anal glands, which are located between the layers of the anal sphincters and drain into the anal canal. If the glands become blocked and an abscess forms, it can begin to tunnel toward the surface of the skin. There may be only one tunnel or tract, or several. Abscesses can recur if they heal over at the surface. As purulent material collects beneath the healed surface, pressure builds, and it breaks through again. Anorectal fistulas are common in those with Crohn's disease. They can also occur with rectal cancer or following radiation therapy.

42. B: With enterocutaneous fistulae (extending from intestines to skin), nutritional support is provided with total parenteral nutrition (TPN) if both the small intestine and colon are involved, but enteral support if only the colon is involved. Fluid restriction and somatostatin help to decrease small bowel secretions. The most frequent causes are Crohn's disease, cancer, anastomotic leak, bowel obstruction, and sepsis. They may develop postoperatively or spontaneously. If excess pressure develops on an anastomosis, a fistula can develop. Fistulae seek weakness in tissues and thus may exit through wounds, incisions, drain sites, or compromised tissue.

43. B: A fistula that drains 300 mL in 24 hours would be classified as a small to medium output fistula. Classification systems help to characterize fistulae and assist in their management and treatment. Sometimes, more than one classification may be used to describe a fistula. Below are volume (drainage) classifications:

- Low-output fistulas drain <150 mL in 24 hours.
- Small to medium output fistulas drain 150 to 500 mL in 24 hours.
- High output fistulas drain >500 mL in 24 hours.

44. A: Intersphincteric. Parks classification for anorectal fistulae include:

- Intersphincteric: extending from the internal sphincter downward to the perineum, up to a high blind tract, or open into the rectum itself (70%).
- Transsphincteric: extending from the internal and external sphincters to the ischiorectal fossa to the perineum (25%).
- Suprasphincteric: crossing the internal sphincter to the external sphincter above the puborectalis muscles and then down to the ischioanal fossa and to the skin (5%).
- Extrasphincteric: extending from the perianal skin through the levator ani muscles and through the rectal wall (1%).
- Horseshoe: partially circling the anus, opening at both ends in the cutaneous tissue.

45. B: Topical corticosteroid cream may be effective in treating peristomal hyperplasia and is less invasive than other treatments. If corticosteroid cream is ineffective, the next step is usually cauterization with silver nitrate. Surgical debridement may be required in severe cases. Resiting may result in development of peristomal hyperplasia at the new site. Peristomal hyperplasia is an overgrowth of granulation tissue about the stoma. It usually results from irritation caused by latex tubes, tube migration, or moisture.

46. D: Care must be taken to use silver nitrate only on the granulation tissue, as it can cause painful burns if it touches other tissue, so the first apply a skin barrier around the tissue to be cauterized. Silver nitrate sticks usually need to be moistened with small amount of sterile water to activate. Silver nitrate is applied by running the tip of the stick in a rolling motion over the tissue to be cauterized. Cauterization is usually required 2 to 3 times weekly until granulation tissue resolves.

47. C: Buried bumper syndrome involves migration of the internal bumper into the gastric mucosa. The most common cause is excessive traction pulling the bumper against the gastric mucosa for extended periods, sometimes causing necrotic lesions and abscesses, so there should be 1.5 cm between the external bumper and skin to prevent excessive traction. Symptoms include partial or complete occlusion of the tube, erythema and swelling about stoma, and pain in the abdominal wall. The bumper may be palpable on examination. In all cases, the tube must be removed, either by external traction or surgical excision with endoscopy.

48. D: Prevention of occlusion in enteral feeding tubes requires proper administration of medications and feedings, and maintaining a regular schedule of flushing. Tubes should be flushed with 30 mL of water at least every 4 hours for continuous feeding, as well as before and after intermittent feedings and administration of medications. Medications should be in liquid form or should be crushed completely. Enteric-coated or delayed-release preparations should be avoided, as they may not be adequately absorbed. Feeding solutions should be liquid in consistency.

49. B: The PEG tube does not have an inflatable balloon, but the tube should be stabilized by pulling gently to ensure that the internal bumper is against the abdominal wall and then sliding the external stabilizer to 1.5 cm above the skin. Replacing the PEG tube is done only if the leakage cannot be otherwise controlled. Routine skin care, including application of barrier ointment or other skin sealant, is necessary to prevent skin breakdown. In some cases, alginates, foam dressing, gauze, or pouching may be necessary.

50. D: Because kidneys are active during the night, urinary output may increase to 2 L, so to prevent the ostomy bag from becoming overfull during the night and pulling away from the skin, a long tube should attach a large overnight urinary drainage bag. The bag can be placed in a container on the floor or hung on the side of the bed. Overnight drainage also helps to keep the urine from constantly bathing the stoma, which causes white, gritty crystals to form.

51. B: A patient with an ileostomy has developed hyponatremia when the sodium value drops to less than 135 mEq:

- Normal value: 135-145 mEq/L.
- Hyponatremia: <135 mEq/L. Critical value: <120 mEq/L.
- Hypernatremia: >145 mEq/L. Critical value >160 mEq/L.

Symptoms of hyponatremia may include:

- Irritability to lethargy to confusion and alterations in consciousness.
- Cerebral edema with seizures and coma.
- Dyspnea to respiratory failure.

52. C: A low-profile percutaneous feeding tube is recommended for pediatric patients because it is less likely become dislodged. The low-profile tube is almost flush with the skin whereas the standard tube protrudes up to 7 inches and can easily be pulled out by a child tugging on the tube or catching it on clothing. Adults may also prefer the low-profile tube because it is easier to conceal with clothing and less inconvenient to manage.

53. A: Providing feedback is an essential element of active listening because it shows the speaker that the listener is paying attention and processing what the person is saying as well as paying respect. Feedback may include nodding the head, restating something the person has said, asking pertinent comments, making comments, and showing agreement. The listener should pay close attention to not only the speaker's words but also to nonverbal communication, including gestures, facial expression, body position, and tone of voice.

54. A: Rotating the tube daily is a measure to prevent buried bumper syndrome with a PEG tube. Additionally, the external fixation device should be about 1 to 2 cm above the surface of the skin so that there is no undue tension. If buried bumper syndrome occurs, the patient will likely experience pain, and fluids may infuse poorly. The PEG tube must be removed and replaced if buried bumper syndrome occurs.

55. D: When using a closed suction system to manage a high-output fistula, the suction catheter is positioned next to the fistula orifice but not inside the orifice because of the danger that the catheter may contaminate the fistula and result in ascending infection. The skin about the fistula should be protected with barrier spray and/or hydrocolloid barrier strips and then the wound base is covered with a few layers of moist gauze to protect the tissue from the suction. The catheter is placed on these layers of gauze and covered with additional moist gauze to secure it in place.

56. B: The tract of a PEG usually matures and heals within 2 to 4 weeks. Once the tract has healed, the original PEG tube can generally be replaced with a balloon gastrostomy tube. Gastrostomy tubes with an internal balloon or mushroom tip, measured markings, and an external disk are easier to stabilize, but internal devices should be checked daily by gently pulling until resistance is felt. External stabilizing devices can be applied to the skin to hold the tube in place. The tube may also be taped to the abdomen or secured with a binder.

57. A: If a patient complains of difficulty keeping a seal of an ostomy appliance because of a bulge on one side of the stoma, the most likely cause is parastomal hernia. The hernia may not be always evident unless the patient coughs or strains when it is small, but over time it may enlarge. The patient should be examined in good light in standing, lying, and sitting position and should be asked to cough, lift the head, and strain as though having a bowel movement. Parastomal hernias are usually managed conservatively with diet, flexible pouching system, and hernia support belts.

58. B: Management of severe stomal stenosis usually requires surgical repair. While dilators were used at one time, dilation should not be used long term although digital dilation may be used in an emergent situation. With mild stenosis, dietary modifications may help to relieve symptoms if the stool is kept softer, but dietary modification alone is not generally adequate for severe stenosis.

59. D: If a patient with a colostomy has a new onset of loose stools, the nurse should initially review the patient's food history because, in most cases, loose stools are caused by dietary changes. Foods/Beverages that may increase loose stools include alcohol, beans, cucumbers, fresh fruits, cruciferous vegetables, bran cereals, whole grains, prunes, raisins, raw vegetables, spicy foods, and milk.

60. C: If an ostomy pouch has a drainable spout, it is usually positioned at 6 o'clock so that gravity aids drainage. This position makes it easy to empty the pouch into a toilet while sitting on the toilet or while sitting in front of the toilet. Ostomy pouches with drainable spouts are typically used for urinary ostomy pouches and fecal ostomies with liquid stool, especially with high output.

61. B: An ostomy pouch with a deodorizing gas filter works best with formed stool. A gas filter contains deodorizing charcoal that is sandwiched between breathable membranes. The gas filter is at the top of the appliance where it is less likely to be contaminated with fecal material because moist material may plug the filter and render it useless. The life expectancy of a filter is 24 to 36 hours. For this reason, some patients choose to also add a gas vent to the pouch.

62. A: When preparing a cut-to-fit ostomy pouch, the patient should be taught to trace the stoma on a piece of plastic wrap by placing the plastic wrap directly over the stoma and tracing the outline with a felt-tip pen and then placing the plastic wrap over the cut-to-fit skin barrier and using it as a template to cut the correct size. Sizing templates are available, but they may not be accurate enough if the stoma is irregular-shaped.

63. D: Stomal retraction is most common in patients who are obese although it may also result when the abdominal wall is thick, there is scar tissue, or the mesentery is short. In obese patients, the fatty mesentery interferes with the mobilization of the bowel and puts tension on the stoma, causing it to retract. A retracted stoma increases the risk of leakage under the appliance. A convex pouching system and a belt may help to elevate the stoma.

64. C: A clear pouch should be used over the stoma in the immediate postoperative period in order to allow stomal assessment. The stoma needs to be assessed frequently for early complications, such as mucocutaneous separation, stomal ischemia and necrosis, and stomal retraction as well as signs of bleeding. The patient may or may not be ready to look at the stoma, and the patient should be allowed to proceed at a pace that is right for the individual.

65. B: If the patient is markedly obese with a very large abdomen, the stoma may need to be sited higher than usual because the patient may have difficulty seeing a stoma that is lower on the abdomen. Another consideration is that stomas often retract in obese patients, and the patient may need to wear a belt to secure an appliance. It's important that the appliance avoid creases and the underside of a fold.

66. A: If, following an emergent traumatic injury, a 25-year old patient required a colectomy and permanent end colostomy, but the patient has become increasingly withdrawn and shows evidence of suicidal ideation, the most appropriate response is to refer the patient for psychological counseling. Most patients have some preparation for fecal diversion preoperatively, but the sudden change in body image that may occur with emergent surgery can be difficult for some patients to process and can lead to depression and even suicide. One study indicated that up 60% of patient have considered suicide after colostomy surgery.

67. D: If a patient develops granulomas at the peristomal skin/stoma juncture, the treatment of choice is usually silver nitrate cauterization, which can easily be done in the office or clinic. Cauterization is usually done one to three times a week for about 4 weeks. Small lesions may eventually disappear without treatment, but

Answer Key and Explanations

lesions must be protected from mechanical trauma as they may bleed. Large lesions may require electrical cauterization.

68. D: Sodium phosphate bowel prep is usually more acceptable to patients than polyethylene glycol preparations because sodium phosphate has low volume, so the patient doesn't have to drink so much unpleasant liquid, such as with polyethylene glycol. Polyethylene glycol is an osmotic laxative while sodium phosphate is a hyperosmotic preparation that may result in dehydration and electrolyte imbalance. Sodium phosphate is available in liquid form or in tablets, which must be taken with a prescribed volume of water. Patients should be advised to drink plenty of liquids when taking sodium phosphate and to avoid use of any other laxatives.

69. C: The two primary concerns of ostomy patients are odor control and leakage. Both of these problems can be observed by others, and the patients often feel embarrassed or shame that others may perceive their bodily functions. The nurse should discuss these issues openly with patients and advise them on methods to avoid odor, such as diet control and use of charcoal filters, and leakage and methods to manage them if they do occur.

70. B: When assessing the postoperative condition of a fecal stoma, the nurse expects the stoma to be deep red in color. If the stoma appears pale or dusky, this may be an indication of inadequate oxygenation. Typically, the stoma is initially edematous, but gross edema is cause for concern. The edema subsides over about 6 weeks postoperatively. A stoma that is flush with the skin increases the difficulty of pouching to prevent leakage.

71. B: Ideally, a stoma, such as for an end ileostomy, should protrude from the skin by approximately 2 to 3 centimeters because this allows a pouch to fit snugly about the stoma and decreases the risk that drainage will leak under the appliance and macerate the skin. Also, this allows a little leeway for the normal retraction and extension of the stoma. If the stoma is too long, on the other hand, it is at risk of trauma with increased irritation and bleeding.

72. C: The ideal site for a stoma is in the rectus abdominus muscle. This vertical muscle is in the front of the abdomen, and placing the stoma in this muscle reduces problems, such as parastomal hernias. The incision is made through the muscle longitudinally in the direction of the fibers. The nurse siting the stoma should look for a flat area (at least 8 cm in diameter) within the muscle and in an area free of scars and away from the beltline.

73. D: Following construction of an Indiana pouch, irrigation is usually carried out with 30 to 60 mL normal saline four times daily. Typically, mucus is produced in the pouch and must be flushed out with irrigation. With each irrigation, the procedure should be repeated 3 or more times until the fluid returns clear of mucus. The irrigations are typically spaced throughout the day although this should be guided by the amount of mucus produced and the patency of the catheter.

74. B: The continent ileostomy (Kock pouch) is currently used primarily as a backup for IPAA failure. The Kock pouch is complex to construct and frequently requires revision, so the IPAA has become more commonly used although the Kock pouch may still be utilized for patients who have an inadequate sphincter, have cancer low in the rectum, or do not want an IPAA. Patients with Crohn's disease of the small intestine are not candidates for the Kock pouch.

75. A: The ileal pouch anal anastomosis (IPAA) is not routinely recommended for patients with Crohn's disease because of the increased risk of pouch failure/pouch-associated fistulae. The IPAA can be performed in a one-stage, two-stage, or three-stage procedure. The IPAA procedure removes the colon and the rectum but retains the anal sphincter, and the ileal pouch is formed to serve as the neorectum. In two-stage and three-stage procedures, a temporary ileostomy is created.

76. C: Patients with a perineal wound should be reminded to avoid using a donut cushion because it causes pulling of the incision and decreased blood flow to the area. The patient should be instructed in methods to reduce pressure on the incisional area, such as by shifting weight from one side to the other. Sitz baths or directing the shower at the perineal wound may help to remove drainage and relieve discomfort.

77. D: If a patient with inflammatory bowel disease presents with hair loss, weight loss, balance problems, decreased energy and fatigue, the nurse should suspect malnutrition. Malnutrition is very common in patients with IBD, with the severity correlating to the extent of lesions that interfere with absorption. Patients may have deficiencies in protein and calories as well as micronutrients (vitamins and minerals).

78. B: The most common surgical procedure for Crohn's disease is removal of the terminal ileum and cecum. Surgical resection is usually limited only the area of involvement because lesions often recur and require further surgical intervention, so as much of the intestines as possible is retained. In some cases, primary anastomosis may be done, but if the patient's condition is poor, then a temporary ileostomy may be created to allow healing; however, in many cases, the patient may eventually require an ileostomy.

79. C: With extensive ulcerative colitis, the distance (measured from the anal verge) of involved tissue is greater than 60 cm. Proctitis, which involves generally only the rectum may extend to only 20 cm; left-sided ulcerative colitis extends 35 to 40 cm from the rectum to the splenic flexure; and pancolitis involves the entire colon. The continuous involvement of the tissue is circumferential but involves does not involve the submucosa or muscle layers.

80. A: If a patient with an IPAA experiences anal burning and loose stools after eating certain foods, the treatment may include bile salt binding agents, such as Colestid and cholestyramine, because the burning can likely be attributed to bile salt diarrhea. Foods that tend to trigger burning include those high in fiber/roughage (raw fruits, vegetable, nuts) and acidic foods, such as citrus fruits and tomatoes.

81. D: If a patient has developed skin irritation about a biliary tube, the best solution is to apply alcohol-free liquid skin barrier. Barrier paste contains alcohol and may cause discomfort and further irritation. Barrier pastes with creams and oils should be avoided. The biliary tube must be secured so that it doesn't dislodge and is generally flushed with 10 mL NS twice daily to maintain patency. If blockage occurs, the patient may develop fever, chills, and pain.

82. B: The most common cause of bladder cancer is smoking (cigarettes, cigars, pipes), which accounts for about 50% of cases, and the risk of getting cancer is at least 4 times higher than in non-smokers. While males have a higher overall incidence of bladder cancer, recent studies show the same proportion of females (50%) as males develop bladder cancer related to smoking. Other causes of bladder cancer include exposure to chemicals, history of radiation to the pelvic area, and chronic irritation.

83. C: If siting both a fecal and a urinary stoma, the urinary stoma should be on a different horizontal plane at least one inch higher than the fecal stoma. When siting the stomas, the nurse should consider the surface areas needed for placement of pouches and the patient's possible need to wear an ostomy belt for one or both ostomies to ensure that a belt would not need to cross over the other stoma or pouch.

84. D: A patient with an ileostomy should be advised that the best way to take fluids is immediately after eating because this allows the food to absorb the liquid while it's still in the stomach and slows passage of the liquid into the small bowel. Patients should be encouraged to avoid carbonated beverages (which increase flatus) and beverages with a high sugar content. Recommended drinks include water, Gatorade, coconut water, and vegetable juice (such as V8).

85. B: Chronic pouchitis develops in about 10% of patients with an IPAA. Various factors may be involved in the development of chronic pouchitis, including cytomegalovirus infection, idiopathic, fungal infection, ischemia, bacterial infection (*Escherichia coli, Clostridioides difficile, Klebsiella, Pseudomonas*), NSAID-induced, autoimmune response, spread of Crohn's disease, and cuffitis. Treatment depends on identifying the underlying cause, which may require endoscopy and biopsy.

Answer Key and Explanations

86. A: If a patient has familial adenomatous polyposis (FAP), the chance of developing colon cancer by age 40 is 100%. FAP is an autosomal dominant disorder resulting from mutation of the APC, a tumor suppressor gene which causes up to thousands of adenomatous polyps to form in the colon and rectum. Cancer may occur at any age, but the average age at diagnosis is 39, most typically in the rectum although the sigmoid and other parts of the colon may be involved. The most common cause of death, however, is periampullary cancer.

87. C: A moderate output enterocutaneous fistula (ECF) is one with output of 200 to 500 mL/24 hours:

- Low output: <200 mL/24 hours.
- Moderate output: 200 to 500 mL/24 hours.
- High output: >500 mL/24 hours.

Output is only one way of categorizing ECFs, as they may also be categorized according to the origin and the etiology. Most ECFs are iatrogenic, with some resulting from leak of an anastomosis and others from trauma associated with surgery.

88. B: Modifiable risk factors for the development of colorectal cancer include high fat/low fat diet. Other modifiable risk factors include lack of exercise and obesity. By making changes in lifestyle, the patient may reduce risk. Non-modifiable risk factors include age (especially older age), disease (such as ulcerative colitis and Crohn's disease), and genetic predisposition.

89. D: If the physician has ordered that a nephrostomy tube be flushed because of mucus and sediment in the urine, the irrigation should be done with 5 to 10 mL of NS. The purpose of flushing is to clear the tube rather than to irrigate the kidney. The saline is instilled into the tube, but not forced, and then drained by gravity. If the tube is so blocked that the saline will not instill, then the physician should be notified immediately.

90. A: Characteristics of ulcerative colitis include superficial mucosal penetration within the colon with continuous areas of involvement but no granulomas or fistulae, perianal disease, or strictures. Pain is usually minimal, but extraintestinal manifestation may occur. Smoking seems to have some protective function for ulcerative colitis although other negative effects of smoking may occur, so it is not recommended as part of treatment.

91. C: The first step in managing stomal trauma is to identify the cause of the trauma and then to take steps to alleviate the problem. In some cases, the size or type of the pouching system may need to be changed, but trauma may also be caused by other things, such as from the seat belt of a car, from wearing clothing or a belt that is too tight, or from engaging in activities, such as football, that risk direct trauma to the stoma.

92. D: If a patient has a proximal enterocutaneous fistula, the primary concern is nutrition as the proximal location of the origin means that calories, proteins, fluids, and electrolytes are lost in the exudate, which can be copious. Patients may need increased fluids and nutrition to compensate, and in some cases total parental nutrition may be necessary. If the origin is distal, then there may be enough small bowel above the fistula for adequate absorption.

93. C: Most cases of metastatic melanoma to the gastrointestinal system occur in the small intestine with only about 15% in the colon. The primary tumor usually originates from a different site. Patients are often asymptomatic, so the tumor is advanced when it is diagnosed; thus, prognosis is often poor. Treatment includes excision although survival is not prolonged with abdominal perineal resection, so this is usually avoided unless needed to relieve intractable pain.

94. B: A patient with a high output ileostomy should avoid drinking excessive hypotonic fluids, such as water, fruit juice, soda, tea, and coffee because they increase the risk of hyponatremia. These fluids have low sodium content and cause increased loss of sodium in the bowel, and much of this sodium is not reabsorbed, leading to hyponatremia. Patients should be encouraged to drink fluids with electrolytes, such as sports drinks (Gatorade®) or vegetable juices.

95. A: If a patient has an IPAA and has become pregnant, the patient should be advised that she may experience increased frequency of stools and fecal incontinence as the pressure of the fetus bears down on the fecal reservoir. Patients with an IPAA can successfully become pregnant and deliver a healthy infant although whether vaginal delivery or Caesarean is preferred is not yet established, but vaginal delivery may put the anal sphincter more at risk.

96. B: A patient is undergoing video capsule endoscopy for Crohn's disease, a primary concern is capsule retention. For the endoscopy, the patient must swallow a capsule that contains a miniature camera that conveys video imaging to a monitor. In some cases with Crohn's disease, a stricture may develop and the capsule can become imbedded in the strictures and deep endoscopy or surgical intervention is needed in order to remove the capsule.

97. D: If an 80-year-old male patient lives with his 72-year-old wife and is about to be discharged with a new colostomy that will require irrigations, but the patient is too frail to carry out the irrigations independently and his wife is still confused about the procedure, the best plan is to refer the patient to a home health agency for assistance. The home health nurse can monitor the patient and continue to educate and supervise the patient's wife until she is more comfortable with the irrigation procedures.

98. B: If, when the urostomy appliance is removed after 4 days, the skin is clear but there is erosion in the peristomal area of the barrier of the appliance, this means that the appliance should be changed more frequently because it is starting to break down. This could mean that urine will begin to seep under the barrier and could result in peristomal skin irritation. Most patients change the urostomy bag once or twice a week.

99. A: If a 64-year-old female client has recently had surgery for colon cancer and has a colostomy, but the client has been resistive to educational efforts and refuses to look at the colostomy, the most appropriate intervention is to remain supportive and encourage the client to express her feelings. Clients cope with a changed body image in different ways, and the client may need extra time to process the changes and to cope emotionally.

100. C: If a Vietnamese immigrant patient had surgery for a bowel resection and colostomy but has not requested pain medicine in the 6 hours after returning from the recovery room to his room on the surgical unit, the nurse should assume the patient is reluctant to complain of pain. Asian patients are traditionally stoic, so the nurse should ask the patient to rate or describe his pain rather than asking if the patient has pain.

101. C: When teaching a patient to irrigate a colostomy, the patient should be advised to use 500 to 1000 mL for the irrigation, beginning with 500 mL at first and then adding more fluid until the right amount for the individual is determined. The bag should be filled with 1000 mL warm water and bag hung so that the bottom of the bag is at shoulder level so that gravity will help the flow of water into the bowel. Patients may sit on the toilet with the irrigation bag between the legs or may sit on a chair or stool in front of the toilet.

102. B: The best choice to protect the skin from drainage is skin barrier spray, which provides a thin, breathable layer of silicone protection from both adhesive and discharge (including enzymes). The barrier spray can be applied to the skin prior to application of a wound management/pouching system. The barrier spray does not sting and can be applied quickly because it dries within seconds. (The same product is available in wipes.)

103. D: When siting the stoma for a woman who is 6 months pregnant, the stomas site should be more lateral than the usual site because of the enlarged abdomen. Following pregnancy, when the abdomen returns to a more normal shape, the lateral stoma will move medially. A stoma placed high on the abdomen will tend to shift downward, and a stoma placed low on the abdomen will tend to shift upward.

104. B: Most bacteria that is ingested orally is eliminated by gastric acidity; therefore, the stomach is relatively sterile. However, bacteria increase throughout the small and large intestine. Bile acids in the duodenum and antibodies decrease bacterial growth of aerobic bacteria. Anaerobic bacteria are plentiful distal to the ileocecal valve and serve essential roles in digestion, but they can become pathogenic if the normal balance is disrupted.

105. B: Absorption of nutrients, electrolytes, vitamins, and minerals takes place primarily in the small intestine. Most absorption occurs in the first 100 cm of the small intestine, primarily the duodenum and jejunum, which have plentiful villi. Of the 8 to 9 L of fluid that are received or produced by the small intestine, 7 to 8 L are reabsorbed, including carbohydrates and minerals. The duodenum neutralizes the gastric contents while pancreatic enzymes continue digestion and bile emulsifies fat. Most fats, proteins, and vitamins as well as a smaller amount of carbohydrates are absorbed in the jejunum.

106. C: Penrose drains are usually kept in a wound postoperatively for 3 to 5 days and are usually slowly removed as the wound heals. The drain may be cut with sterile scissors as it is advanced, being sure to place a sterile safety pin near the end to prevent the drain from migrating into the wound. The longer the drain is in place, the greater the risk of developing an ascending infection from the drain.

107. A: Up about 70% of colorectal lymphomas are located in the cecum/ascending colon because this area has a large amount of lymphoid tissue. Onset of symptoms is usually in the 50s to 70s. Because the disease is usually systemic, treatment may include radiation and chemotherapy, but surgery is not usually indicated except for focal lesions or complications, such as perforations. Patients may present with nonspecific symptoms, abdominal pain, and/or abdominal mass

108. D: If a patient is diagnosed with rectal cancer, the TNM (tumor size, nodal status, and metastatic spread) classification that generally indicates the need for transanal excision only is T1N0. T1 indicates that the tumor has invaded the mucosa and the submucosa, and N0 indicates no nodal spread and, therefore, no metastasis. Tis (in situ) would indicate only invasion of the mucosa but not the submucosa.

109. A: Most electrolyte loss occurs through urine because essential electrolytes (sodium, chloride, potassium, calcium, phosphate, bicarbonate, hydrogen, and magnesium) are regulated by the kidneys. Normally, food and food intake provide an adequate electrolyte balance, but disease or surgical interventions (such as ileostomy) may result in electrolyte imbalance that can be life threatening, so the electrolyte balance must be carefully monitored and replacement therapy provided as needed.

110. C: If a colonoscopy shows a fragmented polyp with invasive cancer, the likely treatment will be colectomy, removal of lymph nodes, and possible diversion. If the polyp is not fragmented and is a single specimen that is able to be completely removed, then only observation is needed with colonoscopy at least every 3 years. If colon cancer is found and the lesion is not obstructing, then diversion may or may not be necessary.

111. B: Carcinoid tumors are most common in African Americans. These slow-growing neuroendocrine tumors generally don't occur until the 50s or 60s and are accompanied by carcinoid syndrome in 10% to 18% of patients. Carcinoid syndrome results in flushing of skin, liquid stools, pain in the abdomen, heart failure (right-sided), and wheezing. Colorectal carcinoid tumors are often asymptomatic and found on colonoscopy.

112. D: Smoking makes patients with Crohn's disease more refractory to treatment. Additionally, smokers are more likely to develop Crohn's disease and to exhibit more severe symptoms and may have more than twice as many flareups; therefore, patients with Crohn's disease need to stop smoking as part of the plan of treatment, but they may need support in order to do so. Female patients tend to have more negative effects from smoking than male patients.

113. A: A patient with Crohn's disease is especially at risk for deficiency of vitamin B12 because the terminal ileum, which is essential for vitamin B12 absorption, is the most commonly involved part of the small intestine and the most commonly resected. Patients should receive preventive vitamin B12. If the ileocecal valve and cecum are removed, the patient may also have deficiency of fat-soluble vitamins and zinc.

114. D: With ulcerative colitis, toxic megacolon is an indication for urgent surgery. Other urgent situations include perforation, uncontrolled bleeding, obstruction, and fulminant attack that is nonresponsive to treatment. Indications for elective surgery include refractory disease, adenocarcinoma, failure to thrive (pediatrics), and chronic steroid dependency because delay in surgery is not immediately life threatening.

115. B: If a patient has a subtotal colectomy with ileostomy and a Hartman's pouch for Crohn's disease, the patient should be told to expect to feel the urge to defecate and pass mucus periodically. This usually occurs about once a day because the pouch continues to produce mucus. With a Hartman's pouch, the anus and rectum stay in place but the top of the rectum is sewn closed. The Hartman's pouch may later be removed if a proctectomy is indicated.

116. A: If a male patient who is 6 weeks postoperative with an IPAA complains of difficulty achieving an erection and engaging in sexual activity and seems quite distressed, the most appropriate referral is to a urologist. During the surgical procedure, sometimes the nerves that affect urination and sexual function become damaged, so the urologist can best make this assessment. In most cases, function resumes within a few months.

117. D: If a patient with Crohn's disease is considering surgery to create an ileostomy, the most important role of the nurse is to provide information about the procedure, including the pros and cons, to help the patient make an informed decision. The nurse could provide literature and pictures to explain the procedure and provide a list of resources, such as the United Ostomy Association of America and Crohn's and Colitis Foundation.

118. B: When a patient undergoing a 3-stage proctocolectomy and IPAA procedure has the end ileostomy changed to a temporary loop ileostomy, the patient is especially at increased risk of dehydration. The loop ileostomy is created more proximally than the end ileostomy, so the stool is very liquid and in large quantities (1000 to 2000 mL/24 hours). Patients should be advised to increase intake of liquids after eating meals and snacks to but avoid drinking on an empty stomach because the fluid will rapidly enter the small intestine.

119. C: If a patient has an ileostomy, the type of food that is most indicated to thicken the stool is starchy foods, which tend to act somewhat like a sponge and absorb liquid. Starchy foods include potatoes, rice, and foods made with flour, such as bread and pasta. Sugary foods are also high in starch, but the calories provide little in the way of nutrition, and since malnutrition is always a concern, they should be avoided.

120. A: A contradiction to negative pressure wound therapy (NPWT) (AKA vacuum-assisted wound closure) for an enterocutaneous fistula is an exposed bowel at the wound base because the suction may result in perforation of the bowel. The tract must have the potential for spontaneous closure, so NPWT is contraindicated if a pseudostoma is evident. NPWT should not be used for a fistula if an abscess is present or if there is a distal obstruction and should be avoided if malignancy is present.

Continence Care

1. A: Moisture-barrier pastes are ointments with powder added to improve absorption and make them more durable and solid, providing a thick skin barrier. Many are zinc oxide-based, making them somewhat difficult to remove. Mineral oil is often used to remove the paste. Some paste products now on the market are transparent so the skin can be monitored. Pastes are frequently used over denuded or excoriated tissue to absorb exudate and protect from drainage, urine, or feces, so they are used for both perianal and periwound tissues. Pastes are usually reapplied with each dressing/disposable brief change without being completely removed.

2. D: About 3 to 4 pints of liquid, including digested food, bile, and digestive enzymes, travel through the small intestine to the colon each day. The colon absorbs more than 90% of the fluid as the stool traverses the bowel. Undigested food takes only about 2 hours to reach the colon, but 2 to 5 days to reach the rectum, allowing time for reabsorption. The urge to defecate is caused when the stool travels from the sigmoid colon to the rectum. The rectosigmoid area provides storage. Eating stimulates contractions in the descending and rectosigmoid colon.

3. C: Phase I: Filling/storing is triggered by emptying the bladder. Neurotransmitters in the brain signal the detrusor muscle to relax and the bladder to expand, drawing urine from the kidney and ureters. When the bladder reaches capacity (8 to 16 ounces), nerves send a signal back to the brain. Voluntarily tightening the external sphincter muscles retains the urine. Phase II: Emptying occurs when the nervous system signals the voiding reflex, and spinal nerves contract the detrusor muscle and relax internal sphincter muscles, allowing urine to flow to the urethra. Relaxing external sphincter muscles allows urination.

4. C: Type 3. The Bristol Stool Form is given to people keeping a bowel diary.

- *Type 1* is separate small, hard lumps of stool that are difficult to pass
- *Type 2* is sausage-shaped, lumpy stool
- *Type 3* is sausage-shaped and lumpy, but with cracks on the surface
- *Type 4* is long, smooth, soft, snake-like stool
- *Type 5* is soft blobs of stool that are easily passed and have clear-cut edges
- *Type 6* is mushy, fluffy pieces of stool with uneven ragged edges
- *Type 7* is watery stool that is entirely liquid with no solid pieces

5. B: Postinfectious irritable bowel syndrome is a chronic bowel inflammation that develops in some people after acute enteritis, characterized by altered bowel habits, usually with chronic diarrhea and abdominal pain. About 2/3 of those with IBS have predominately diarrhea, while a fourth alternate between constipation and diarrhea, and the remaining have primarily constipation. Onset of symptoms is often abrupt. Symptoms often persist for years, with 40% still reporting symptoms after 6 years. Treatment is usually with antidiarrheals and a low fiber diet.

6. A: Rectoceles (rectal prolapses) can cause chronic constipation and difficulty in passing stool because of weakening of the muscles, contributing to fecal incontinence. Untreated, rectoceles can cause inflammation, ulceration, and fistula formation. Pessaries may reduce the prolapse. Surgical repair may not correct all symptoms, especially underlying damage to the muscles, and can result in surgical trauma to the rectum or sphincters, adding to the risk of incontinence. Rectoceles occur when the muscles between the wall of the vagina and rectum weaken and the rectum prolapses or protrudes into the back wall of the vagina.

7. B: While some fecal material may leak through fistulae, the primary cause of fistula-associated incontinence is inflammation and tissue damage. Fistulas involving the anus, rectum, or vagina, and the perineal tissue can result in damage to intestinal and pelvic floor muscles, nerves, and sphincters. Anorectal fistulas, the most common type, usually result from an abscess and may have one or more tunnels connecting the rectum and the skin around the anus. Fistulas may also result from trauma, disease, or radiation.

417

8. D: With MS, the myelin sheath and underlying nerve fibers in the brain, eyes, and spinal cord are damaged or destroyed, sometimes affecting nerves that control bowel movements, causing constipation and fecal incontinence. With PD both voluntary and involuntary muscle control may be compromised, sometimes resulting in loss of sphincter control and fecal incontinence. MD is a group of genetic disorders that cause progressive weakening and atrophy of muscles. Fecal incontinence is a frequent problem with some types of MD: ALS affects the motor neurons, resulting in muscle atrophy and weakness, sometimes causing incontinence.

9. D: Q-tip test measures mobility and axis position of the urethra to assess urinary incontinence in women.

Procedure:

- The patient lies in supine position.
- A cotton swab (Q-tip), sterile and lubricated with anesthetic gel, is inserted through the urethra to the bladder and then pulled back to the bladder neck.
- Supine, the patient strains as though urinating. The angle of the swab is measured when straining and again when resting.
- Standing, the patient again strains, and the angles are measured.
- A positive result is a Q-tip angle of 30°or more at maximal straining, indicating urethral hypermobility.

10. A: Provocative stress maneuver (urinary cough test) is a noninvasive test to determine if coughing will cause urinary stress incontinence in women. The test is done with the woman in supine position. Follow this procedure.

- The patient, with a full bladder, lies in a supine position with legs apart and coughs multiple times. Leakage of urine confirms stress incontinence.
- The patient then stands with one leg on stool and holds a pad or paper towels over the perineum and coughs. A wet stain confirms stress incontinence.

11. C: The mini-mental state exam (MMSE) requires the patient to carry out specified tasks.

- Counting backward from 100 by 7s or spelling "world" backward
- Remembering and later repeating the names of 3 common objects
- Naming items as the examiner points to them
- Providing the location of the examiner's office, including city, state, and street address
- Repeating common phrases
- Copying a picture of interlocking shapes
- Following simple 3-part instructions, such as picking up a piece of paper, folding it in half, and placing it on the floor

12. D: Anal manometry measures the pressure of the sphincter muscles, the degree of sensation in the rectum, and whether the neural reflexes that control normal bowel movements are intact. Anal wink (anocutaneous reflex), reflexive contraction of the anus in response to gentle stroking or stimulation of the skin around the rectum, and bulbocavernosus reflex, reflexive contraction of the anus in response to natural or electrical stimulation of the bulbocavernosus muscle of the penis, are used to determine if there is an interruption or defect in the reflex arc. Endoanal ultrasound is used to diagnose perianal fistulas and abscesses and to assess sphincter damage.

13. A: Foods that cause gas include cabbage, broccoli, kale, onions, turnips, brussel sprouts, asparagus, dried beans, fish, eggs, and strong cheeses. Foods that cause diarrhea or loosening of stool include apple juice, prune juice, fresh fruit, raw vegetables, spicy foods, and fried foods. Foods that cause constipation or thickening of stool include applesauce, bananas, cheese, creamy peanut butter, potatoes, rice, pasta, and marshmallows.

Foods that cause obstruction include dried fruits, fruits with skin, nuts, popcorn, whole corn, bean sprouts, celery, and large servings of raw fruits or vegetables.

14. C: Underwear soaked with overflow down legs is estimated to equal 30 to 60 mL volume of incontinence. A bladder diary is kept for 3 to 5 days and includes all urinations and incontinence.

- Time of urination.
- Amount of urination estimated (small, medium, or large) or measured.
- Fluid intake (amount and time).
- Estimate of incontinence (A small volume of less than 30 mL is enough to wet underwear. A moderate volume of 30 to 60 ml is enough to soak underwear with overflow down the legs. A large volume of more than 60 mL is usually enough to soak clothes and run onto floor or furniture.)
- Characterization of incontinence by activity and sensation of urge.

15. B: Anal sphincter electromyography (EMG) assesses muscle contractions to determine if the sphincter muscles are contracting properly. Drugs such as muscle relaxants and both cholinergic and anticholinergic preparations can affect the outcome of the test. This is the procedure.

- With the patient lying on the left side, insert a small lubricated sponge or plug electrode into the anal canal. Alternately, needle electrodes may be used.
- The patient must lie still during the procedure, or the results will be affected.
- The electrical activity of the anal sphincter muscles is recorded on a computer screen while the patient tightens the muscles, then relaxes them and pushes.

16. C: The normal specific gravity of urine is 1.015 to 1.025 with a pH of 4.5 to 8 (average 5 to 6). Urine should be pale yellow or amber, and clear or slightly cloudy. Odor should be slight. Bacteria may give urine a foul odor, depending on the organism, and some foods, such as asparagus, may cause odor. Urine should be free of sediment, glucose, ketones, protein, blood, bilirubin, and nitrates. Urobilinogen ranges from 0.1 to 1 unit.

17. A: During a 24-hour pad test, the pads are weighed before use, and when damp, are sealed in plastic bags and stored. At the end of the 24-hour period, the pads are weighed to determine the total volume of urine lost through incontinence. A shorter version of the test requires the patient to drink 500 mL of liquid, apply a pre-weighed incontinence pad after a half hour, and then engage in some mild to moderate exercise or activity for an hour. Then the pad is weighed to determine the degree of incontinence.

18. D: Cystometry assesses bladder capacity and pressure, including how full the bladder is when the urge to urinate is felt. Electromyography measures activity of the muscles in and around the urethral sphincter. Uroflowmetry measures the flow rate of urine, including the speed of urination and the volume. Pressure flow study measures the amount of bladder pressure that is needed to urinate and the flow rate at different pressures. Leak point pressure measures the bladder pressure at the point where leakage of urine occurs.

19. A: A reduced Valsalva leak point pressure indicates stress incontinence. Valsalva Leak point pressure (VLPP) measures the pressure at which bladder pressure overcomes urethral resistance without contraction of the detrusor muscle of the bladder wall. Use this procedure to check.

- Insert a 6 to 10 Fr. microtip pressure transducer catheter into the bladder.
- Insert rectal probe to monitor intraabdominal pressure.
- The patient sits or stands during the testing.
- Instill the bladder with saline or contrast material at 50 ml min to total of 200 ml.
- Ask patient (sitting or standing) to make a progressive Valsalva motion, bearing down with a closed glottis or coughing, until incontinence.

20. B: When fitting a pessary, a finger should be able to pass easily between the vaginal wall and the pessary. Pessaries are plastic or silicone removable prosthetic devices that are placed in the vagina for management of pelvic muscle support defects, such as cystocele and rectocele. Fitting a pessary may require trial and error to arrive at the correct size and style. The type of pessary is determined by the problem the pessary is intended to correct and the type of muscle weakness or prolapse present. The largest comfortable pessary is the optimum choice for effectiveness.

21. A: Chronic pelvic pain syndrome of unknown etiology (unknown cause or origin) is characterized by persistent or recurrent episodes of pelvic pain that is associated with urinary, sexual, bowel, or gynecological dysfunction, despite lack of evident infection or other pathology. The pain must be continuous or recurrent for 6 months or more. In males, it is often associated with perineal (including anal) and penile pain (often referred to as chronic prostatitis). The distribution and intensity of pain can vary considerably from one individual to another and may involve many different organs and structures.

22. C: Anticholinergics, such as oxybutynin or tolterodine, reduce urinary frequency and incontinence is patients with MS. Almost all MS patients develop difficulty with urination, including frequency, urgency, and incontinence. Some may respond to dietary modification, including avoidance of caffeine or other substances that cause diuresis, such as tea and alcohol. Scheduled voiding may be helpful, but some patients must control incontinence with intermittent straight catheterization every few hours, especially as muscles become increasingly weak and spasticity increases with progression of the disease.

23. D: The average age for menopause is 51. When menopause occurs, ovaries no longer produce eggs, ovulation and menstruation stop, and hormone levels of estrogen and progesterone fall. Estrogen maintains the lining of the bladder and the urethra and stimulates the flow of blood to the pelvic area. As levels of estrogen begin to drop with menopause, the muscles are less well-nourished and the lining of the bladder and urethra may become dry and irritated. The sphincter muscles may lose tone as well.

24. A: Obesity is a primary factor in developing urinary incontinence because of increased stress on muscles, which causes them to weaken and stretch. The increased abdominal mass exerts direct pressure on the bladder. Diuretics may contribute to existing urinary dysfunction, because increased urinary flow stimulates bladder contractions. HPV may result in cervical cancer or genital warts. Oral contraceptives reduce the risk of stress and urgency incontinence as well as overactive bladder because the hormones have a protective effect.

25. D: Social function includes support from family or friends, the need for a caregiver, financial resources, mistreatment or abuse, the ability to drive, and the presence of advance directives. Psychological function includes anxiety, worry, grief, and depression. Those with depression may be at increased risk of physical disability or may neglect self-care. Sensory function includes presence of cataracts, glaucoma, myopia, presbyopia, astigmatism, macular degeneration, or eye disorders that make it difficult for people to read medication labels or perform self-care. Hearing should be evaluated in both ears for hearing deficits and waxy buildup in the ear canals.

26. A: The environmental factor that may most contribute to incontinence in a person with reduced mobility is distance from the bathroom or difficult access to the bathroom, such as when the bathroom is on the second floor. In this case, a urinal (male) or a portable commode should be placed within easier access. Rugs in the hallway and poor lighting may slow the person and increase risk of falls. Toilets should be raised to the appropriate level for the person, with arm supports or grab rails, to facilitate getting on and off the toilet.

27. C: Artificial sweeteners (aspartame, saccharine) are bladder irritants. Other bladder irritants include

- Caffeine, which occurs naturally in coffee beans, tea leaves, and cocoa beans, is added to many soft drinks, and is found in chocolate drinks, candy, and many drugs (Excedrin®, Anacin®, Fiorinal®), by increasing detrusor muscle contractions, resulting in urinary urgency and frequency.
- Citrus foods, such as orange juice, and many other highly acidic fruits.
- Spicy foods, such as Mexican or Chinese food, horseradish, and chili peppers.

28. D: "The knack," a preventive use of Kegel exercises, is using precisely-timed muscle contractions to prevent stress incontinence. It is "the knack" of squeezing up before bearing down. Women learn to contract the pelvic floor muscles right before and during events that usually cause stress incontinence. For example, if a woman feels a cough or sneeze coming, she immediately contracts the pelvic floor muscles and holds until the stress event is over. This contraction augments support of the proximal urethra, reducing the amount of displacement that usually takes place with compromised muscle support, thereby preventing incontinence.

29. A: "Quick flicks" help to treat urinary incontinence by increasing contractility. This procedure utilizes Kegel (pelvic floor) exercises. The patient rapidly contracts and relaxes the pelvic floor muscles, usually in sets of 10 or 20, repeated 10 times, so each set includes up to 200 quick flicks. "Slow squeeze," contracting over a count of 2 to 4, holding for 3 to 4 seconds, and then relaxing is used to increase endurance. Most people with incontinence should do both types of exercises.

30. C: The most important factor in decreasing constipation is to increase dietary fiber and fluids. Exercise also helps to reduce constipation by increasing motility, but some people may be physically limited in their ability to exercise. Stool softeners may also help reduce constipation, but are not a substitute for dietary management. Laxatives should be avoided, as overuse may result in a cycle of constipation and diarrhea.

31. C: Liquid stool often leaks around a fecal impaction, resulting in incontinence. The pressure of the stool often causes hemorrhoids to become engorged. Fecal impaction occurs when the hard stool moves into the rectum and becomes a large, dense, immovable mass that cannot be evacuated, even with straining, usually as a result of chronic constipation. In addition to abdominal cramps and distention, the person may feel intense rectal pressure and pain, accompanied by a sense of urgency to defecate. Nausea and vomiting may also occur.

32. D: Food sources of soluble fiber include bananas, starches (potatoes, bread), cheese, dried beans, nuts, apples, oranges, and oatmeal. Soluble fiber dissolves in liquids to form a gel-like substance. This is one reason liquids are so important in conjunction with fiber in the diet. Soluble fiber slows the movement of stool through the gastrointestinal system. Insoluble fiber changes little with the digestive process and increases the speed of stool through the colon, so too much can result in diarrhea. Food sources of insoluble fiber include seeds, skins of fruits and vegetables, and nuts. Oat bran contains both soluble and insoluble fiber.

33. B: Defecation should be scheduled for 20 to 30 minutes after a meal, when there is increased motility. Scheduled defecation is usually at the same time daily, but for some people it is done only 3 to 4 times weekly, depending on individual bowel habits. Stimulation is necessary. Drinking a cup of hot liquid may work, but initially many require rectal stimulation with a gloved finger. Some people require rectal suppositories, such as glycerin, but stimulus suppositories or enemas should be avoided if possible. The patient should be sitting upright with knees elevated slightly, if possible, and leaning forward during defecation.

34. D: The initial step in controlling occasional urinary incontinence is scheduled urination, in which the patient is asked to urinate at scheduled intervals. Fluids should not be limited, as dehydration can impair wound healing. Foley catheters should be avoided if at all possible because they pose considerable risk of urinary and systemic infections. Anticholinergic medications can be used if other efforts fail and if incontinence is due to muscle spasms.

35. B: Black, tarry stools may occur from digested blood from the upper gastrointestinal tract or from iron supplements, black dye (licorice), or Pepto-Bismol®. Clay-colored stools may indicate lack of sufficient bile or use of antidiarrheals, such as Kaopectate®. Orange stools may be caused by medications (Rifadin®, Rimactane®) or beta-carotene in pills or foods, such as apricots, carrots, sweet potatoes, pumpkin, and mangoes. Green stools may be caused by leafy vegetables or green dye in foods. With diarrhea, it's possible that the bile didn't break down when the stool moved quickly through the colon, causing a green color. Bright yellow stools may indicate bile obstruction.

36. C: Desmopressin® at bedtime reduces urinary production for 5 to 6 hours. Antidepressants, such as Imipramine, relax the bladder and tighten the urethral sphincter, and anticholinergics (such as oxybutynin) reduce instability of the detrusor muscle. Tamsulosin (Flomax®) may reduce nocturnal enuresis in males with benign prostatic hypertrophy. Other treatments for nocturnal enuresis include behavior modifications such as bladder training, scheduled urination, fluid restriction, and dietary modifications. Conditioning therapy with enuresis alarms may be helpful, especially for primary nocturnal enuresis.

37. C: A test to determine correct size of vaginal weights is to begin inserting the lightest weight cone into the vagina, requiring the pelvic muscles to tighten to hold it in place. If the patient can hold it in place for one minute, progress to the next higher weight, increasing the weights incrementally to determine the heaviest weight that can be held for one minute. Exercise with the vaginal weights is usually done two times a day for 15 minutes until the heaviest weight can be held.

38. D: Bladder training, a behavioral therapy, has an improvement rate of about 75% for urge incontinency, so it is the treatment of choice. Scheduled urination should be done, gradually increasing time between urinations, along with strategies to delay urination. People who have dementia or caregivers may need prompted urination in order to maintain a schedule. Medications are usually given only if behavioral therapy is unsuccessful. Surgical treatment is not recommended for urge incontinence. Reducing caffeine and other bladder irritants may reduce contractions.

39. C: Because all treatments can have adverse effects, treatment for BPH usually begins conservatively with medications. Alpha-blockers (such as tamsulosin and alfuzosin) relax the prostatic and bladder neck muscles to facilitate urination, and 5-alpha-reductase inhibitors (such as finasteride and dutasteride) help prevent further enlargement and may shrink the prostate. If medical treatments do not provide relief of symptoms, then prostatectomy or less invasive procedures, such as high-intensity focused ultrasound, transurethral needle ablation, or microwave and thermotherapy (water-induced) may be indicated.

40. A: The treatment of choice for a male with detrusor sphincter dyssynergia (most commonly related to spinal cord injury or multiple sclerosis) is insertion of a urethral stent (UroLume®), because the procedure is less invasive than an external sphincterectomy, and urethral stents are reversible. Long-term catheterization poses the risk of infection and urethral trauma, and urinary diversion poses more risks. Detrusor sphincter dyssynergia occurs when involuntary contractions of the detrusor muscle coincide with involuntary contraction of the external urethral sphincter, resulting in obstruction that may cause vesicourethral reflux, hydronephrosis, sepsis, kidney stones, and renal failure.

41. C: Conservative treatment for DHIC is most common and includes bladder training with scheduled urination, or prompted urination, and if necessary, Credé maneuver and double voiding. Anticholinergics may worsen DHIC: Other treatment includes diet modifications to eliminate bladder irritants. While intermittent clean catheterization may be needed, long-term catheterization increases the risk of infection. Detrusor hyperactivity with impaired contractile function (DHIC) is characterized by overactive detrusor contractions during the storage phase but underactive contractions during urination, resulting in both frequency and residual urine in bladder. It is common with neurological impairment from trauma or with diseases such as Parkinson's or multiple sclerosis.

42. A: A fecal pouch is an external pouching devise that is applied to intact skin to protect the anus and perianal area from contamination and irritation caused by fecal incontinence. The fecal pouch can manage a volume of ≤500 mL of liquid or semi-liquid stool. The bag is attached with adhesive for a secure fit and is changed every 24 to 72 hours or if leakage occurs. A fecal containment system is used with >500 mL of liquid or semi-liquid stool daily. Disposable underwear is used for ambulatory patients. Refastenable briefs may not be adequate to prevent maceration of skin.

43. C: The best solution for helping a patient with mild dementia remember to urinate is an alarm system that sets off a bell, beep, or flashing light at regularly set intervals. While disposable underwear may also be useful, the patient should be encouraged to maintain scheduled urination to reduce incontinence and risk of skin

Answer Key and Explanations

irritation. Catheterization should be avoided, because of risk of trauma and infection and difficulty in self-care. A telephone reminder may not be practical as a long-term solution.

44. D: A penile clamp should be released on a regular schedule of every 2 hours to prevent complications. Penile clamps apply pressure around the penis to compress the urethra and prevent incontinence. It is clamped about halfway down the penis shaft and has soft foam on the inside of the clamp. The clamp is released at least every 2 hours to prevent circulatory restriction and to allow for urination. It is very important that the clamp not be placed too tightly, because it can cause strictures, skin breakdown, or even necrosis.

45. C: The urethral plug (such as the FemSoft TM) may prevent stress incontinence during strenuous exercise. The plugs are for one-time use and must be removed and replaced every 3 to 4 hours. An alternative is the external urethral patch (such as the Impress SoftpatchTM), but it may be more easily dislodged. Absorbent pads contain fluids but don't prevent incontinence. Valved catheters are intended for long-term use and are usually changed about every 28 days. Tampons are intended for menstrual flow, but some women find that tampons provide pressure against the urethra, preventing mild incontinence.

46. B: Biofeedback aims to increase sensory perception and control of the muscles of defecation. A sensor is placed in the rectum or around the external sphincters. An electromyograph sensor or intraanal manometric pressure probe may be inserted into the anus. Strength training uses manometry to measure pressure of the anal sphincters during contraction and relaxation. Coordination exercises are done to ensure that the internal and external anal sphincters are working in concert. The person receives instant feedback from a visual or auditory response regarding the ability to sense fullness in the rectum and to contract and relax the sphincter muscles.

47. D: Phosphate (Fleet®) enemas come prepackaged for one-time use with about 120 mL of solution. They stimulate contractions and, because they are hypertonic, draw fluid back into the intestines. Frequent use can result in hyperphosphatemia (>4.5 mEq/L) when too much phosphate is absorbed into the bloodstream. Symptoms include tachycardia, muscle cramping, hyperreflexia, tetany, nausea, and diarrhea. Hypocalcemia (<8.2 mg/dL) can also result. Symptoms include tetany, tingling, seizures, altered mental status, and ventricular tachycardia.

48. A: With augmentation cystoplasty, a section of the colon is removed, shaped, and sutured into the bladder wall to expand the bladder capacity. With the sling procedure for women, abdominal, donor, or synthetic tissue is placed under the urethra, acting like a hammock and compressing the urethra to prevent leakage. With TVT, a mesh tape is placed under the urethra, acting like a hammock. With retropubic suspension, the urethra and bladder neck are repositioned and secured.

49. B: While catheters at home may be reused after washing and drying, sterilization is more effective in preventing infection. At-home sterilization can be done by boiling the catheters and equipment for 10 minutes, pouring off liquid, and placing catheters in sealable plastic bags. An alternate method is to place the clean and dry catheters and equipment on a paper towel in the microwave with a glass of water and to microwave on high for 6 minutes. The glass of water in the microwave will provide steam.

50. A: The amplitude of the electrical current must be sufficiently strong to elicit the anal wink, or it will be ineffective. The patient may experience pain if ramping (speed at which the current reaches the muscles) is too fast. The frequency rate may vary, but is usually set at 50 Hz to increase strength for stress incontinence and 13 Hz to relax muscles for urge incontinence. The ratio of on to off for electrical stimulation should be 1:1 (minimal) to 1:2 (most common), for example 5 seconds with current on and 10 seconds with current off.

51. B: For female patients undergoing anal sphincteroplasty, the most common problem in the postoperative period is difficulty urinating, and this may continue for days or even weeks while healing takes place. The ability to urinate is evaluated after surgery, and if patients are unable to initiate flow, then they may require an indwelling catheter or learn to carry out clean intermittent catheterization if able to do so until they can urinate independently.

52. A: The first indication that a patient may develop fecal incontinence is flatus incontinence. If a patient is unable to prevent the loss of flatus through the anus, over time some stool may begin to be expelled with the flatus, and the sphincter may continue to weaken. Therefore, with any indication of flatus incontinence, the patient should undergo testing to determine if interventions are appropriate in order to prevent further deterioration.

53. D: If a patient is diagnosed with detrusor external sphincter dyssynergia (DESD), the nurse expects the treatment plan to include clean intermittent catheterization. Patients with DSD have suprasacral lesions that result in inability to voluntarily control urination as well as loss of bladder-sphincter coordination although the reflex arc remains intact, so the detrusor muscle contracts when the bladder is full, but the sphincter may contract at the same time.

54. A: If a patient has quit smoking and has been chewing sugar free gum and snacking on carrots, nuts, and celery all day to control cravings but has developed recurrent diarrhea, the most likely cause of the diarrhea is sugar free chewing gum. Many sugar free chewing gums contain sorbitol, which can cause flatus and has a laxative effect, especially if the person is chewing multiple pieces of gum throughout the day. Additionally, people tend to swallow more air while chewing gum, which increases bloating.

55. B: If using ultrasound scanning to decrease obsessive toileting for a patient with overactive bladder the patient should be urged to delay urination if the bladder volume is less than 100 mL to 150 mL. Patients with obsessive toileting often have volumes of 50 to 75 mL. It's important to engage the patient in the scanning process, showing them the results and explaining what that means. If the volume is small, the patient should be encouraged to try to delay voiding for at least 15 minutes.

56. C: Patients with fecal incontinence often try to self-manage for years before discussing the problem with healthcare providers primarily because they feel shame and embarrassment about the incontinence. Some patients may also be unaware that there are options to control incontinence. Healthcare providers should directly ask patients if they have had any problem with urinary and/or fecal incontinence, especially those at increased risk, such as patients with diabetes.

57. B: The most common cause of fecal incontinence in females is obstetric trauma, especially if associated with perineal tears (third and fourth degree), instrumental delivery, breach delivery, or epidural anesthesia. Those at increased risk include primiparas and grand multiparas and those who receive oxytocin during the second stage of labor to speed labor and delivery.

58. A: When treating urge urinary incontinence with pelvic floor electrical stimulation, the frequency rate, pps/Hz, should be set at 13 pps/Hz. If treating stress incontinence, 50 pps/Hz is utilized. The on/off time refers to the ratio of time the muscle is exposed to current and is at rest. This on/off ratio is usually 1:2, but at no times should the on time exceed the off time because inadequate recovery time could lead to muscle fatigue.

59. D: If a patient is undergoing bladder training and is trying to resist the urge to urinate for one-hour periods but feels a strong urge to urinate after 40 minutes, the patient should be advised to practice distraction techniques, such as relaxation and deep breathing exercises. As preparation for bladder training, the patient should practice various distraction techniques to determine which are most effective. Often, the strong urge to urinate will pass if the patient is able to avoid urinating because the volume of urine is likely small with frequent voiding.

60. C: If the urinalysis is positive for leukocyte esterase, this usually indicates pyuria because it indicates the presence of white blood cells (an indication of infection). Vaginal secretions and trichomonas infection may give an inaccurate test result, and high protein and vitamin C levels may provide a false negative. Other indications of a urinary infection include presence of nitrite and RBCs (bleeding results from irritation caused by infection). If a urea-splitting organism is present, the pH may increase.

61. A: The pessary that is most appropriate for treatment for cystocele stress urinary incontinence is the Gehring with knob. The knob applies pressure to the cystocele. Gehrung pessaries are U-shaped and provide support under the bladder and keep the uterus from descending. The Gehring pessary is more successful than many pessaries in keeping the cystocele from slipping out of place. When inserted, the pessary should provide a bridge to hold the bladder in place.

62. B: Smoking increases the risk of urinary incontinence, especially stress incontinence, and the more the patient smokes, the more the impact, especially if the person smokes more than 20 cigarettes daily. While smoking can worsen all forms of incontinence, it is believed that the cough associated with smoking tends to increase the risk of early development of stress incontinence through weakening the pelvic floor muscles. Smoking also increases the risk of developing bladder cancer.

63. D: Reservoir incontinence is associated with decreased colonic or rectal capacity, which may occur with chronic rectal ischemia or irritable bowel syndrome. Reservoir incontinence may also occur after previous surgical repair of the rectum as well as from prolapse of pelvic organs into the rectal vault. Those with irritable bowel syndrome may have decreased tolerance to capacity. In some cases, increased capacity (such as with megacolon) may also lead to incontinence because evacuation may be inadequate, leading to impaction.

64. C: Proctography (AKA defecography) is the test used to determine the amount of fecal material the rectum can accommodate and how effectively the stool is expelled. For the procedure, the patient must drink a container of 500 mL of barium liquid about an hour prior to imaging. With the patient in left Sims position, a catheter is inserted into the rectum and barium (sometimes thickened with other materials) injected until the patient has the urge to defecate at which time the patient is seated on a special commode beside a fluoroscope which takes x-ray images during defecation. For females, a small catheter is inserted into the vagina and about 5 mL of barium injected to help to distinguish the organs on the films.

65. D: For patients with fecal incontinence, the most troubling physical effect is generally urgency. Patients are often fearful of going out in public or socializing with others because they fear that they will experience urgency and be unable to find a bathroom in time to avoid incontinence. The feeling of urgency may come on very abruptly, so the patient often experiences anticipatory anxiety that interferes with the ability to socialize with others.

66. B: Simethicone (Mylicon®, Gas-X®) may relieve flatus incontinence and can be purchased by patients OTC. Beano®, an enzyme-based product, may also help to reduce gas. Patients should also be educated about foods that produce gas, such as beans and cruciferous vegetables (cabbage, Brussels sprouts, cauliflower, broccoli), and carbonated beverages. Lactose, found in dairy products, may also cause gas in some individuals.

67. C: If, during an interview, older patients fail to mention urinary incontinence, it is often because they believe incontinence is a natural part of aging, a common myth. Therefore, they often delay seeking medical help for the problem until it is severe enough to seriously impact their lives. Others may believe that there is no effective treatment. Some may feel embarrassed about urinary incontinence and associate it with hygiene problems, preferring to use absorbent pads rather than to face the shame of discussing the problem.

68. B: If a patient with no previous fecal incontinence has developed a sudden onset of slow leakage of stool and a feeling of rectal discomfort, the patient should be assessed for fecal impaction. With impaction, a hard mass of stool forms in the colon or rectum and the body attempts to compensate by decreasing absorption of liquid from the stool above the impaction, and this liquid stool then often leaks around the impaction. If the impaction is in the rectum, the pressure may impair sphincter control, resulting in leakage.

69. A: The most common cause of urinary obstruction in older males is benign prostatic hyperplasia (BPH). The symptoms do not necessarily correlate with the size of the enlargement. Typical indications include frequency and urgency, difficulty initiating stream, weak or intermittent stream, and leakage of urine. Risk factors for BPH include older age, family history of prostatic hyperplasia, diabetes, heart disease, beta blockers, and obesity.

70. D: If, following a urethral bulking injection of silicone polymers (Macroplastique®), the patient develops urinary retention, the recommended intervention is intermittent catheterization. Urinary retention is common for the first few days until swelling subsides, but an indwelling catheter may put too much pressure on the implants and result in leakage of urine. For intermittent catheterization, a small gauge catheter should be utilized to ensure that trauma is minimized. Macroplastique® is very viscous so it is injected with a high-pressure injection gun into the mid-urethra at the 6, 10, and 12 o'clock positions.

71. C: Anal endoscopic sonography is generally the imaging test of choice for identification of the specific type of fecal incontinence that a patient has and has often replaced electromyography, which required that needles be inserted into the muscles of the sphincter. Anal endoscopic sonography is able to identify the type of damage that has occurred to the sphincters. Patients are generally asked to take a colon prep to ensure the rectum is empty prior to the ultrasound.

72. A: Since the patient has only occasional stress incontinence and has been doing Kegel exercises, the gerontological nurse should recommend the use of the "knack," which is precisely-timed contractions of the pelvic floor muscles immediately before and during a stressful event (such as a cough or sneeze) to prevent incontinence. This maneuver helps to provide support to the urethra. The knack is effective for mild to moderate urinary incontinence and can decrease incontinence by 70% to 98%.

73. D: If a female patient complains of new onset of urinary incontinence, the medication that may be implicated is the alpha blocker (alpha-adrenergic antagonists), doxazosin (Cardura®), which can cause reduced bladder outlet resistance. Alpha blockers may increase incontinence in females by up to 5 times. Other medications often implicated in incontinence include clonidine, methyldopa, antipsychotics, diuretics, ARBs, CCBs, ACEIs, estrogens, hypnotics, antidepressants, and hydroxychloroquine.

74. B: The most common complication after midurethral sling surgery to correct stress incontinence is urinary retention. Some patients also may experience new onset of urgency. These symptoms usually recede over time. Less common complications include erosion of the mesh into the urethra, urinary obstruction, and infection. Pain should be mild to moderate after the procedure. Severe pain may indicate hematoma or injury to muscle or nerve.

75. C: If a patient is taking mirabegron (Myrbetriq®) for treatment of overactive bladder with urgency, frequency, and urinary leakage, the patient's blood pressure should be routinely assessed because the most common adverse effect of mirabegron is hypertension. Other adverse effects may include cold and flu symptoms, dry mouth, back and joint pain, headaches, cystitis, and UTI. While mirabegron works similarly to oxybutynin, it tends to have fewer adverse effects and may be used for patients with glaucoma.

76. B: A clotting disorder is a contraindication to the use of an internal bowel management system, especially if the patient is taking anticoagulants or antiplatelet drugs. The internal balloon may cause irritation to the tissue with bleeding, and bleeding can also occur if the internal portion is inadvertently pulled out. Other contraindications include inadequate sphincter tone, anal stenosis, ischemic mucosa, hemorrhoids (severe), and fecal impaction.

77. C: If urinary incontinence is associated with atrophic vaginitis, treatment may include topical estrogen cream or vaginal ring (Estring®), which provides a steady dose of estradiol over a 90-day period after insertion. Vaginal cream is applied with a slide-in applicator and is used daily for several weeks and then three times weekly. Oral estrogen is not advised because of adverse effects associated with the oral preparation. Atrophic vaginitis is common in postmenopausal women because the vaginal wall begins to atrophy because of the diminished supply of estrogen.

78. A: While causes for fecal incontinence may vary, the dietary modification that is most indicated to help patients control the fecal incontinence is increased fiber. This may be accomplished through dietary fiber (whole grains, fruits, vegetables) or the use of high fiber bulking agents, such as psyllium (Metamucil®), but patients must have an adequate fluid intake or constipation may occur. The patient may benefit from a regular toileting program. In some cases, fecal incontinence is associated with excessive use of laxatives.

79. B: If, when adjusting the amplitude for pelvic floor stimulation, the anal wink is absent, this indicates nontherapeutic stimulation; that is, the current is not resulting in contraction of the sphincter, which likely indicates denervation of the pelvic floor. In that case, electrical stimulation of the pelvic floor muscles will not be a successful treatment, and other alternatives must be considered.

80. C: If a patient has been wearing a pessary but has developed chronic constipation associated with the pessary, the best solution is to change to a different size or type of pessary. Patients often need to change pessaries 2 to 3 times before the correct fit and comfort level is achieved, so patients should be encouraged to report any problems that arise, such as constipation, which usually occurs when the pessary applies too much pressure to the rectum.

81. A: The internal fecal management system should be used for no more than 29 consecutive days. Indications for the internal fecal management system include fecal incontinence (4-5/12 hrs) of liquid to semi-liquid stool, expectation of liquid stool for more than 3 days, and possible contamination of wound from fecal material. Patients who are completely ambulatory are not good candidates because they will likely not retain the device.

82. D: If a post-menopausal patient has a vaginal balloon (Eclipse® system) inserted to control fecal incontinence, the patient should be advised to remove the device for cleaning weekly. If women are pre-menopausal, they should remove the device daily during menses. The vaginal balloon, which has tubing attached, is inserted into the vagina like a tampon, with the tube hanging out of the vagina. A pump is attached to the tubing to inflate and deflate the balloon. The balloon is deflated when the patient needs to defecate.

83. A: When reviewing a patient's management of clean intermittent catheterization, carrying out intermittent catheterization only 3 times daily may indicate increased risk of complications. Intermittent catheterization should be done 4 to 6 times daily in order to ensure that the bladder volume does not exceed 400 mL. Infrequent catheterization may result in bladder distention and stagnant urine, increasing the risk of infection. The bladder should be completely emptied with each catheterization, and total urine volume should not fall below 1200 mL/day.

84. D: The saline infusion test is given to assess capacity to retain stool by simulating diarrhea. A small catheter is inserted into the rectum and taped in place and then the patient is seated on a commode and warm saline solution is infused at the rate of 60 mL/min while the patient is instructed to tighten the sphincters and hold the fluid as long as possible. At the first leakage of 15 mL or more, the volume of liquid infused is noted. Usually about 800 mL to 1500 mL of NS is infused and a patient with normal sphincter control can usually hold most of the liquid.

85. B: If a patient with Parkinson's disease has increasing urinary incontinence, has fallen 3 times in recent months, suffers from depression, and exhibits functional decline, these problems would best be categorized as geriatric syndromes, which is the occurrence of disease along with age-related conditions. Diseases that are often associated with geriatric syndromes also include diabetes mellitus, peripheral arterial disease, cerebrovascular disease, and Alzheimer's. Common problems associated with geriatric syndromes include cognitive impairment, urinary incontinence, depression, falls, fractures, and functional decline.

86. C: The normal functional capacity of the bladder is 400 to 600 mL. Beyond that, the bladder may become distended and uncomfortable, and the risk of overflow urinary incontinence increases. As the bladder fills, the detrusor muscle of the bladder wall stretches, allowing the bladder to expand. The internal muscle layer of the bladder, the urothelium, contains sensory processes. The sphincter mechanism controls the flow of urine into the urethra, which is about 3 to 4 cm long in females and 20 cm in males.

87. A: If a family member complains that an 80-year-old patient with multiple health problems repeatedly urinates on the floor during the night on the way to the bathroom, which is down the hall, the best solution is likely a bedside commode as this appears to be functional incontinence. Because of the arthritis, the patient probably must move slowly and is, therefore, unable to hold the urine for the time it takes to reach the bathroom.

88. D: The best time for scheduled evacuation is 20 to 30 minutes after a meal because eating stimulates motility. The scheduled time (usually daily but may be 3-4 times weekly, depending on individual habits) should be at the same time each day, so work hours or activities should be considered. Stimulation may include drinking hot liquid or rectal stimulation (inserting a gloved, lubricated finger into the anus and running it around the rim of the sphincters). The best position for defecation is upright and leaning forward with knees elevated slightly. The patient should massage the abdomen, strain, and attempt to tighten abdominal muscles and relax sphincters if possible.

89. B: If a patient has developed urinary incontinence and has been researching all different treatment options and comes with a list of questions for the physician, the type of coping strategy this exemplifies is behavioral adaptation because the patient is actively seeking solutions to mitigate the condition. Those utilizing behavioral adaptation are interested in finding the cause of a problem and dealing directly with the cause and likely to feel in control and informed.

90. C: If a patient is undergoing the balloon (50 mL) expulsion test to assess defecatory disorders, the normal time to expel the balloon is 1 minute. If the patient requires more than 3 minutes, this is an indication of dyssynergic defecatory muscle action. For this test, a balloon is inserted into the rectum and filled with 50 mL of air or water and then the patient is asked to expel the balloon and the time needed to expel is recorded.

91. B: If an outbreak of *Clostridioides difficile* has resulted in 20 patients in a medical-surgical unit becoming infected, the breakdown in process that likely caused the outbreak related to inadequate handwashing. *C. difficile* is commonly spread through spores in the feces which contaminate the hands of healthcare workers and transfer to environmental surfaces. Alcohol-based hand scrubs do not adequately kill the spores, so when infections with *C. difficile* are suspected or confirmed, then handwashing should be done consistently with soap and water.

92. A: The patient's socioeconomic status is likely to have the greatest impact on a patient's access to quality healthcare. Patients with low income may not be able to afford insurance or may have insurance with a very large deductible or restrictions in coverage. Patients may be unable to qualify for Medicaid because of assets or because their income is slightly above the cutoff level. Patients may be unable to afford prescription drugs or prescribed treatments, and this may negatively impact their health outcomes.

93. C: While all of these (education, cost, follow-up) are important, the most important factor in ensuring compliance with the treatment regimen is the therapeutic relationship between the patient and the healthcare provider. If the patient feels trust, and the healthcare provider takes the time to discuss patient concerns (such as convenience and cost) and explain both the need for the treatment and the consequences of failing to comply, some of the problems that arise with compliance may be avoided.

94. B: If a patient has impaired mobility and often cannot get to the toilet in time, this is an example of functional incontinence, which can include any physical or psychological problem that interferes with the patient's ability to self-toilet even though the person may be aware of the need to do so. Possible physical problems that may result in functional incontinence include impaired vision, environmental barriers (stairways, poor lighting, long distance), cognitive impairment, musculoskeletal disorders, and neurological disorders.

95. D: If a 76-year-ld female patient complains of nocturnal enuresis but denies having any problem during the daytime, the likely contributing cause is nocturnal polyuria. Water excretion tends to shift with older age with about 33% (and up to 50% in some people) of urine production occurring during the night coupled with decreased release of antidiuretic hormone during the night. Also, during the daytime, fluid tends to increase in extracellular spaces, but this fluid is released more quickly into the bloodstream during the night when the patient is in supine position.

96. C: Overactive bladder (OAB) in males is most often associated with bladder outlet obstruction. However, this is rarely the case with females because of a much shorter urethra. Bladder outlet obstruction in males is most often caused by benign prostatic hyperplasia, which compresses the urethra and causes difficulty with urination and increased risk of urinary infection, which further impairs urination. About half of those with BPH also have detrusor overactivity. BPH primarily affects males over age 60.

97. A: If a patient with urinary incontinence shows the nurse a small notebook that lists all of the available toilets in the shopping area of the town, this is an example of toilet mapping. The patient wants to be sure to know where all bathrooms are located in case of urgent need. Patients attempting to deal with urinary incontinence without medical assistance often result in multiple strategies to manage incontinence, including restricting activities outside of the home because of the fear of incontinence.

98. B: Strategies for defensive urination include urinating on a scheduled basis, such every 2 hours and before activities that may increase incontinence, like exercise. If urinary incontinence is severe, patients may find they need to urinate more and more frequently in order to prevent or control incontinence, and this can become not only time-consuming but exhausting and burdensome. Patients often combine this strategy with fluid restriction, increasing the risk of urinary infection, which in turn worsens incontinence.

99. C: The activity that may be used to assess fine motor skills includes picking up pencils from a table top and placing the pencils in a cup. Other assessments include the box and block test in which blocks are moved from one section of a box to another section and the 9-hold peg test in which pegs are picked up, placed in a peg-board, removed, and returned to the original container. The activities are timed.

100. D: If a 4-year-old male patient has developed retentive encopresis with leakage of stool, the primary interventions are scheduled toileting and dietary changes. While positive reinforcement (praise, rewards) and stool softeners may help to encourage the child to cooperate and to facilitate bowel function, scheduling toileting after meals and increasing fiber in the diet are essential. The child may also need to increase fluid intake and decrease intake of food high in fat and simple carbohydrates as these slow the movement of fecal material through the digestive tract.

101. B: Dehydration/Delirium. PRAISED mnemonic for reversible causes of urinary incontinence:

P	Pharmaceuticals/Psychological problems
R	Restricted mobility/Retention
A	Atrophic urethritis/Vaginitis
I	Infection (urinary), symptomatic
S	Stool impaction
E	Excessive urinary output (from endocrine or cardiovascular disease, excessive fluid intake, pedal edema)
D	Dehydration/Delirium (and other confusion-inducing states)

102. A: If a patient with severe urge incontinence is learning to manage urgency and feels a strong urge to urinate, the patient should walk slowly to the bathroom. Rushing to the bathroom often results in increasing the contractions of the bladder muscles, so the patient is more likely to have an episode of incontinence. Initially, when a patient is trying to avoid rushing, the patient should be situated near a bathroom to reduce anxiety and encourage compliance.

103. C: As part of the bowel diary the patient is provided a Bristol stool form (which contains pictures and descriptions) in order to help to identify the type of stool passed:

- Type 1: Separate small hard lumps of stool that are difficult to pass.
- Type 2: Sausage-shaped lumpy stool.
- Type 3: Sausage-shaped and lumpy but with cracks on the surface.
- Type 4: Long, smooth, soft, snake-like stool.
- Type 5: Soft blobs of stool that are easily passed and have clear-cut edges.
- Type 6: Mushy, fluffy pieces of stool with uneven ragged edges.
- Type 7: Watery stool that is entirely liquid with no solid pieces.

104. D: The most common type of urinary incontinence in long-term care facilities is urge incontinence. Urge incontinence is often associated with impaired cognition or physical impairment and is common with neurological disorders, such as MS, SCI, CVA, and Parkinson's disease. Some things may serve as triggers, for example, a patient may feel increased urge to urinate when approaching the patient's room or bathroom, a condition referred to "key-in-the-lock" because the person unconsciously associates the action of returning to the room or bathroom with urinating.

105. A: Reflex incontinence is urinary leakage that occurs without a warning sensation when the bladder contracts involuntarily (often with a large volume of urine excreted) without any feeling of urgency because of damage to the nerves. Reflex incontinence may be associated with MS, SCI, or other neurological disorder. Reflex incontinence is similar to urge incontinence even though the patient lacks the sensation of urgency, so treatment for reflex incontinence is similar.

106. C: Normal micturition is controlled by the central nervous system, including an area in the pons referred to as the pontine micturition center, the central relay. While micturition is an autonomic reflex, urinating is under voluntary control mediated by the spine and brain. Contraction of the bladder is controlled by the sacral micturition center (S2-S4). The cerebral cortex inhibits the sacral micturition center. Therefore, neurological disorders or damage to different parts of the brain may affect different aspects of micturition.

107. B: If a patient is learning pelvic floor exercises to increase muscle strength, for the first week or two, the patient should aim to be able to tighten and hold for 5 seconds. Exercises should be done at least 3 times daily. They may be done, for example, while lying down in the morning and evening and while sitting midday.

- *1-2 weeks:* Tighten 1 second, relax 5. Repeat 10 times.

  Then tighten 5 seconds and relax 10. Repeat 10 times.

- *3-4 weeks:* Tighten 5-10 seconds and relax 10. Repeat 20 times.
- *5-6 weeks:* Tighten 8-10 seconds and relax 10. Repeat 20 times.

108. B: For a patient with dementia who forgets where the bathroom is and doesn't recognize the bathroom if the door is shut, resulting in periodic urinary incontinence, the best solution is likely prompted voiding and assisting the patient to locate the bathroom. Placing a picture of a toilet on the bathroom door or painting the bathroom a distinctive color may help the patient to recognize the bathroom, but the patient may still need prompting because of the dementia.

109. D: In a healthy person, the normal frequency of urination during waking hours is every 2 to 6 hours, and can vary depending on such factors as ambient temperature, activity level, and fluid intake. If, however, a person continually urinates every 2 hours, this would be considered abnormal, as most people urinate between 4 and 10 times in a 24-phour period. Children urinate more frequently than adults because the capacity of their bladders is less.

110. A: If a patient complains that it takes at least 60 seconds to initiate urinary flow, as part of assessment the nurse considers that the normal duration is 15 seconds. Urine hesitancy is common in males, especially those with prostatic hyperplasia. Other causes may include surgical trauma, childbirth, infection, neurological impairment (MS, CA), disorder of bladder muscle, shy bladder syndrome (inability to urinate when others are present), tumor, or medications (anticholinergics/antimuscarinics, antidepressants.

111. C: A patient is considered to have chronic constipation if the patient has bowel movements fewer than 3 times per week. Constipation is usually characterized by a number of different complaints: hard stool, need to strain, feeling of rectal fullness and blockage, need to splint, and inability to completely empty rectum. The most common form of constipation is normal-transit constipation in which the stool traverses the colon in the usual time but is hard and difficult to pass.

112. D: If a patient needs to increase fiber in the diet, unprocessed wheat bran provides the most concentrated form of dietary fiber as it contains 40% fiber. Bran may be added to other foods, such as cereals, ice cream, fruit, and puddings, and is often combined with applesauce and prune juice (which has a laxative effect) in a mixture and given to patients (4 to 5 tablespoons) daily in order to prevent constipation. Processed bran in cereals is less effective.

113. B: Prompted voiding is appropriate for a patient having <4 episodes of urinary incontinence in 12 hours (during waking hours). Prompted voiding includes verbal toileting reminders and positive feedback. Prompted voiding begins with a 3-day trial period during which patients are asked if they are wet or dry and then checked and feedback provided. Patients are then asked if they want to use the toilet and if refusing to do so, are prompted 3 times. The trial period helps to assess the patients' awareness of continence and the need to urinate.

114. A: Bisacodyl laxative tablets are classified as stimulants, which stimulate nerve endings to increase intestinal motility. Stimulants generally work within 1 to 6 hours but should not be taken long-term or frequently because they may cause damage to the bowel and result in electrolyte imbalances. Simulants should not be taken with warfarin (may decrease effectiveness of warfarin) or with dairy products or antacids (may decrease effectiveness of the stimulant).

115. C: Caffeine may increase intestinal fluid secretion and liquid stools, which may increase incidence of fecal incontinence. Patients should be advised to avoid fluids and foods high in caffeine, such as caffeinated beverages (tea, coffee, cola drinks) and chocolate. Foods high in starch (pasta, potatoes, sweets, beans) and cruciferous vegetables (Brussels sprouts, cabbage) and spicy foods may increase production of gas, which can also increase the risk of flatus-associated fecal incontinence.

116. B: Upon the digital rectal exam for a male patient, a hard lump is felt in the prostate, likely indicating a tumor. The exam may be carried out with the patient in left lateral Sims position or standing and leaning forward against an examining table. The prostate should extend about 1 cm into the rectum and be about 3.5 cm in width. The prostate should feel smooth and firm. If a lump is felt, then a biopsy is usually done to confirm presence of tumor/malignancy.

117. A: If a bedbound patient is incontinent of frequent loose stools and wears adult briefs but has developed incontinence-associated skin damage (IASD), the best solution is likely a fecal containment device because this prevents fecal material from coming in contact with the skin and allows air to circulate. IASD is more common with fecal or mixed fecal/urinary incontinence than with just urinary incontinence because of the enzymes found in the fecal material.

118. C: When utilizing habit training for a patient with urinary incontinence and toileting is scheduled every 3 hours, the best response to a patient who has the urge to urinate in 2.5 hours is to ask the patient to try to wait 30 minutes (the entire 3 hours) before urinating. Often the urge to urinate will subside if the patient waits for a period of time. With habit training, the established schedule for urinating is based on the patient's own pattern of urination.

119. A: If the nurse notes an itchy red oozing rash in the labial folds, under abdominal rolls, in the underarms, and under the breasts of a very obese patient, this most likely indicates intertriginous dermatitis. This often develops in areas of the skin that lack adequate circulation of air and where the skin rubs together, causing friction and irritation. Moisture, such as from perspiration, urine, or feces may worsen the condition. Infection is common, especially with yeast, such as *Candida*, but bacteria and other types of fungi may be implicated.

120. B: The most common psychiatric comorbidity with urinary incontinence is depression, which is commonly found in older adults, especially those with chronic illness. Up to 25 to 50% of those with urinary incontinence experience sexual dysfunction (often because they are afraid of experiencing incontinence during coitus), and many feel that the quality of their lives is negatively impacted. They may experience feelings of shame and humiliation and actively avoid social situations, further adding to their isolation and feelings of depression.

How to Overcome Test Anxiety

Just the thought of taking a test is enough to make most people a little nervous. A test is an important event that can have a long-term impact on your future, so it's important to take it seriously and it's natural to feel anxious about performing well. But just because anxiety is normal, that doesn't mean that it's helpful in test taking, or that you should simply accept it as part of your life. Anxiety can have a variety of effects. These effects can be mild, like making you feel slightly nervous, or severe, like blocking your ability to focus or remember even a simple detail.

If you experience test anxiety—whether severe or mild—it's important to know how to beat it. To discover this, first you need to understand what causes test anxiety.

Causes of Test Anxiety

While we often think of anxiety as an uncontrollable emotional state, it can actually be caused by simple, practical things. One of the most common causes of test anxiety is that a person does not feel adequately prepared for their test. This feeling can be the result of many different issues such as poor study habits or lack of organization, but the most common culprit is time management. Starting to study too late, failing to organize your study time to cover all of the material, or being distracted while you study will mean that you're not well prepared for the test. This may lead to cramming the night before, which will cause you to be physically and mentally exhausted for the test. Poor time management also contributes to feelings of stress, fear, and hopelessness as you realize you are not well prepared but don't know what to do about it.

Other times, test anxiety is not related to your preparation for the test but comes from unresolved fear. This may be a past failure on a test, or poor performance on tests in general. It may come from comparing yourself to others who seem to be performing better or from the stress of living up to expectations. Anxiety may be driven by fears of the future—how failure on this test would affect your educational and career goals. These fears are often completely irrational, but they can still negatively impact your test performance.

Elements of Test Anxiety

As mentioned earlier, test anxiety is considered to be an emotional state, but it has physical and mental components as well. Sometimes you may not even realize that you are suffering from test anxiety until you notice the physical symptoms. These can include trembling hands, rapid heartbeat, sweating, nausea, and tense muscles. Extreme anxiety may lead to fainting or vomiting. Obviously, any of these symptoms can have a negative impact on testing. It is important to recognize them as soon as they begin to occur so that you can address the problem before it damages your performance.

The mental components of test anxiety include trouble focusing and inability to remember learned information. During a test, your mind is on high alert, which can help you recall information and stay focused for an extended period of time. However, anxiety interferes with your mind's natural processes, causing you to blank out, even on the questions you know well. The strain of testing during anxiety makes it difficult to stay focused, especially on a test that may take several hours. Extreme anxiety can take a huge mental toll, making it difficult not only to recall test information but even to understand the test questions or pull your thoughts together.

Effects of Test Anxiety

Test anxiety is like a disease—if left untreated, it will get progressively worse. Anxiety leads to poor performance, and this reinforces the feelings of fear and failure, which in turn lead to poor performances on subsequent tests. It can grow from a mild nervousness to a crippling condition. If allowed to progress, test anxiety can have a big impact on your schooling, and consequently on your future.

Test anxiety can spread to other parts of your life. Anxiety on tests can become anxiety in any stressful situation, and blanking on a test can turn into panicking in a job situation. But fortunately, you don't have to let anxiety rule your testing and determine your grades. There are a number of relatively simple steps you can take to move past anxiety and function normally on a test and in the rest of life.

Physical Steps for Beating Test Anxiety

While test anxiety is a serious problem, the good news is that it can be overcome. It doesn't have to control your ability to think and remember information. While it may take time, you can begin taking steps today to beat anxiety.

Just as your first hint that you may be struggling with anxiety comes from the physical symptoms, the first step to treating it is also physical. Rest is crucial for having a clear, strong mind. If you are tired, it is much easier to give in to anxiety. But if you establish good sleep habits, your body and mind will be ready to perform optimally, without the strain of exhaustion. Additionally, sleeping well helps you to retain information better, so you're more likely to recall the answers when you see the test questions.

Getting good sleep means more than going to bed on time. It's important to allow your brain time to relax. Take study breaks from time to time so it doesn't get overworked, and don't study right before bed. Take time to rest your mind before trying to rest your body, or you may find it difficult to fall asleep.

Along with sleep, other aspects of physical health are important in preparing for a test. Good nutrition is vital for good brain function. Sugary foods and drinks may give a burst of energy but this burst is followed by a crash, both physically and emotionally. Instead, fuel your body with protein and vitamin-rich foods.

Also, drink plenty of water. Dehydration can lead to headaches and exhaustion, especially if your brain is already under stress from the rigors of the test. Particularly if your test is a long one, drink water during the breaks. And if possible, take an energy-boosting snack to eat between sections.

Along with sleep and diet, a third important part of physical health is exercise. Maintaining a steady workout schedule is helpful, but even taking 5-minute study breaks to walk can help get your blood pumping faster and clear your head. Exercise also releases endorphins, which contribute to a positive feeling and can help combat test anxiety.

When you nurture your physical health, you are also contributing to your mental health. If your body is healthy, your mind is much more likely to be healthy as well. So take time to rest, nourish your body with healthy food and water, and get moving as much as possible. Taking these physical steps will make you stronger and more able to take the mental steps necessary to overcome test anxiety.

Mental Steps for Beating Test Anxiety

Working on the mental side of test anxiety can be more challenging, but as with the physical side, there are clear steps you can take to overcome it. As mentioned earlier, test anxiety often stems from lack of preparation, so the obvious solution is to prepare for the test. Effective studying may be the most important weapon you have for beating test anxiety, but you can and should employ several other mental tools to combat fear.

First, boost your confidence by reminding yourself of past success—tests or projects that you aced. If you're putting as much effort into preparing for this test as you did for those, there's no reason you should expect to fail here. Work hard to prepare; then trust your preparation.

Second, surround yourself with encouraging people. It can be helpful to find a study group, but be sure that the people you're around will encourage a positive attitude. If you spend time with others who are anxious or cynical, this will only contribute to your own anxiety. Look for others who are motivated to study hard from a desire to succeed, not from a fear of failure.

Third, reward yourself. A test is physically and mentally tiring, even without anxiety, and it can be helpful to have something to look forward to. Plan an activity following the test, regardless of the outcome, such as going to a movie or getting ice cream.

When you are taking the test, if you find yourself beginning to feel anxious, remind yourself that you know the material. Visualize successfully completing the test. Then take a few deep, relaxing breaths and return to it. Work through the questions carefully but with confidence, knowing that you are capable of succeeding.

Developing a healthy mental approach to test taking will also aid in other areas of life. Test anxiety affects more than just the actual test—it can be damaging to your mental health and even contribute to depression. It's important to beat test anxiety before it becomes a problem for more than testing.

Study Strategy

Being prepared for the test is necessary to combat anxiety, but what does being prepared look like? You may study for hours on end and still not feel prepared. What you need is a strategy for test prep. The next few pages outline our recommended steps to help you plan out and conquer the challenge of preparation.

STEP 1: SCOPE OUT THE TEST

Learn everything you can about the format (multiple choice, essay, etc.) and what will be on the test. Gather any study materials, course outlines, or sample exams that may be available. Not only will this help you to prepare, but knowing what to expect can help to alleviate test anxiety.

STEP 2: MAP OUT THE MATERIAL

Look through the textbook or study guide and make note of how many chapters or sections it has. Then divide these over the time you have. For example, if a book has 15 chapters and you have five days to study, you need to cover three chapters each day. Even better, if you have the time, leave an extra day at the end for overall review after you have gone through the material in depth.

If time is limited, you may need to prioritize the material. Look through it and make note of which sections you think you already have a good grasp on, and which need review. While you are studying, skim quickly through the familiar sections and take more time on the challenging parts. Write out your plan so you don't get lost as you go. Having a written plan also helps you feel more in control of the study, so anxiety is less likely to arise from feeling overwhelmed at the amount to cover.

How to Overcome Test Anxiety

STEP 3: GATHER YOUR TOOLS

Decide what study method works best for you. Do you prefer to highlight in the book as you study and then go back over the highlighted portions? Or do you type out notes of the important information? Or is it helpful to make flashcards that you can carry with you? Assemble the pens, index cards, highlighters, post-it notes, and any other materials you may need so you won't be distracted by getting up to find things while you study.

If you're having a hard time retaining the information or organizing your notes, experiment with different methods. For example, try color-coding by subject with colored pens, highlighters, or post-it notes. If you learn better by hearing, try recording yourself reading your notes so you can listen while in the car, working out, or simply sitting at your desk. Ask a friend to quiz you from your flashcards, or try teaching someone the material to solidify it in your mind.

STEP 4: CREATE YOUR ENVIRONMENT

It's important to avoid distractions while you study. This includes both the obvious distractions like visitors and the subtle distractions like an uncomfortable chair (or a too-comfortable couch that makes you want to fall asleep). Set up the best study environment possible: good lighting and a comfortable work area. If background music helps you focus, you may want to turn it on, but otherwise keep the room quiet. If you are using a computer to take notes, be sure you don't have any other windows open, especially applications like social media, games, or anything else that could distract you. Silence your phone and turn off notifications. Be sure to keep water close by so you stay hydrated while you study (but avoid unhealthy drinks and snacks).

Also, take into account the best time of day to study. Are you freshest first thing in the morning? Try to set aside some time then to work through the material. Is your mind clearer in the afternoon or evening? Schedule your study session then. Another method is to study at the same time of day that you will take the test, so that your brain gets used to working on the material at that time and will be ready to focus at test time.

STEP 5: STUDY!

Once you have done all the study preparation, it's time to settle into the actual studying. Sit down, take a few moments to settle your mind so you can focus, and begin to follow your study plan. Don't give in to distractions or let yourself procrastinate. This is your time to prepare so you'll be ready to fearlessly approach the test. Make the most of the time and stay focused.

Of course, you don't want to burn out. If you study too long you may find that you're not retaining the information very well. Take regular study breaks. For example, taking five minutes out of every hour to walk briskly, breathing deeply and swinging your arms, can help your mind stay fresh.

As you get to the end of each chapter or section, it's a good idea to do a quick review. Remind yourself of what you learned and work on any difficult parts. When you feel that you've mastered the material, move on to the next part. At the end of your study session, briefly skim through your notes again.

But while review is helpful, cramming last minute is NOT. If at all possible, work ahead so that you won't need to fit all your study into the last day. Cramming overloads your brain with more information than it can process and retain, and your tired mind may struggle to recall even previously learned information when it is overwhelmed with last-minute study. Also, the urgent nature of cramming and the stress placed on your brain contribute to anxiety. You'll be more likely to go to the test feeling unprepared and having trouble thinking clearly.

So don't cram, and don't stay up late before the test, even just to review your notes at a leisurely pace. Your brain needs rest more than it needs to go over the information again. In fact, plan to finish your studies by noon or early afternoon the day before the test. Give your brain the rest of the day to relax or focus on other things, and get a good night's sleep. Then you will be fresh for the test and better able to recall what you've studied.

STEP 6: TAKE A PRACTICE TEST

Many courses offer sample tests, either online or in the study materials. This is an excellent resource to check whether you have mastered the material, as well as to prepare for the test format and environment.

Check the test format ahead of time: the number of questions, the type (multiple choice, free response, etc.), and the time limit. Then create a plan for working through them. For example, if you have 30 minutes to take a 60-question test, your limit is 30 seconds per question. Spend less time on the questions you know well so that you can take more time on the difficult ones.

If you have time to take several practice tests, take the first one open book, with no time limit. Work through the questions at your own pace and make sure you fully understand them. Gradually work up to taking a test under test conditions: sit at a desk with all study materials put away and set a timer. Pace yourself to make sure you finish the test with time to spare and go back to check your answers if you have time.

After each test, check your answers. On the questions you missed, be sure you understand why you missed them. Did you misread the question (tests can use tricky wording)? Did you forget the information? Or was it something you hadn't learned? Go back and study any shaky areas that the practice tests reveal.

Taking these tests not only helps with your grade, but also aids in combating test anxiety. If you're already used to the test conditions, you're less likely to worry about it, and working through tests until you're scoring well gives you a confidence boost. Go through the practice tests until you feel comfortable, and then you can go into the test knowing that you're ready for it.

Test Tips

On test day, you should be confident, knowing that you've prepared well and are ready to answer the questions. But aside from preparation, there are several test day strategies you can employ to maximize your performance.

First, as stated before, get a good night's sleep the night before the test (and for several nights before that, if possible). Go into the test with a fresh, alert mind rather than staying up late to study.

Try not to change too much about your normal routine on the day of the test. It's important to eat a nutritious breakfast, but if you normally don't eat breakfast at all, consider eating just a protein bar. If you're a coffee drinker, go ahead and have your normal coffee. Just make sure you time it so that the caffeine doesn't wear off right in the middle of your test. Avoid sugary beverages, and drink enough water to stay hydrated but not so much that you need a restroom break 10 minutes into the test. If your test isn't first thing in the morning, consider going for a walk or doing a light workout before the test to get your blood flowing.

Allow yourself enough time to get ready, and leave for the test with plenty of time to spare so you won't have the anxiety of scrambling to arrive in time. Another reason to be early is to select a good seat. It's helpful to sit away from doors and windows, which can be distracting. Find a good seat, get out your supplies, and settle your mind before the test begins.

When the test begins, start by going over the instructions carefully, even if you already know what to expect. Make sure you avoid any careless mistakes by following the directions.

Then begin working through the questions, pacing yourself as you've practiced. If you're not sure on an answer, don't spend too much time on it, and don't let it shake your confidence. Either skip it and come back later, or eliminate as many wrong answers as possible and guess among the remaining ones. Don't dwell on these questions as you continue—put them out of your mind and focus on what lies ahead.

Be sure to read all of the answer choices, even if you're sure the first one is the right answer. Sometimes you'll find a better one if you keep reading. But don't second-guess yourself if you do immediately know the answer. Your gut instinct is usually right. Don't let test anxiety rob you of the information you know.

If you have time at the end of the test (and if the test format allows), go back and review your answers. Be cautious about changing any, since your first instinct tends to be correct, but make sure you didn't misread any of the questions or accidentally mark the wrong answer choice. Look over any you skipped and make an educated guess.

At the end, leave the test feeling confident. You've done your best, so don't waste time worrying about your performance or wishing you could change anything. Instead, celebrate the successful completion of this test. And finally, use this test to learn how to deal with anxiety even better next time.

> **Review Video: <u>Test Anxiety</u>**
> Visit mometrix.com/academy and enter code: 100340

Important Qualification

Not all anxiety is created equal. If your test anxiety is causing major issues in your life beyond the classroom or testing center, or if you are experiencing troubling physical symptoms related to your anxiety, it may be a sign of a serious physiological or psychological condition. If this sounds like your situation, we strongly encourage you to seek professional help.

Online Resources

Due to our efforts to try to keep this book to a manageable length, we've created a link that will give you access to all of your online resources:

mometrix.com/resources719/cwocn

It's Your Moment, Let's Celebrate It!

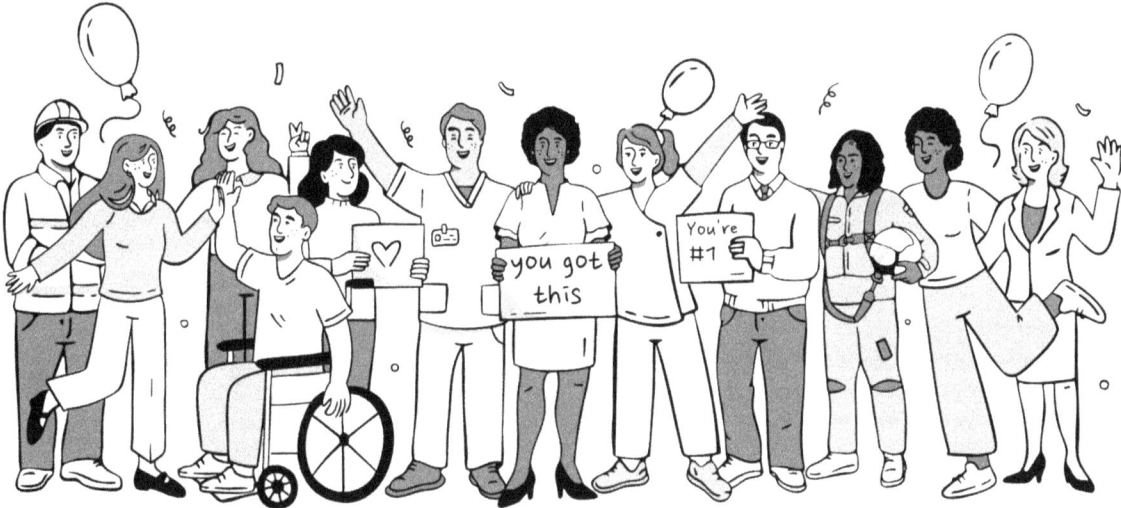

Share your story @mometrixtestpreparation